D0848701

The Nazi Doctors
and the
Nuremberg Code

THE NAZI DOCTORS AND THE NUREMBERG CODE

Human Rights in Human Experimentation

Edited by

George J. Annas
Michael A. Grodin

New York   Oxford
OXFORD UNIVERSITY PRESS
1992

Oxford University Press

Oxford   New York   Toronto
Delhi   Bombay   Calcutta   Madras   Karachi
Kuala Lumpur   Singapore   Hong Kong   Tokyo
Nairobi   Dar es Salaam   Cape Town
Melbourne   Auckland

and associated companies in
Berlin   Ibadan

Copyright © 1992 by Oxford University Press, Inc.

Published by Oxford University Press, Inc.,
200 Madison Avenue, New York, New York 10016

Oxford is a registered trademark of Oxford University Press

All rights reserved. No part of this publication may be reproduced,
stored in a retrieval system, or transmitted, in any form or by any means,
electronic, mechanical, photocopying, recording, or otherwise,
without the prior permission of Oxford University Press.

Library of Congress Cataloging-in-Publication Data
The Nazi Doctors and the Nuremberg Code:
human rights in human experimentation /
edited by George J. Annas, Michael A. Grodin.
p.   cm.   Includes bibliographical references and index.
ISBN 0-19-507042-9
1. Human experimentation in medicine—Moral and ethical aspects.
I. Annas, George J. II. Grodin, Michael A.
R853.H8N87 1992 174'.28—dc20 91-17391

9 8 7 6 5 4 3 2 1

Printed in the United States of America
on acid-free paper

This book is dedicated to the victims of Nazi medical experimentation and to all whose human rights have been violated in the conduct of human experimentation

Foreword

When the editors came to meet with me to discuss this project, I immediately saw its extraordinary importance. I think the Nuremberg Code, given its origins and its role in protecting human rights, is one of the most urgent and meaningful codes related to the dark era of Nazi experimentation on human beings. But I wanted to try to enlarge its scope. It is not only medicine and human experimentation that are called into question: The areas of scholarship, learning, education and culture must also be reexamined in the light of what happened. That doctors participated in the planning, execution, and justification of the concentration camp massacres is bad enough, but it went beyond medicine. Like a cancer of immorality, it spread into every area of spiritual, cultural, intellectual endeavor. Thus, the meaning of what happened transcended its own immediate limits.

I was personally interested not in Mengele, whom I remember, or other physicians whom I also remember from their selections, but in the *Einsatzkommandos*. Years after the end of World War II, like every other survivor, I began reading as much as I could in any language I knew—anything that was available in that period on that subject. One of the shocks of my adult life occurred when I realized that the *Einsatzkommandos* were headed by men with college degrees, and often with Ph.D.s or M.D.s. The other shock was when I discovered Roosevelt's nonassistance to the people in danger.

I couldn't understand these men who had, after all, studied for 8, 10, 12, or 14 years in German universities, which then were the best on the Continent, if not in the world. Why did their education not shield them from evil? This question haunted me.

I then developed an interest in a very small, yet significant, area. It had to do with a man whom I admire, Shimon Dubnow, one of the greatest historians in Eastern Europe. He wrote a definitive history including the years 1939–1940. Every person today, I am sure, who reads about that period knows the famous story of when he was led, together with other Jews in Riga, to the execution. He turned to his fellow Jews, saying, "Jews, remember, remember (in Yiddish: *schreibt un verschreibt*), write down everything." This injunction became a kind of testament that every survivor, every Jew, wanted to follow by becoming a witness.

I also liked Dubnow because he had a warm attitude toward Hasidism. I then began reading more about him. At one point, I opened the *Encyclopedia Judaica*. Doing some research on him, I found a strange notation. Some sources say that he was killed in Riga by a former pupil of his, who had become a member of the Gestapo in Riga. That caught my attention. How is it possible for a professor to be killed by his former student, now a Gestapo officer? It sounded too incredible to be true. I began checking. It took more than a year to track down every piece of evidence and information. I discovered that Dubnow, the great Shimon Dubnow, was actually a Bundist, a territorialist. He was against Zionism. He believed in Jewish culture and survival in Europe and, therefore, he did not want to go anywhere. He wanted to stay in Eastern Europe and work for Jewish culture, cultural autonomy, and cultural sovereignty. He could have come to America. He was invited here, and to London and Palestine, but he wanted to live there. He died there, standing alongside the Chief Rabbi of Riga.

What happened to him? As a professor in Germany in the 1920s, teaching not only Jewish history but also Oriental studies, he had a student named Johann Siebert, who later became the head of the Gestapo in Riga. When Siebert heard that Dubnow was living in the Riga ghetto, he often came to taunt him. To mock him. He would say, "Well, Professor, are you still a humanist? Do you still believe in humanism? Do you still believe in the fate of the human species?" Dubnow would say, "Yes, I do." Dubnow had been writing a continuation of Jewish history; witnesses describe his working at night.

His writings are probably buried somewhere in the former ghetto of Riga; we don't know where. One day they *will* be discovered. In Jewish history, nothing is really forgotten. If we could wait 2,000 years to discover the manuscripts of Qumran, we would find these documents, too. Dubnow kept on writing until one of the last transports was taken out to be killed. He could have been saved even then. He refused; he wanted to stay with the community. Johann Siebert noticed him. "Do you still see yourself as a humanist?" He said, "Yes." "Are you still an historian?" "Yes." "Well, in that case," said Siebert, "let me tell you that yesterday in the nearby forest, we killed Jews and Russians," and he gave a number. So, Dubnow said, "How many did you say?", and he made him repeat the figure. And Dubnow took out a piece of paper with a pencil and said, "Let me write it down." And he did. Siebert, in a rage, killed Dubnow, and the Chief Rabbi. From a witness, we have learned that the snow became red and the blood of Dubnow united with the blood of the Chief Rabbi.

I was preoccupied by Siebert. What kind of man was Dubnow, if one of his students could become a Gestapo officer? What, then, is the role and goal of teaching? What is the role of the student? What can happen to culture, to education? So, you see why we must go beyond the topic of medicine and the Nuremberg Code. But then, medicine may be a broader topic than I thought. Isn't an educator also a doctor? A doctor of the mind, of the soul. An artist is perhaps also a doctor. We all are, therefore, pupils who try to help, to cure, to appease, if not to redeem. But then the question remains open to this day. I hope that you have come up with better answers than I. How is it possible? How was it possible? I really do not have the answer.

All I could think of in my sleepless nights was that somehow the method of education in those times and places was not what I would have liked it to be. The emphasis on abstraction was too strong. When you take an idea or a concept and turn it into an abstraction, that opens the way to take human beings and turn *them*, also, into abstractions. When human beings become abstractions, what is left? I think that somehow those who, in the 1920s or 1930s, studied how to reduce life and the mystery of life to abstractions, were perhaps not equipped to resist the temptation of evil, for to them, it wasn't evil. They did not think that what they were doing was wrong. They were convinced that what they did was good.

I once read a dissertation — from the University of California, I think — by a psychiatrist who maintains that the sense of morality was not impaired in these killers. They knew how to differentiate between good and evil. Their sense of *reality* was impaired. Human beings were not human beings in their eyes. They were abstractions. This is the legacy of the Nuremberg Tribunal and the Nuremberg Code. The respect for human rights in human experimentation demands that we see persons as unique, as ends in themselves.

So maybe this is a lesson, a fragment, a part, a spark of a lesson that we could learn: When we teach, we must not see *any* person as an abstraction. Instead, we must see in every person a universe with its own secrets, with its own treasures, with its own sources of anguish, and with some measure of triumph.

Elie Wiesel

Preface

Discussions of human rights in human experimentation consistently begin with the Nuremberg Code. Nonetheless, little has been written about the Code itself, and references to it are invariably followed by attempts to justify deviation from its uncompromising principles. This book attempts to fill the existing void by bringing together the major historical documents regarding the Code. Equally important, we have brought together scholars from diverse disciplines to examine the modern relevance of the Code's message of the primacy of human rights in human experimentation. The book's title stresses the roots of the Code in Nazi brutality; the subtitle stresses the Code's continuing relevance.

Both of us have approached this work from our own background and history. One of us (GJA) is a health lawyer and bioethicist who coauthored a book entitled *Informed Consent to Human Experimentation* for the National Commission for the Protection of Human Subjects in the mid-1970s, and has focused his research on human rights in health care for the past two decades. The other editor (MAG), a physician and bioethicist, is the son of a Jewish clergyman whose interests have focused on the interface of science and technology and the humanities, and who has been the chairman of the Human Studies Committee of the Department of Health and Hospitals of the City of Boston for the past decade. This text is the culmination and integration of almost two decades of our study and work.

When we began this project four years ago, we expected to find many books devoted to the Nazi Doctors, the Doctors' Trial and the Nuremberg Code. We located only a few texts that even touched on the medical trials. Writings by Robert Proctor, Bruno Müller Hill, Michael Kater, Robert Jay Lifton, and William Siedelman focused primarily on Nazi physicians and racial medicine. The only two books specifically on the Doctors' Trial are the official German account, *Wissenschaft ohne Menschlichkeit* by Alexander Mitscherlich and Fred Mielke, 1949, and François Bayle's *Croix Gammeé Contre Caducée*, 1950. There has been virtually no discussion of the history, scope, and implications of the Nuremberg Code itself in the literature.

The official set of English transcripts of the Doctors' Trial is stored in the U.S. National Archives in Washington, D.C. Twenty-two complete or partial copies of the official record of all of the Nuremberg trials were shipped upon their completion to various U.S. institutions, including West Point, Columbia University, Cornell University, Duke University, and Harvard University. Copies of the official record in German are in the Nuremberg Staat Archiv.

We attempted to contact anyone who had participated in the medical trial, as well as some survivors of the medical experiments. The judges are all dead. James McHaney, the chief prosecutor, is in a nursing home in Arkansas. Telford Taylor, who delivered the powerful opening statement, is currently a professor at Cardozo Law School in New York and was helpful. The two physicians who acted as expert witnesses for the prosecution (Leo Alexander and Andrew Ivy) are both deceased. Fortunately, Alexander had donated all of his papers to Boston University's Mugar Library. Interviews with the few concentration camp survivors we located were the most painful of all. Survivors spoke of their dehumanizing experiences, of their treatment as subjects, and of murder. We were able to interview two women who had been experimented on as "guinea pigs" for Josef Mengele's twin experiments.

After a year of reviewing the transcripts and exhibits from the trial, and interviewing those few participants we could locate, we concluded that our project required the integration of many disciplines. Thus, as part of our project we decided to convene an international meeting to serve as a forum for scholarly interchange, clarification, and reexploration of the Nuremberg Doctors' Trial and Code. The meeting was held at Boston University in December 1989 and was sponsored by Boston University's Law, Medicine and Ethics Program in cooperation with its B'nai B'rith Hillel Foundation. Many of the participants in that dialogue were asked to write chapters for this book, and all have been extremely generous in their contributions and enthusiasm. We also recruited a group from the World Health Organization to put the Code into an international law perspective.

In addition to those already mentioned, we would especially like to acknowledge the help of Lawrence Altman in locating material on Leo Alexander; Albert Haas, a physician and prisoner in Dachau concentration camp; and John Fried, the former consultant to the judges of the Tribunal, for sharing their experiences with us. The librarians at the International and Foreign Law Library of Harvard Law School, especially Jeanette Yackle; the librarians at the Boston University libraries, especially Dan Freehling, and the Boston Medical Library, as well as the staffs of the United States Archives, the World Health Organization, and the Archives of the American Medical Association were all very cooperative. The research meeting was made possible by the work of Mary Lou McClellan, as well as Barry Manuel, Barbara Alpert, Mary Hill, and Betty Russell, all of Boston University. Mary Lou McClellan was also primarily responsible for the preparation of the manuscript with assistance from Aida Valentin. We also feel privileged to have been able to work with our editor, Jeffrey House, who has always demonstrated a commitment to the subject matter and helped keep us focused on it, and the skillful copyediting of Stanley George.

Other individuals who have made significant contributions to this book include: Joel Alpert, Alexander Capron, William Curran, Ray D'Addario, Erwin Deutsch, Daniel Deykin, Benjamin Freedman, Linda Hunt, Susan Lederer, James McHaney, Robert Neville, Rabbi Joseph Polak, Alan Rosen, Hans Martin Sass, Norman Scotch, William Seidelman, Evelyne Shuster, John Silber, and Herman Wigodsky. Portions of chapters 10 and 11 were funded by a 1987 grant from the U.S. Dept. of Veterans Affairs Cooperative Studies Program, and chapter 16 was partially funded by a grant from the American Foundation for AIDS Research.

We are, of course, happy to have completed this book. Nonetheless, it should be emphasized that the promise of the Nuremberg Code has not been realized, and the project to protect human rights in human experimentation is an ongoing one that even a half century after the promulgation of the Nuremberg Code remains in its infancy.

Boston, 1992   George J. Annas
                                                                   Michael A. Grodin

Contents

Primary Documents and Background Information

Contributors

Marcia Angell, M.D.
Executive Editor
New England Journal of Medicine

George J. Annas, J.D., M.P.H.
Edward R. Utley Professor of
Health Law, and Director, Law,
Medicine and Ethics Program
Boston University Schools of
Medicine and Public Health

Zbigniew Bankowski, M.D.
Secretary-General
Council for International
Organization of Medical
Sciences, World Health
Organization

Arthur L. Caplan, Ph.D.
Professor and Director
Center for Biomedical Ethics
University of Minnesota

Robert F. Drinan, S.J., J.D.
Professor of Law
Georgetown University Law School

Sev. S. Fluss, M.S., Dip. Ag.
Chief, Health Legislation
World Health Organization

Leonard H. Glantz, J.D.
Professor of Health Law and
Associate Director
Boston University School
of Public Health

Michael A. Grodin, M.D.
Associate Professor of Medical
Ethics and Associate
Director, Law, Medicine and
Ethics Program
Boston University Schools of
Medicine and Public Health

Jay Katz, M.D.
John A. Garver Professor of Law
and Psychoanalysis
Yale University Law School

Eva Mozes-Kor, B.S.
Founder and President
Children of Auschwitz Nazi
Deadly Lab Experiments
Survivors (CANDLES)

Ruth Macklin, Ph.D.
Professor of Bioethics
Department of Epidemiology and
Social Medicine
Albert Einstein College of Medicine

Wendy K. Mariner, J.D., M.P.H.
Associate Professor of Health Law
Boston University Schools of
Medicine and Public Health

Sharon Perley, B.A.
School of Law '92
New York University

Robert N. Proctor, Ph.D.
Associate Professor of History
Penn State University

Christian Pross, M.D.
West Berlin Chamber of Physicians

**Françoise Simon, Docteur
en Droit**
Technical Officer, Health
Legislation
World Health Organization

Telford Taylor, LL.B., LL.D.
Professor of Law
Benjamin Cardozo School of Law

Elie Wiesel
Andrew W. Mellon Professor
in the Humanities
Boston University

The Nazi Doctors
and the
Nuremberg Code

THE NUREMBERG CODE

1. The voluntary consent of the human subject is absolutely essential.

This means that the person involved should have legal capacity to give consent; should be so situated as to be able to exercise free power of choice, without the intervention of any element of force, fraud, deceit, duress, over-reaching, or other ulterior form of constraint or coercion; and should have sufficient knowledge and comprehension of the elements of the subject matter involved as to enable him to make an understanding and enlightened decision. This latter element requires that before the acceptance of an affirmative decision by the experimental subject there should be made known to him the nature, duration, and purpose of the experiment; the method and means by which it is to be conducted; all inconveniences and hazards reasonably to be expected; and the effects upon his health or person which may possibly come from his participation in the experiment.

The duty and responsibility for ascertaining the quality of the consent rests upon each individual who initiates, directs or engages in the experiment. It is a personal duty and responsibility which may not be delegated to another with impunity.

2. The experiment should be such as to yield fruitful results for the good of society, unprocurable by other methods or means of study, and not random and unnecessary in nature.

3. The experiment should be so designed and based on the results of animal experimentation and a knowledge of the natural history of the disease or other problem under study that the anticipated results will justify the performance of the experiment.

4. The experiment should be so conducted as to avoid all unnecessary physical and mental suffering and injury.

5. No experiment should be conducted where there is an *a priori* reason to believe that death or disabling injury will occur; except, perhaps, in those experiments where the experimental physicians also serve as subjects.

6. The degree of risk to be taken should never exceed that determined by the humanitarian importance of the problem to be solved by the experiment.

7. Proper preparations should be made and adequate facilities provided to protect the experimental subject against even remote possibilities of injury, disability, or death.

8. The experiment should be conducted only by scientifically qualified persons. The highest degree of skill and care should be required through all stages of the experiment of those who conduct or engage in the experiment.

9. During the course of the experiment the human subject should be at liberty to bring the experiment to an end if he has reached the physical or mental state where continuation of the experiment seems to him to be impossible.

10. During the course of the experiment the scientist in charge must be prepared to terminate the experiment at any stage, if he has probable cause to believe, in the exercise of the good faith, superior skill, and careful judgment required of him, that a continuation of the experiment is likely to result in injury, disability, or death to the experimental subject.

1

Introduction

GEORGE J. ANNAS
MICHAEL A. GRODIN

This book grew out of our continuing work on the ethics and law of human experimentation. The themes of patients' rights and the protection of human subjects of research have led us to broader public policy considerations. Since all contemporary debate on human experimentation is grounded in Nuremberg, it is the goal of this project to explore the history, context, and implications of the Doctors' Trial at Nuremberg and the impact of the Nuremberg Code on subsequent codes of research ethics and international human rights. The Nuremberg Code was an attempt to formulate a universal natural law standard for human experimentation. This book explores the origin and influence of the code for human rights in the United States and throughout the world.

The most important historical forum for questioning the permissible limits of human experimentation was the trial of Nazi physicians in post–World War II Nuremberg, Germany. The trial provided the occasion for a substantive analysis of ethical standards. The physicians and professors prosecuted at Nuremberg represent a frightening example of medicine gone wrong. The extent of human experimentation, atrocities, and murders that were recorded during the trials is inescapable. Most relevant, however, was the focus on universal ethical codes within the context of a criminal trial.

After the war, the United States and its allies were involved in a succession of criminal trials. Perhaps the most famous Nuremberg trial involved the military officers of the Third Reich. Other trials involved soldiers, industrialists, and politicians. The Doctors' Trial, although less well known, is perhaps the most disturbing chapter of Nazi ideology. How could physician healers have turned into murderers? This is among the most profound questions in medical ethics. To understand the Nuremberg Code, one must understand the setting and circumstances of these Nuremberg trials.

The Doctors' Trial, also known as the "Medical Case," was tried at the Palace of Justice in postwar Nuremberg Germany. The trial was Case No. 1 of Military Tribunal I and was officially designated United States of America v. Karl Brandt et al. The trial was conducted under U.S. military auspices according to the Moscow Declaration on German Atrocities (November 1, 1943, signed by Roosevelt, Churchill, and Stalin), Executive Order 9547 (May 2, 1945, signed by Truman), and the London Agreement (August 8, 1945, signed by the United States, the French Republic, the United Kingdom, and the Union of Soviet Socialist Republics). The Charter of the International Military Tribunal was drawn up, and Control Council Law No. 10 established a uniform legal basis in Germany for the prosecution of war criminals and other similar offenders other than those dealt with by the International Military Tribunal. Signed on December 20, 1945, Control Council Law No. 10 established the articles for the punishment of persons guilty of war crimes, crimes against peace, and crimes against humanity.[1]

President Truman provided for the representation of the United States in preparing and prosecuting charges of atrocities and war crimes in January 1946. The military government in the U.S. zone of Germany set out the organization and powers of certain military tribunals in October 1946 and February 1947. Military Tribunal I was constituted on October 25, 1946. The judges designated as members of Tribunal I to hear Case No. 1 were Walter Beals, Harold Sebring, Johnson Crawford, and Victor Swearingen. The chief of counsel for the prosecution was Brigadier General Telford Taylor. The chief prosecutor was James McHaney.

The Tribunal for the Doctors' Trial convened 139 times following the indictment and arraignment of the 23 defendants. The prosecution's opening statement was made on December 9, 1946, and the judgment was delivered some 8 months later, on August 19, 1947. There were a total of 85 witnesses, 1,471 documents, and 11,538 pages of transcript. The Tribunal reviewed prosecution and defense exhibits, which included documents, photographs, affidavits, interrogations, letters, maps, and charts. On August 20, 1947, the death sentence was imposed on Karl Brandt, Rudolf Brandt, Karl Gebhardt, Joachim Mrugowsky, Victor Brack, Wolfram Sievers, and Waldemer Hoven.

Counts 2 and 3 of the guilty verdict were for war crimes and crimes against humanity. The human experimentation carried out by the Nazi physicians included both war-related and non-war-related activities. The judgment contains the documented proof of crimes and proceeds to the question of the permissibility of medical experimentation. The judgment concludes with enumeration of a 10-point code of human experimentation ethics that is now known as the Nuremberg Code.

That the Nuremberg Code is relevant to modern medical research cannot be doubted. A few contemporary events illustrate its relevance. In the May 17, 1990, *New England Journal of Medicine*, Robert Berger, a surgeon and

Holocaust survivor, published an article focusing on the Nazi data obtained from the hypothermia experiments at the Dachau, Germany, concentration camp in 1942 and 1943. This article highlighted the continued debate on the science and on appropriate use and citation of unethically obtained research data from human experimentation by Nazi physicians.[2]

In the October 18, 1990, issue of *Nature*, there is a report of a World Health Organization official investigating claims that an untested AIDS treatment was being administered to children, mostly orphans, in violation of international research ethics, in a hospital in Bucharest, Romania.[3]

On December 21, 1990, the U.S. Food and Drug Administration published a new regulation permitting the Commissioner to determine that the requirement for obtaining informed consent from all human subjects prior to the use of an experimental drug or vaccine could be waived for Desert Shield participants when it was not feasible in "certain battlefield or combat-related" situations. The regulation further noted that the term "combat-related" might mean only the threat of combat. The request for this regulation came from the U.S. Department of Defense, which claimed that "military combat is different."[4] In October 1990, the World Medical Association called on its physician members to stop all research on chemical weapons and germ warfare experiments.[5]

In November 1991 it was suggested that the AIDS epidemic may have originated from malaria experiments in which humans were directly innoculated with chimpanzee or mangabey blood.[6] Most of these experiments — both pre- and post-Nuremberg — violated precepts of the Nuremberg Code. In 1991, French officials admitted that AIDS-contaminated blood was knowingly used for blood transfusions and the production of factor 8 (for hemophiliacs) in 1985.[7] Although not technically an "experiment" (criminal charges have been filed against the physicians involved), the decision to permit this contaminated blood to be used violated two major points of the Nuremberg Code.

Less than one year after the reunification of Germany, in the fall of 1991, it was revealed that East German scientists and physicians had for more than a decade been using "men, women, and children as human guinea pigs in a state-sponsored research program intended to perfect steroid hormone drugs" in an effort "to develop compounds that would boost the performance of East German athletes . . . "[8] The investigation is ongoing as this book goes to press, but it appears that research was conducted on children without their consent (or that of their parents), and that permanent damage was done to many of the athletes. For now, however, according to Lutz Nover of the Institute for Plant Biochemistry in Halle, a longtime opponent of the Communist regime, "No one is asking about ethics."[9]

All of these contemporary events are concerned with the nature, scope, and limits of medical research and the legal justification and ethical standards for the conduct of human experimentation. The search for universal international codes of research ethics has had a disturbing history. Virtually all scholarly inquiries into the content, and the universality of ethical and legal norms of human experimentation, are divided into a pre-Nuremberg and a post-Nuremberg era. Abuses of human subjects by the medical and scientific communities have served as a focal point for reassessment and promulgation of ongoing standards. No atrocities, however, can be compared to the human experimentation carried out by Nazi medical doctors during the Second World War.

The chief of counsel for the prosecution, Brigadier General Telford Taylor, delivered the opening statement at the Nuremberg Tribunal:

> The defendants in this case are charged with murder, tortures and other atrocities committed in the name of medical science. The victims of those crimes are numbered in the hundreds of thousands. A handful are still alive; a few of the survivors will appear in this courtroom. But most of these miserable victims were slaughtered outright or died in the course of the tortures to which they were subjected.
>
> For the most part they are nameless dead. To their murderers, these wretched people were not individuals at all. They came in wholesale lots and were treated worse than animals.

The Nuremberg Code set the general agenda for all future ethical and legal questions pertaining to the conduct of human experimentation. What are the individual and societal values that justify science and technology? What are the source and the imperative of the quest for knowledge? Who decides on the limits of the scientific endeavor? Who determines the benefits and who sets the research agenda? How are responsibility and culpability determined? If controls and regulations are needed, should they be established at the level of law or ethical code? Who has the expert authority to carry out human experimentation? What roles, interests, goals, judgments, and standard of competence must investigators adhere to? How willing are we to risk human life to serve individual or societal ends? What are the limits of acceptable consequences and harm to human subjects? How is harm assessed, and what is the distinction between therapeutic and non-therapeutic research? How central a role should informed consent play in the acceptability of human experimentation? What are the roles of professional, private, and public institutions? What added safeguards might be necessary to protect vulnerable populations such as minors, the incompetent, and the disenfranchised? Is it ever justifiable to use prison populations as research subjects? Who should monitor the research process? And finally, how should society deal with human rights abuses in human experimentation?

This book is an attempt to answer some of these questions. It is divided into four major parts, each of which focuses on the interplay of history and human experimentation. A central theme is the pivotal role Nuremberg has played and continues to play in the ethics, law, and ethos of the protection of human subjects in medical research. The common theme is the attempt to understand the context, origins, and significance of the Nuremberg Code for today and tomorrow.

Part I focuses on the Nazi doctors and their medical experiments. One cannot understand the context of Nuremberg without a foundational knowledge of the nature of prewar German medicine, and how social Darwinism and notions of racial hygiene meshed with Nazi ideology to foster the atmosphere necessary to carry out these human atrocities. This part addresses the extent of German physicians' knowledge of and complicity in human experimentation. The victims' perspective serves as the grounding for all further explorations of human rights and dignity.

Part II consists partly of edited primary documents from the Doctors' Trial itself, including the prosecution's opening statement, and the final judgment, which contains the Nuremberg Code. An excerpt from the German official court observers covers the sentencing and aftermath of the trial. This part also outlines the historical origins of codes of research ethics and details the sources of the Nuremberg Code itself.

Part III analyzes the role of the Nuremberg Code in international and U.S. law. The Code's influence on later international regulations and directives is traced. Despite the fact that the Code was promulgated by U.S. judges in a U.S. military tribunal, it has rarely been cited in U.S. courts. In fact, only a few human experimentation cases have ever been tried in a court of law. The use of the Code as a basis for legislation and regulation is also addressed, with special attention to its influence on the regulation of research on fetuses and prisoners.

Part IV attempts to put the ethical principles of the Nuremberg Code in the context of modern medical research. This part addresses the centrality of informed consent, suggesting that without consent there is no other rationale to justify human experimentation. Two chapters address the specific ethical concerns of relativism, and the justification for the modern invocation of Holocaust metaphors in the context of medical ethics and research. The responsibility of scientific publications and editorial reviews in monitoring the ethics of human experimentation is analyzed. Finally, the application of the Nuremberg Code and its principles to the increasing complexity of modern therapeutic research is discussed.

In a concluding chapter we ask, where do we go from here? Among other things, we endorse past calls for an international covenant on nontherapeutic human experimentation. We also discuss the more refined and difficult task of developing a consensus of the appropriate ethical norms for nontherapeutic research with incompetent subjects and for the limits of therapeutic research.

The theme of human rights in human experimentation is a universal one. The need to respect the humanity and self-determination of all humans is central to the ethos not only of medicine and human experimentation but of all civilized societies. This may be the simplest and yet most profound conclusion of our project.

N O T E S

1. *The Declaration on German Atrocities, Executive Order 9547*, and the *London Agreement of 8 August 1945* are reproduced here. *Control Council Law No. 10* appears at p. 317.

DECLARATION ON GERMAN ATROCITIES
[Moscow Declaration]
Released November 1, 1943

THE UNITED KINGDOM, the United States and the Soviet Union have received from many quarters evidence of atrocities, massacres and cold-blooded mass executions which are being perpetrated by the Hitlerite forces in the many countries they have overrun and from which they are now being steadily expelled. The brutalities of Hitlerite domination are no new thing and all the peoples or territories in their grip have suffered from the worst form of government by terror. What is new is that many of these territories are now being redeemed by the advancing armies of the liberating Powers and that in their desperation, the recoiling Hitlerite Huns are redoubling their ruthless cruelties. This is now evidenced with particular clearness by monstrous crimes of the Hitlerites on the territory of the Soviet Union which is being liberated from the Hitlerites, and on French and Italian territory.

Accordingly, the aforesaid three allied Powers, speaking in the interests of the thirty-two [thirty-three] United Nations, hereby solemnly declare and give full warning of their declaration as follows:

At the time of the granting of any armistice to any government which may be set up in Germany, those German officers and men and members of the Nazi party who have been responsible for, or have taken a consenting part in the above atrocities, massacres, and executions, will be sent back to the countries in which their abominable deeds were done in order that they may be judged and punished according to the laws of these liberated countries and of the free governments which will be created therein. Lists will be compiled in all possible detail from all these countries having regard especially to the invaded parts of the Soviet Union, to Poland and Czechoslovakia, to Yugoslavia and Greece, including Crete and other islands, to Norway, Denmark, the Netherlands, Belgium, Luxemburg, France and Italy.

Thus, the Germans who take part in wholesale shootings of Italian officers or in the execution of French, Dutch, Belgian, or Norwegian hostages or of Cretan peasants, or who have shared in the slaughters inflicted on the people of Poland or in territories of the Soviet Union which are now being swept clear of the enemy, will know that they will be brought back to the scene of their crimes and judged on the spot by the peoples whom they have outraged. Let those who have hitherto not imbrued their hands with innocent blood beware lest they join the ranks of the guilty, for most assuredly the three allied Powers will pursue them to the uttermost ends of the earth and will deliver them to their accusers in order that justice may be done.

The above declaration is without prejudice to the case of the major criminals, whose offences have no particular geographical localisation and who will be punished by the joint decision of the Governments of the Allies.

[Signed]
Roosevelt
Churchill
Stalin

EXECUTIVE ORDER 9547

PROVIDING FOR REPRESENTATION OF THE UNITED STATES IN PREPARING AND
PROSECUTING CHARGES OF ATROCITIES AND WAR CRIMES AGAINST THE LEADERS
OF THE EUROPEAN AXIS POWERS AND THEIR PRINCIPAL AGENTS AND ACCESSORIES

By virtue of the authority vested in me as President and as Commander in Chief of the Army and Navy, under the Constitution and statutes of the United States, it is ordered as follows:

1. Associate Justice Robert H. Jackson is hereby designated to act as the Representative of the United States and as its Chief of Counsel in preparing and prosecuting charges of atrocities and war crimes against such of the leaders of the European Axis powers and their principal agents and accessories as the United States may agree with any of the United Nations to bring to trial before an international military tribunal. He shall serve without additional compensation but shall receive such allowance for expenses as may be authorized by the President.

2. The Representative named herein is authorized to select and recommend to the President or to the head of any executive department, independent establishment, or other federal agency necessary personnel to assist in the performance of his duties hereunder. The head of each executive department, independent establishment, and other federal agency is hereby authorized to assist the Representative named herein in the performance of his duties hereunder and to employ such personnel and make such expenditures, within the limits of appropriations now or hereafter available for the purpose, as the Representative named herein may deem necessary to accomplish the purposes of this order, and may make available, assign, or detail for duty with the Representative named herein such members of the armed forces and other personnel as may be requested for such purposes.

3. The Representative named herein is authorized to cooperate with, and receive the assistance of, any foreign Government to the extent deemed necessary by him to accomplish the purposes of this order.

Harry S. Truman

The White House,
May 2, 1945.
(F.R. Doc. 45-7256; Filed, May 3, 1945; 10:57 a. m.)

LONDON AGREEMENT OF 8 AUGUST 1945

AGREEMENT by the Government of the UNITED STATES OF AMERICA, the Provisional Government of the FRENCH REPUBLIC, the Government of the UNION OF SOVIET SOCIALIST REPUBLICS for the Prosecution and Punishment of the MAJOR WAR CRIMINALS of the EUROPEAN AXIS.

WHEREAS the United Nations have from time to time made declarations of their intention that War Criminals shall be brought to justice;

AND WHEREAS the Moscow Declaration of the 30th October 1943 on German atrocities in Occupied Europe stated that those German Officers and men and members of the Nazi Party who have been responsible for or have taken a consenting part in atrocities and crimes will be sent back to the countries in which their abominable deeds were done in order that they may be judged and punished according to the laws of these liberated countries and of the free Governments that will be created therein;

AND WHEREAS this Declaration was stated to be without prejudice to the case of major criminals whose offenses have no particular geographical location and who will be punished by the joint decision of the Governments of the Allies;

Now THEREFORE the Government of the United States of America, the Provisional Government of the French Republic, the Government of the United Kingdom of Great Britain and Northern Ireland and the Government of the Union of Soviet Socialist Republics (hereinafter called "the Signatories") acting in the interests of all the United Nations and by their representatives duly authorized thereto have concluded this Agreement.

Article 1. There shall be established after consultation with the Control Council for Germany an International Military Tribunal for the trial of war criminals whose offenses have no particular geographical location whether they be accused individually or in their capacity as members of organizations or groups or in both capacities.

Article 2. The constitution, jurisdiction and functions of the International Military Tribunal shall be those set out in the Charter annexed to this Agreement, which Charter shall form an integral part of this Agreement.

Article 3. Each of the Signatories shall take the necessary steps to make available for the investigation of the charges and trial the major war criminals detained by them who are to be tried by the International Military Tribunal. The Signatories shall also use their best endeavors to make available for investigation of the charges against and the trial before the International Military Tribunal such of the major war criminals as are not in the territories of any of the Signatories.

Article 4. Nothing in this Agreement shall prejudice the provisions established by the Moscow Declaration concerning the return of war criminals to the countries where they committed their crimes.

Article 5. Any Government of the United Nations may adhere to this Agreement by notice given through the diplomatic channel to the Government of the United Kingdom, who shall inform the other signatory and adhering Governments of each such adherence.

Article 6. Nothing in this Agreement shall prejudice the jurisdiction or the powers of any national or occupation court established or to be established in any allied territory or in Germany for the trial of war criminals.

Article 7. This agreement shall come into force on the day of signature and shall remain in force for the period of one year and shall continue thereafter, subject to the right of any Signatory to give, through the diplomatic channel, one month's notice of intention to terminate it. Such termination shall not prejudice any proceedings already taken or any findings already made in pursuance of this Agreement.

IN WITNESS WHEREOF the Undersigned have signed the present Agreement.

DONE in quadruplicate in London this 8th day of August 1945 each in English, French and Russian, and each text to have equal authenticity.

For the Government of the United States of America
Robert H. Jackson
For the Provisional Government of the French Republic
Robert Falco
For the Government of the United Kingdom of Great Britain
and Northern Ireland
Jowitt, C.
For the Government of the Union of Soviet Socialist Republics
I. Nikitchenko
A. Trainin

2. L. Altman, "Nazi Data on Hypothermia Termed Unscientific," *New York Times*, May 17, 1990, p. B11, and R. Berger, "Nazi Science — The Dachau Hypothermia Experiments," *New England Journal of Medicine* 322 (1990): 1435–1440. Also see M. Angell, "The Nazi Hypothermia Experiments and Unethical Research Today," *New England Journal of Medicine* 322 (1990): 1462–1465.

3. S. Dickman and P. Aldhous, "WHO Concern Over New Drug," *Nature* 347 (1990): 606.

4. Department of Health and Human Services, Food and Drug Administration, "Informed Consent for Human Drugs and Biologics: Determination That Informed Consent Is Not Feasible: Interim Rule and Opportunity for Public Comment," *Federal Register* 55: 52814–52816 (1990). Also see G. Annas and M. Grodin, "Our Guinea Pigs in the Gulf," *New York Times* (January 8, 1991), p. A22, and J. Foreman, "Ethicists Assail Plan to Give Troops Unapproved Vaccine," *Boston Globe* (January 9, 1991), p. 1D.

5. World Medical Association, "Declaration on Chemical and Biological Weapons," adopted by the 42nd World Medical Assembly, Rancho Mirage, California, October 1990.

6. C. Gilks, "AIDS, Monkeys and Malaria," *Nature* 354 (1991): 262.

7. D. L. Breo, "Blood, Money, and Hemophiliacs — The Fatal Story of France's 'AIDSgate'," *Journal of the American Medical Association* 266 (1991): 3477–3482.

8. S. Dickman, "East Germany: Science in the Disservice of the State," *Science* 254 (1991): 26–27.

9. Ibid.

I

THE NAZI DOCTORS
AND THE
MEDICAL EXPERIMENTS

This part addresses the nature, source, and scope of Nazi medical experimentation. In his preface, Elie Weisel asks how medical doctors could have performed such murderous crimes against humanity. The crimes themselves, however, must be seen in conjunction with Nazi ideology and eugenic beliefs.

In Chapter 2, historian Robert Proctor argues that Nazi experimentation is rooted in the pre-1933 racial hygiene movement. He argues that, far from being passive pawns or a small minority in the Nazi effort, physicians were instrumental in formulating, and took the lead in carrying out, the Nazi racial hygiene program. The Nazi theory, based on a social Darwinist view of genetics and racial purity, meshed perfectly with the Nazi ideology. Physicians became leaders in the National Socialist Party and were honored for their work.

Christian Pross, a German physician and historian, has been instrumental in uncovering the extent of Nazi physicians' involvement in human experimentation. In 1989, he organized an exhibit for the West German Medical Society that was the first formal recognition of Nazi medical involvement by this society since the Nuremberg war crimes trials. In Chapter 3, Pross highlights the broad nature of physician involvement, from professor to common practitioner. He also discusses the attempts to cover up and rewrite this period of medical history.

Eva Mozes-Kor is a survivor of the infamous Mengele twin experiments. Ms. Kor is the president and founding member of an international organization called CANDLES — Children of Auschwitz Nazi Deadly Lab Experiments Survivors. Mengele, the "Angel of Death," was one of the most notorious of the Nazi physicians. Eyewitness accounts summarize the cold and murderous brutality of this M.D.-Ph.D. "man of science." Some of his most horrifying work involved genetically-related experiments performed on children who were twins, many of whom he personally killed. In an affidavit, one of his prison assistants, Dr. Miklos Nyiszli, described how Mengele killed fourteen Gypsy twins:

> In the work room next to the dissecting room, fourteen Gypsy twins were waiting and crying bitterly. Dr. Mengele didn't say a single word to us, and prepared a 10 cc and a 5 cc syringe. From a box he took Evipal and from another box he took chloroform, which was in 20 cc glass containers, and put these on the operating table. After that the first twin was brought in . . . a fourteen year old girl. Dr. Mengele ordered me to undress the girl and put her head on the dissecting table. Then he injected

the Evipal into her right arm intravenously. After the child had fallen asleep, he felt for the left ventricle of the heart and injected 10 cc of chloroform. After one little twitch the child was dead, whereupon Dr. Mengele had her taken into the corpse chamber. In this manner all four-teen twins were killed during the night.[1]

Dr. Nyiszli first observed this method of killing when it was used on four pairs of twins, all under 10 years of age. Mengele was inter-ested in them because three of the pairs had different-colored eyes. He had them killed, and their eyes and other organs removed and shipped to the Kaiser Wilhelm Institute in Berlin, marked "War Ma-terials — Urgent."

In Chapter 4, Eva Mozes-Kor gives her personal account of Men-gele and the extent of human experimentation. Ms. Kor describes the types of experimentation and the human horror and tragedy of those atrocities. And she sets an ethical agenda for the progress of medical research from the perspective of a victim of Nazi experimentation.

NOTES

1. G. L. Posner and J. Ware, *Mengele: The Complete Story* (New York: McGraw-Hill, 1986), p. 39.

2

Nazi Doctors, Racial Medicine, and Human Experimentation

ROBERT N. PROCTOR

> Only a good person can be a good physician.
>> Rudolf Ramm, the leading Nazi medical ethicist, 1942

The human experimentation carried out by physicians in Nazi concentration camps can be understood only within the context of the German militarized state and the racial hygiene movement.[1] Profound and disturbing questions arise concerning how and why physicians were able to engage in these medical crimes and atrocities. How could men and women sworn to the Hippocratic oath, trained as professionals in the world's most advanced scientific culture, come to commit crimes that even today stand as exemplars of evil?

My interest in these questions is part of a larger interest in what can be called the "political history of science": How do political formations shape the structure of science? Why do scientists support or resist the emergence of a particular political order? How does this pattern of support or resistance differ from discipline to discipline? Why do governments find it in their interest to support one kind of science and not another? And how are the theories or methods in a particular science shaped by the larger political order?

The well-established fact of medical complicity in Nazi crimes[2] does not fit well with traditional views of how scientists or other professionals establish and maintain norms of conduct. It used to be argued (by both logical positivists and many liberal sociologists) that science is either *inherently democratic* (that is, it depends on and contributes to democratic political formations) or, at worst, *apolitical*, and that the politicization of science implies its destruction. Science, in this view, must have only itself as a goal and a guide; science in the service of "interests" is no longer science. There is a political view implicit in this judgment — namely, that science grows only in the soil of democracy and that social forces hostile to democracy will be hostile to science. Such a view holds that science in a totalitarian regime is fated to be suppressed. The possibility that science (or medicine) might contribute to fascist movements is ruled out.

The point I would like to make here, however, is that this conclusion is not borne out when we look at medicine under the Nazis. Biomedical scientists played an active and leading role in the initiation, administration, and execution of each of the major Nazi racial programs. In this sense, science (especially biomedical science) under the Nazis cannot be seen simply as an essentially *passive and apolitical* scientific community responding to *external* political forces. This model of science as passive and apolitical in the face of Nazi racial politics underestimates the extent to which political initiatives arose from within the medical community and the extent to which medicine was an integral part of the Nazi program. It is a mistake, in other words, to view the relation of physicians and the state in this period as essentially one of hostility. Certain forms of medicine were indeed suppressed, but others did quite well.

EARLY RACIAL HYGIENE

The kind of science I focus on is what was known as *racial hygiene*. At the end of the nineteenth century, German social Darwinists, fearing a general "degeneration" of the human race, set about to establish a new kind of hygiene—a racial hygiene (*Rassenhygiene*) that would turn the attention of physicians away from the individual or the environment and toward the human germ plasm. In the eyes of its founders (Alfred Ploetz and Wilhelm Schallmayer), racial hygiene was supposed to complement personal and social hygiene; racial hygiene would provide long-run preventive medicine for the "German germ plasm" by combatting the disproportionate breeding of "inferiors," the celibacy of the upper classes, and the threat posed by feminists to the reproductive performance of the family.[3]

Interestingly, the early racial hygiene movement was primarily nationalistic and meritocratic rather than anti-Semitic or Nordic supremacist. Eugenicists worried more about the indiscriminate use of birth control (by the "fit") and the provision of inexpensive medical care (to the "unfit") than about the breeding of superior with inferior races or many of the other themes we associate with the Nazis. Anti-Semitism played a relatively minor role in early racial hygiene. In fact, for Alfred Ploetz, Jews were to be classed along with the Nordics as one of the superior, "cultured" races of the world.[4]

By the mid-1920s, however, this situation had changed, and the right-wing faction of racial hygiene had merged with National Socialism. The conservative, anti-Semitic J. F. Lehmann Verlag took over publication of the *Archiv für Rassen- und Gesellschaftsbiologie* (the main racial hygiene journal) shortly after World War I, and Nazi ideologues begin to incorporate eugenics rhetoric into their propaganda. By the mid-1920s, biology (especially *biological determinism*) had begun to play an important role in Nazi ideology. Fritz Lenz (one of Germany's most prominent racial hygienists) praised Hitler in 1930 as "the first politician of truly great import who has taken racial hygiene as a serious element of state policy." Hitler himself was lauded as the "great doctor of the German people" (he once called his revolution "the final step in the overcoming of historicism and the recognition of purely biological values").

Biological imagery was important in Nazi literature in several ways. SS journals spoke of the need for "selection" to replace "counterselection," borrowing their language directly from the social Darwinian racial hygienists. Nazi leaders commonly referred to National Socialism as "applied biology"; indeed, it was Lenz who originally coined this phrase in the 1931 edition of his widely read textbook on human genetics.[5] The Nazi state was itself supposed to be organic (*biologisch*) in two separate senses: in its suppression of dissent (the organic body does not tolerate a battle between one part and another) and in its emphasis on "natural" modes of living. Nature and natural modes of living were highly prized by Nazi philosophers. Women were not supposed to wear makeup, and legislation was enacted early in the Nazi period to protect endangered species. Hitler did not smoke or drink, nor would he allow anyone to do so in his presence.

Given the importance of biology in Nazi discourse, it is not surprising that doctors were among those most strongly attracted to the Nazi movement. It is frightening to see how early and eagerly they joined. In 1929 a number of physicians formed the National Socialist Physicians' League to coordinate Nazi medical policy and purify the German medical community of "Jewish Bolshevism." The organization was an immediate success, with nearly 3,000 doctors, representing 6 percent of the entire profession, joining the League by January 1933—that is, *before* the rise of Hitler to power. Doctors in fact joined the Nazi Party earlier and in greater numbers than any other professional group. By 1942, more than 38,000 doctors had joined the Nazi Party, representing about half of all doctors in the country. In 1937, doctors were represented in the SS seven times more often than the average for the employed male population; doctors assumed leading positions in German government and universities.

PAWNS OR PIONEERS?

One often hears that National Socialists distorted science, and that doctors perhaps cooperated more with the Nazi regime than they should have done, but that by 1933 it was too late, and scientists had no alternative but to cooperate or flee. There is certainly some truth in this, but I think it misses the more important point: that medical scientists were the ones who *invented* racial hygiene in the first place. Most of the 20-odd university institutes for racial hygiene were established at German universities before the Nazi rise to power, and by 1932 racial hygiene had become an orthodox fixture in the German medical community. The major expansion in this occurred *before* Hitler came to power; most of the 15-odd journals of racial hygiene, for example, were established long before the rise of National Socialism.

Racial hygiene was recognized as the primary research goal of two separate institutes of the prestigious Kaiser Wilhelm Gesellschaft: the Kaiser Wilhelm Institute for Anthropology in Berlin (1927–1945), directed by Eugen Fischer, and the Kaiser Wilhelm Institute for Genealogy in Munich (1919–1945), directed by the psychiatrist Ernst Rüdin. Both institutes helped train SS physicians; both helped construct the "genetic registries" later used to round up Jews and Gypsies. Twin studies—that is, of identical twins raised apart—were among the leading preoccupations of these and other racial institutes; their purpose was to sort out the relative influences of nature and nurture in human character and institutions.[6] Racial hygienists were convinced that many human behaviors were at root genetic—crime, alcoholism, wanderlust, even divorce. Studies of how twins behave in different environments were supposed to prove the ultimate genetic origins of racial and social differences. In 1939, Interior Minister Wilhelm Frick ordered all twins born in the Reich to be registered with Public Health Offices for the purpose of genetic research.

The largest such institution, however, was Otmar von Verschuer's Frankfurt Institute for Racial Hygiene. This institute had 67 rooms and several laboratories; this was where Josef Mengele did his doctoral research on the genetics of cleft palate, working under Verschuer. Mengele was subsequently appointed assistant to Verschuer at Berlin and provided "experimental materials" to the Institute (including eyes, blood, and other body parts) from Auschwitz as part of a study on the racial specificity of blood types funded by the Deutsche Forschungsgemeinschaft. This, I should note, was one of the reasons blood groups were so actively studied in the 1930s. When Otto Reche founded the German Society for Blood Group Research in 1926, one of the reasons he gave was to see if he could find a reliable means of distinguishing Aryans from Jews in the test tube.

Scientists, in other words, were not simply pawns in the hands of Nazi officials. But without a strong state to back them, racial hygiene was relatively impotent. It was not until 1933 that the programs of the pre-Nazi era gained the support of officials willing to move aggressively in this area.

THE STERILIZATION LAW

What were the practical results of Nazi racial hygiene? Three main programs—the Sterilization Law, the Nuremberg Laws, and the euthanasia operation—formed the heart of the Nazi program of medicalized "racial cleansing."[7] I shall deal with each in turn.

On July 14, 1933, the Nazi government passed the Law for the Prevention of Genetically Diseased Offspring, or "Sterilization Law," allowing the forcible sterilization of anyone suffering from "genetically determined" ill-nesses, including feeblemindedness, schizophrenia, manic depression, epi-lepsy, Huntington's chorea, genetic blindness, deafness, and "severe alcohol-ism." The measure was drawn up after a series of meetings by several of Germany's leading racial hygienists, including Lenz, Ploetz, Rüdin, Himm-ler (who had been active in breeding chickens prior to 1933), Gerhard Wagner, and Fritz Thyssen, the industrialist.

In 1934, 181 Genetic Health Courts and Appellate Genetic Health Courts were established throughout Germany to adjudicate the Sterilization Law. The courts were usually attached to local civil courts and presided over by two doctors and a lawyer, one of whom had to be an expert on genetic pathology. Doctors throughout the Reich were required to register every case of genetic illness known to them and could be fined 150 RM for failing to register any such defective.[8] Physicians were also required to undergo train-ing in genetic pathology at one of the numerous racial institutes established throughout the country. The German Medical Association founded a jour-nal, *Der Erbarzt* (*The Genetic Doctor*), to help physicians determine who should be sterilized. The journal included a regular column to which physi-cians could write to ask whether a patient with, say, a club foot or hearing disorder should be sterilized.

Estimates of the total number of people sterilized in Germany range from 350,000 to 400,000. Compared with the demands of some racial hygienists, this number was relatively modest. Lenz, for example, had argued that as many as 10–15 percent of the entire population were defective and ought to be sterilized.

As a consequence of the Sterilization Law, sterilization research and engi-neering rapidly became one of the largest medical industries. Medical sup-ply companies designed new and improved sterilization equipment; medical students wrote more than 180 doctoral theses exploring new methods and consequences of sterilization. There were obvious incentives for developing more rapid techniques, especially since, for women, the standard tubal liga-ture involved a hospital stay of more than a week. The most important of these techniques was a nonsurgical procedure involving scarification of the fallopian tubes through injections of supercooled carbon dioxide. In 1943, the gynecologist Carl Clauberg announced to Himmler that, using such a technique and with a staff of 10 men, he could sterilize as many as 1,000 women per day. Experiments were also done on sterilization by X-rays, a technique also used in the United States at this time.

I should also mention that it was the United States that provided the most important model for German sterilization laws. By the late 1920s, some 15,000 individuals had been sterilized in the United States—most while incarcerated in prisons or homes for the mentally ill. German racial hygien-ists throughout the Weimar period expressed their envy of American achievements in this area, warning that unless the Germans made progress in this field, America would become the world's racial leader. After World War

I, the Nazi sterilization program was never considered to have been a criminal program. It would have been difficult to do so, given the sterilization laws in many other countries.

THE CONTROL OF WOMEN

Racial domination and the elimination of the weak and unproductive were not the only forms of oppression in the Nazi regime. One aspect of Nazi ideology that has come under increasing scrutiny in recent years is the masculine and *machismo* nature of that ideology. Nazi medical philosophers were quite explicit about their feelings on this matter. A 1933 editorial by the National Socialist Physicians' League announced that the National Socialist movement was "the most *masculine* movement to have appeared in centuries."

One of the initial thrusts of Nazi policy was to take women out of the workplace and return them to the home, where they were to have as many children as possible. Fritz Lenz, for example, argued that any woman with fewer than 15 children by menopause should be considered "pathological." The government was more modest, pushing what it called the *four-child family* ideal. On December 16, 1938, Hitler announced the establishment of the "Iron Cross of German Motherhood," awarded in bronze for four children, silver for six, and gold for eight. After 1938 all public officials (including professors) were required to marry or resign; medical journals published the names of unmarried or childless colleagues. At the same time that forced sterilization and abortion were instituted for individuals of "inferior" genetic stock, sterilization and abortion for healthy German women were declared illegal and punishable (in some cases by death) as a "crime against the German body." As one might imagine, Jews and others deemed racially suspect were exempted from these restrictions. On November 10, 1938, a Lüneberg court legalized abortion for Jews. A decree of June 23, 1943, allowed abortions for Polish workers, but only if they were not judged "racially valuable."[9]

Nazi population policy, directed to what Interior Minister Wilhelm Frick called "the solution to the woman question," was remarkably successful. The birth rate jumped from 14.7/1,000 in 1933 to 18/1,000 in 1934, representing what Friedrich Burgdörfer called an unprecedented achievement in world population history and a victory in the "war of births."

It is not well known, but there is one final aspect of gender that has escaped most discussions of the Holocaust. In Germany in 1939, there were substantially more Jewish women than Jewish men; indeed, the ratio was roughly 14 women for every 10 men (men had presumably managed to emigrate in greater numbers). Gisela Bock points out that among German Jews killed in concentration camps (including most of the 167,000 Jews living in Germany in 1941), some 60 percent were women. Women also outnumbered men among the Gypsies killed at Auschwitz.[10]

THE NUREMBERG LAWS

In the fall of 1935, Hitler signed into law the so-called Nuremberg Laws — excluding Jews from citizenship and preventing marriage or sexual relations between Jews and non-Jews. A further measure, the Marital Health Laws, required couples to submit to a medical examination before marriage to see if "racial pollution" might be involved.

I will not go into detail here on the operation of these laws; the story has been told elsewhere.[11] Important for our purposes, though, is the fact that the Nuremberg Laws were considered public health measures and were administered primarily by physicians. In early 1936, when the Marital Health Laws went into effect, responsibility for administering them fell to marital counseling centers attached to local public health offices. The Nuremberg Laws, along with the Sterilization Law, were two of the primary reasons expenditures and personnel for public health actually *expanded* under the Nazis.

I should also note that, as with the Sterilization Law, here, too, German racial theorists learned from the Americans. In fact, Nazi physicians on more than one occasion argued that German racial policies were relatively "liberal" compared with the treatment of blacks in the United States. Evidence of this was usually taken from the fact that, in several southern states, a person with 1/32nd black ancestry was legally black, whereas if someone were 1/8th Jewish in Germany (and, for many purposes, 1/4th Jewish), that person was legally Aryan (a 1/4th Jew, for example, could marry a full-blooded German). Nazi physicians spent a great deal of time discussing American miscegenation legislation; German medical journals reproduced charts showing the states in which blacks could or could not marry whites, could or could not vote, and so forth.[12]

Sadly, there is yet another area where Nazi physicians were able to draw support from their American colleagues. In 1939, Germany's leading racial hygiene journal reported the refusal of the American Medical Association to admit black physicians to its membership; 5,000 black physicians had petitioned to join the all-white American body but were turned down. German physicians only one year before, in 1938, had barred Jews from practicing medicine (except on other Jews); Nazi racial theorists were thereby able to argue that Germany was "not alone" in its efforts to preserve racial purity.[13]

EUTHANASIA, GENOCIDE, AND EXPERIMENTATION

In early October 1939, Hitler issued orders that certain doctors be commissioned to grant a "mercy death" (*Gnadentod*) to patients judged "incurably sick by medical examination." By August 1941, when the first phase of the euthanasia plan was brought to a close, more than 70,000 patients from German mental hospitals had been killed in an operation which provided a rehearsal for the subsequent destruction of Jews, homosexuals, Communists, Gypsies, Slavs, and prisoners of war.

The idea of ending "lives not worth living" did not begin with the Nazis, but had been discussed in the legal and medical literatures since the end of the First World War. And not just in Germany. In 1935, the same year Egas Moniz invented the lobotomy, the French-American Nobel Prize winner Alexis Carrel suggested in his book, *Man the Unknown*, that the criminal and the mentally ill should be "humanely and economically disposed of in small euthanasia institutions supplied with proper gases." Six years later, as German psychiatrists were sending the last of their patients into the gas chambers, an article appeared in the *Journal of the American Psychiatric Association* calling for the killing of retarded children, "nature's mistakes."[14] Journals as diverse as *American Scholar* and the *Journal of the American Institute of Homeopathy* debated the merits of forcible euthanasia — at least until reports of wholesale Nazi exterminations began to appear in American newspapers in 1941 and 1942.[15]

The fundamental argument for forcible euthanasia was economic: euthanasia was justified as a kind of "preemptive triage" to free up beds. This became especially important in wartime. I want to stress this: things can happen in war that would not be tolerated in peacetime. The onset of the euthanasia operation was consciously timed to coincide with the invasion of Poland. The first gassings of mental patients occurred at Posen, in Poland, on October 15, 1939, just 45 days after the invasion of that country, marking the beginning of the Second World War. In Germany itself, after August 1941, euthanasia became part of normal hospital routine. Handicapped infants were regularly put to death; persons requiring long-term psychiatric care and judged incurable suffered the same fate. Euthanasia operations were sometimes coordinated with bombing raids: elderly or otherwise infirm individuals were killed in order to make room for war-wounded (patients capable of productive work were usually spared).[16] Psychiatrists eventually worried that their aggressive efforts to eliminate Germany's mental defectives would render their own skills useless. Professor O. Wuth, chief physician for the army, pondered in the midst of the war that with so many mental patients being eliminated by euthanasia, "who will wish to study psychiatry when it becomes so small a field?"[17]

The importance of war can also be seen in the fact that during the First World War, half of all German mental patients starved to death (45,000 in Prussia alone, according to one estimate); they were simply too low on the list to receive rations. In the Nazi period, the starvation of the mentally ill, the homeless, and other "useless eaters" became official state policy after a prolonged propaganda campaign to stigmatize the mentally ill and handicapped as having lives not worth living.

One should recall that the euthanasia program was planned and administered by leading figures in the German medical community. When the first experiments to test gases for killings took place in Brandenburg Hospital in January 1940, Viktor Brack, head of the operation, emphasized that such gassings "should be carried out only by physicians." Brack cited the motto: "The needle belongs in the hand of the doctor."

It is also important to appreciate both the *banality* and the *popularity* of the euthanasia operation. In 1941, for example, the psychiatric institution of Hadamar celebrated the cremation of its ten-thousandth patient in a special ceremony, where everyone in attendance — secretaries, nurses, and psychiatrists — received a bottle of beer for the occasion. The operation was also popular *outside* the medical community. Parents were made to feel shame and embarrassment at having to raise an abnormal or malformed child. Hospital archives are full of letters from parents requesting their children be granted euthanasia.

Historians exploring the origins of the Nazi destruction of lives not worth living have only in recent years begun to stress the link between the euthanasia operation, on the one hand, and the "final solution," on the other. And yet the two programs were linked in both theory and practice. The most important theoretical link was what might be called the "medicalization of anti-Semitism," part of a broader effort to reduce a host of social problems — unemployment, homosexuality, crime, "antisocial behavior," and others — to medical or, ideally, *surgical problems*.

In the late 1930s, German scientists proposed a number of solutions to the "Jewish question." The agronomist Hans Hefelmann suggested exporting all Jews to Madagascar. Philip Bouhler, head of Nazi party Chancellory, proposed sterilizing all Jews by X-rays. Dr. Viktor Brack, the SS colonel, recommended sterilization of the 2 to 3 million Jews capable of work, who might be put to use in Germany's factories. German medical authorities also devoted themselves to this problem. During the early war years, the official journal of the German Medical Association (*Deutsches Ärzteblatt*) published a regular column on "Solving the Jewish Question."

The ultimate decision to *gas* the Jews emerged from the fact that the technical apparatus already existed for the destruction of the mentally ill. In the fall of 1941, with the completion of the bulk of the euthanasia operation, the gas chambers at psychiatric hospitals were dismantled and shipped east, where they were reinstalled at Majdanek, Auschwitz, and Treblinka. The same doctors, technicians, and nurses often followed the equipment. In this sense, there was continuity in both theory and practice between the destruction of the lives not worth living in Germany's mental hospitals and the destruction of Germany's ethnic and social minorities.

Given the effort to destroy entire peoples, and given the medical complicity in Nazi racial crime, it is hardly surprising that physicians attempted to exploit concentration camp inmates as subjects in human experimentation. The experiments chronicled in the Nuremberg trials were carried out for various reasons. Physicians forced people to drink seawater to find out how long a man might survive without fresh water. At Dachau, Russian prisoners of war were immersed in icy water to see how long a pilot might survive when shot down over the English Channel and to find out what kinds of protective gear or rewarming techniques were most effective. Prisoners were placed in vacuum chambers to find out how the human body responds when pilots are forced to bail out at high altitudes.

There were many other experiments. At Fort Ney, near Strasbourg, 52 prisoners were exposed to phosgene gas (a biowarfare agent) in 1943 and 1944 to test possible antidotes;[18] at Auschwitz, physicians experimented with new ways to sterilize or castrate people as part of the plan to repopulate Eastern Europe with Germans.[19] Physicians performed limb and bone transplants (on persons with no medical need) and, in at least one instance, injected prisoners' eyes with dyes to see if eye color could be permanently changed. At Buchenwald, Gerhard Rose infected prisoners with spotted fever to test experimental vaccines against the disease; at Dachau, Ernst Grawitz infected prisoners with a broad range of pathogens to test homeopathic preparations. Nazi military authorities were worried about exotic diseases German troops could contract in Africa or Eastern Europe; physicians in the camps reasoned that the "human materials" at their disposal could be used to develop remedies. Hundreds of people died in these experiments; many of those who survived were forced to live with painful physical or psychological scars.

Contrary to postwar apologies, doctors were never forced to perform such experiments. Physicians volunteered—and in several cases, Nazi officials actually had to restrain overzealous physicians from pursuing even more ambitious experiments.[20] The logic governing the use of prisoners for terminal human experiments was similar to that underlying efforts to eliminate lives not worth living. In the Nazi view of the world, there were superior and inferior races, worthies and unworthies, healthy and diseased. If it required the deaths of 20 or 100 Russian prisoners to increase the chances of saving 1 German pilot, this was, in the Nazi scale of values, a justified investment. Concentration camp inmates were valued as slave labor, and when that labor was exhausted, they were not even worth keeping alive. They were lives without value, and their death implied a saving. Doctors acting in this situation were not without values. Their values were clear (Nordic supremacy, total war demands extreme measures, Jews are vermin, etc.), and they acted in accordance with those values.

CONCLUSION

Most leading German physicians supported the Nazis. Why? Physicians commonly boasted that their profession had shown its allegiance earlier, and in greater strength, than any other professional group. But why?

First of all, we should recall that the medical profession at this time was quite conservative. Before 1933, the leadership of the profession was dominated by the *Deutschnationalen*—a German nationalist party that subsequently threw its support to Hitler. Not all physicians, of course, were conservative. The profession was politicized and polarized after the economic collapse in the late 1920s and early 1930s; physicians moved from the center to the left or (more often) to the right. Socialists and Communists, however, were always a minority in the German medical community. By the end of 1932, the National Socialist Physicians' League was twice as large as the Association of Socialist Physicians (3,000 vs. 1,500 members). In the Reichstag elections leading to the Nazi seizure of power, nine physicians were elected to represent the Nazi Party; only one physician was elected to represent the socialists.

Apart from this conservatism, it is possible to argue that there was a certain ideological affinity between medicine and Nazism at this time. Many physicians were attracted by the importance given to *race* in the Nazi view of the world; physicians were intrigued by the Nazi effort to *biologize* or *medicalize* a broad range of social problems, including crime, homosexuality, the falling birth rate, the collapse of German imperial strength, and the Jewish and Gypsy "problems."

The Nazis, in turn, were able to exploit both the intimacy and the authority of the traditional physician–patient relationship. Crudely stated, they could do things with doctors that would have been much harder without them. Doctors served as executioners; doctors performed "selections" (of people to be killed) in the camps. Himmler recognized the special role of physicians in this regard. On March 9, 1943, the Reichsführer of the SS issued an order that henceforth only physicians trained in anthropology could perform selections at concentration camps.[21] Medicine also served as a *disguise*. In Buchenwald 7,000 Russian prisoners of war were executed in the course of supposed "medical exams," using a device disguised as an instrument to measure height.

There is a further element. The rise of the Nazis coincides with a period of concern about what was widely known as the "crisis" in modern science and medicine: a crisis associated with the increasing specialization and bureaucratization of science, a crisis traced alternatively to capitalism, Bolshevism, materialism, or any of a host of other real or apparent threats to human health. The Nazis promised to restore Germany to a more natural (*biologische*) way of living, a future with "more Goethe and less Newton."

In such a climate, Jews became a convenient scapegoat for all that was wrong in modern medicine. This was especially easy because Jews were in fact quite prominent in the German medical profession; 60 percent of Berlin's physicians, for example, were either Jewish or of Jewish ancestry. It was hard to name an area where opportunistic professionals were able to profit so much from exclusion of their Jewish colleagues.

And in a certain sense, the medical profession might even be said to have *prospered* under the Nazis. The medical community grew substantially under the Nazis despite the banishment of the Jews and Communists. It may even be true that physicians achieved a higher status in the Nazi period than at any time before or since. During the 12 years of Nazi rule, for example, the office of *Rektor* (president) at German universities was occupied by physicians 59 percent of the time; this contrasts with 36 percent for the decade prior to the rise of the Nazis and 18 percent for the two decades following the Nazi period. Doctors also prospered financially under the Nazis. In 1926, lawyers earned an average annual salary of 18,000 RM compared with only 12,000 RM for physicians. By 1936 doctors had reversed this trend and were earning 2,000 RM more than lawyers.

Biomedical science was *not*, in other words, simply destroyed by the Nazis; the story is more complex. If you go to the New York Academy of Medicine, or Stanford's Lane Library, or any other major medical library, you can find more than 150 German medical journals published continuously throughout the Nazi period—more than 100 meters of shelf space of journals! In fact, some 30-odd new medical journals begin publication during the Nazi period. Several of them are still published today.

The Nazis suppressed some areas and encouraged others. They supported extensive research on ecology, public health, cancer, behavioral genetics, and (of course) racial and sociobiology.[22] The Nazi government funded research on the effects of exposure to X-rays and heavy metals; some of the first reliable studies on the health effects of asbestos were done in this period. The Nazis were among the first to initiate bans on smoking in public buildings;[23] Nazi leaders organized unprecedented support for midwifery, homeopathy, and a number of other areas of heterodox medicine. Nazi physicians recognized the importance of a diet high in fruit and fiber, and in the early war years managed to have enacted a law requiring every German bakery to produce whole-grain bread. Nazi physicians restricted the use of DDT and denied women tobacco rationing coupons on the grounds that nicotine could harm the fetus. Racial hygiene itself was supposed to provide "long-run," preventive care for the German germ plasm, complementing shorter-term social and individual hygiene.[24]

I have stressed the continuity with pre-1933 traditions; space limits preclude a discussion of the important postwar continuities. Let me simply note, in conclusion, four points. First, it is important to appreciate not just the extent to which the Nazis were able to draw on the imagery and authority of science, but also the extent to which Nazi ideology informed the practice of science. Second, scientists were not bystanders or even pawns: many (not all, but not a few) helped to construct the racial policies of the Nazi state. It is probably as fair to say that Nazi racial policy emerged from *within* the scientific community as to say that it was imposed *on* that community. Third, it is commonly said that the Nazis politicized science, and that much of what went wrong under the Nazis can be traced to this politicization. The argument I have made here is that one can't consider the experience of the medical profession in terms of a simple "use and abuse" model of science. Among physicians, there were as many volunteers as victims; no one had to *force* physicians to support the regime. Hans Hefelmann testified to this effect in the euthanasia trial at Limburg in 1946: "no doctor was ever ordered to participate in the euthanasia program; they came of their own volition."

The Nazis did not have to politicize science; in fact, it is probably fair to say that the Nazis *depoliticized* science in the sense that they destroyed the political diversity that had made Weimar medicine and public health the envy of the world (with their local outpatient clinics, self-help networks, etc.). Nazism was itself supposed to transcend politics: the German state was to be a *Volksstaat*, not a *Parteistaat*; National Socialism was to be a movement, not a party. The Nazis medicalized politics as much as they politicized medicine; problems of racial, sexual, or social deviance were transformed into "surgical problems" in need of surgical solutions.

Finally, I do not want to leave the impression that the horrors of this period can be attributed to anything inherent in science or medicine, or even in technocracy or the rule of professional elites. It took a powerful state to concentrate and unleash the destructive forces within German medicine, and without that state, science would have remained impotent in this sphere. In the midst of a war engineered by an aggressive, expansionistic state, Nazi ideologues were able to turn to doctors to carry out acts that have come to be regarded as the embodiment of evil.

Rudolf Ramm, the Nazi medical ethicist whose words I cited at the beginning of this chapter, noted in his 1942 book on medical ethics that physicians will often encounter patients who complain of the treatment they have received from another doctor. Ramm advised that physicians should *always take the side of the other doctor*, turning a blind eye to whatever incompetence or malpractice their colleagues may be accused of.[25] Today one hopes that "professional ethics" means more than vigilance in the defense of the honor of the profession against its critics. Or at least that professional honor will always be understood to include a requirement that professionals act in an ethical and socially responsible manner. Elaborating on this ethic has become the painful task of physicians ever since Nuremberg, though hopefully we will never be so vain as to think that the job is finished.

NOTES

1. This paper has appeared in a similar form in Lester Embree and Tim Casey, eds., *Lifeworld and Technology* (Washington, D.C., 1989). For further documentation see my *Racial Hygiene: Medicine under the Nazis* (Cambridge, Mass., 1988).

2. See Robert J. Lifton, *Nazi Doctors* (New York, 1986); Michael H. Kater, *Doctors Under Hitler* (Chapel Hill, N.C., 1989); Hendrik van den Bussche, ed., *Medizinische Wissenschaft im "Dritten Reich"* (Hamburg, 1989); Heidrun Kaupen-Haas, ed., *Der Griff nach der Bevölkerung* (Nördlingen, 1986); Benno Müller-Hill, *Murderous Science: Elimination by Scientific Selection of Jews, Gypsies, and Others, Germany 1933–1945* (1984) (New York, 1988); Karl Heinz Roth, ed., *Erfassung zur Vernichtung, von der Sozialhygiene zum "Gesetz über Sterbehilfe"* (West Berlin, 1984); Achim Thom and Horst Spar, eds., *Medizin im Faschismus* (East Berlin, 1983); also my *Racial Hygiene*.

3. The earliest English-language history of German racial hygiene is a secret Office of Strategic Services report compiled in 1944 or 1945; see Report No. 3114.7, "Principal Nazi Organization Involved in the Commission of War Crimes, Nazi Racial and Health Policy," U.S. Office of Strategic Services, Research and Analysis

Branch, "R and A Reports," Hoover Institution Archives. The document is unsigned, though Oscar Weigart may have been the author. The report reviews the history of the Gesellschaft für Rassenhygiene, noting both the overlap with the Pan German League and the significance of the early takeover of the *Archiv für Rassen- und Gesellschaftsbiologie* by the J. F. Lehmann Verlag and of *Volk und Rasse* and the *Archiv* by the Reichsausschuss für Volksgesundheitsdienst in 1933. The report credits the Gesellschaft für Rassenhygiene with having provided Hitler with his racial ideology.

4. Alfred Ploetz, *Die Tüchtigkeit unserer Rasse und der Schutz der Schwachen* (Berlin, 1895).

5. Fritz Lenz, *Menschliche Auslese und Rassenhygiene (Eugenik)*, 3rd ed. (Munich, 1931), p. 417.

6. See Chapter 4 by Eva Kor.

7. There was also the "Law Against Habitual Criminals" (*Gesetz gegen Gewohnheitsverbrecher*), passed on November 24, 1933, providing for castration of criminals age 21 and over sentenced to at least 6 months for sexual assault. See Ludwig Lotz, *Der gefährliche Gewohnheitsverbrecher* (Leipzig, 1939).

8. Physicians, dentists, nurses, midwives, and directors of mental institutions were all required to register anyone suffering from infirmities named in the law. Children under the age of 14 were not to be forcibly sterilized, but a petition for sterilization could be issued for anyone over the age of 10. See the *Reichsgesetzblatt* 1 (1933): 1021. Local health offices were empowered to inspect municipal and private institutions to guarantee that everyone falling within the rubric of the law would be brought before the courts. On February 25, 1935, the Genetic Health Courts were granted powers to disbar any attorney who persisted too vigorously in arguing that their clients should not be sterilized. See the *Reichsgesetzblatt* 1 (1935): 289.

9. Matthias Hamann, "Die Morde an polnischen und sowjetischen Zwangsarbeitern in deutschen Anstalten," in Götz Aly et al., eds., *Aussonderung und Tod: Die klinische Hinrichtung der Unbrauchbaren* (Berlin, 1985), p. 131.

10. Gisela Bock, *Zwangssterilisation im Nationalsozialismus* (Opladen, 1986), p. 13.

11. See my *Racial Hygiene*, 1988, chap. 6.

12. See, for example, *Neues Volk* (March 1, 1936), p. 9. A 1926 Indiana law declared null and void marriage between white persons and "Persons having one-eighth or more of negro blood." Virginia's "Pure-Race Law" allowed anyone with 1/16th Indian ancestry to pass as white but required that anyone with even a trace of Negro blood be considered Negro, "though he be white as snow." See Joseph C. Carroll, "The Race Problem," *Sociology and Social Research* 11 (1927): 267. By 1940, 30 U.S. states had passed legislation barring miscegenation in one form or another; most of these laws were not repealed until after World War II (California's law, for example, was declared unconstitutional by the state supreme court in 1948). See Ashley Montagu, *Man's Most Dangerous Myth* (New York, 1952), pp. 304–305.

13. See "Keine Negerärzte in der amerikanischen Standesorganisation," *Archiv für Rassen- und Gesellschaftsbiologie* 33 (1939–1940): 276; also 33 (1939–1940): 96. In 1930 there were 5,000 licensed black physicians among a population of 13,000,000 American blacks. The appeal by America's black physicians was placed at the annual meeting of the American Medical Association in St. Louis; it was rejected. America's leading medical organization remained essentially a segregated body until the mid-1950s.

14. Foster Kennedy, "The Problem of Social Control of the Congenitally Defec-

tive: Education, Sterilization, Euthanasia," *American Journal of Psychiatry* 99 (1942): 13–16 (see also 141–143).

15. See my *Racial Hygiene*, 1988, pp. 179–189. On the murder of mentally ill persons in French hospitals under Vichy, see Max Lafont, *L'Extermination douce* (Ligné, 1987).

16. As a memo of July 5, 1943, put it, "total war" precluded the use of hospital beds for the aged or infirm. See Götz Aly, "Medizin gegen Unbrauchbare," in Aly et al., *Aussonderung und Tod: Die klinische Hinrichtung der Unbrauchbaren* (Berlin, 1985), pp. 56–74.

17. Müller-Hill, *Murderous Science*, p. 42.

18. These were the experiments that Lee Thomas, a head of the U.S. Environmental Protection Agency, barred from an EPA report in March 1988. See Philip Shabecoff, "Head of E.P.A. Bars Nazi Data in Study of Gas," *Boston Globe* (March 23, 1988), p. 4.

19. Gerhard Baader, "Menschenexperimente," in Fridolf Kudlien, ed., *Ärzte im Nationalsozialismus* (Cologne, 1985), pp. 178–180.

20. There is little evidence for the claim, made recently by Alan C. Nixon in his defense of using Nazi data, that "German scientists were rather reluctant party members, going along with the Nazis' demands in order to save their lives in an impossible situation." See his "If the Data's Good, Use It — Regardless of the Source," *The Scientist* (November 14, 1988), p. 8. In fact, there were far more volunteers than victims among scientists.

21. Müller-Hill, *Murderous Science*, p. 18.

22. One of the earliest uses of the term *sociobiology* in English can be found in the Nazi criminologist Hans von Hentig's book, translated into English as *The Criminal and His Victim, Studies in the Sociobiology of Crime* (New Haven, Conn., 1948).

23. In 1939 the city of Dresden enacted a law prohibiting smoking in all public buildings. See the *Archiv für Rassen- und Gesellschaftsbiologie* 33 (1939–1940): 274.

24. See my *Racial Hygiene*, chap. 8. For evidence of early racial hygienist concerns about lead poisoning, see E. Abramowski, "Bleivergiftung und Rasse," *Archiv für Rassen- und Gesellschaftsbiologie* 8 (1911): 542ff.

25. Rudolf Ramm, *Ärztliche Rechts- und Standeskunde* (Berlin, 1942), pp. 88–89.

3

Nazi Doctors, German Medicine, and Historical Truth

CHRISTIAN PROSS

One purpose of research during the past decade has been to destroy German postwar legends of Nazism. This work has contributed to a better and deeper understanding of health policy in Nazi Germany, and of the motives and actions of Nazi physicians, by uncovering new, hitherto unknown material and by putting old material into a new context. Anti-Semitism and racism can no longer be identified as the sole driving forces behind Nazi politics, nor can the Nazi power elite be viewed as a small group of deviant monsters who misled a supposedly passive constituency. What for us today appears contradictory in the nature of Nazism was the reason for its success: the connection between destruction and modernization. Auschwitz cannot be seen without the Volkswagen plant in Wolfsburg, or the SS regime of terror without the social security, health, and recreation programs provided by the Nazi trade union Deutsche Arbeitsfront. The so-called *Neue deutsche Seelenheilkunde* (new German psychotherapy) for the "superior" members of the *Volk* complemented the mass sterilizations of the "inferior." The destruction of the latter created social guarantees for the former, and thus secured the standard of living of the productive community of a conformist petit burgeoisie and working class at the expense of excluded minorities.

Along with the homeless, the beggars, the inmates of insane asylums, and the Jews of the East European ghettos, the German authorities eliminated the visible poor, nonproductive people who caused the state expenses during their lifetime. Their mistreatment and liquidation provided housing, employment, assets, and old-age pensions for others. In this sense, the National Socialist *Volksgemeinschaft* (community of the people) really existed. Health policy in Nazi Germany — scientifically labeled as "hereditary and race hygiene" — was a concept of rule. It unified German population, economic, and social policies to achieve one goal: the final solution of the social question. On the whole, the functionaries of the Nazi state were extraordinarily young, and they consciously relied on the results of scientific research. This elite did away with rusty old structures and started to put their political utopias—such as the concept of a common *Gesundheitspflicht* (obligation for health)—into practice. To clean the body of the *Volk* from everything sick, alien, and disturbing was one of the dreams of the German intelligentsia.

In addition to the well-known "euthanasia Aktion T4"—the killing of the mentally ill and the handicapped in 1940 and 1941—there is a hitherto unknown chapter of mass murder, consisting of the ways in which other "useless" members of society were singled out, sent to killing hospitals, starved to death, or killed by injections. The "useless" consisted of "antisocials" or *Gemeinschaftsfremde* (alien to the community), as the Nazis called them: maladjusted adolescents, sick foreign slave laborers, and civilians who had suffered psychic breakdowns, became disoriented after air-raid attacks, and posed a threat to public order and discipline. The planning and executing forces were labor offices, health administration authorities, city mayors, and others who organized the killings. Their rationale was, for example, to provide beds for physically wounded soldiers and civilians in the phase of "total war" by emptying mental hospitals, foster homes, and institutions for the handicapped. These issues were only marginally dealt with in the Doctors' Trial and the postwar trials against euthanasia doctors, because the prosecuting authorities were interested primarily in evidence of individual guilt, not in the overall context and the network in which the doctors had functioned.

There was also a connection between murder and modernization in German psychiatry. The reforms envisioned by the protagonists of euthanasia, who were activists on behalf of an intensive therapy and rehabilitation program for the "superior" members of the *Volk*, demanded the destruction of the "inferior" incurable patients. To reduce the size of the hospitals, to differentiate the inner structure, to shorten the duration of inpatient care, to simplify the reimbursement of costs, to create a variety of outpatient care facilities, and to do systematic research on the causes of mental disease was part of the professional ethos and identity of these doctors who executed mass murder not simply for its own sake. They had been among the leaders of psychiatric reform in the Weimar period, and in 1941–1942 they believed they had achieved the goal of their plans, which had been massively promoted and accelerated by the euthanasia program. As unfinished as their plans were in 1945, the military defeat of German fascism did not make them disappear.

National Socialism removed barriers that in a democratic system would at least have considerably impeded quick reforms and radical scientific experiments. It offered certain researchers and reformers unusual chances. At the same time, a modern social strategy and science gave National Socialism the chance to rationalize its irrational ideology and to legitimize its crimes as scientifically and economically reasonable. These scientific procedures did not require any *Gleichschaltung* (synchronization). Their inner form, guided by their abstract interest, complied with the logic of Nazi rule.

THE ORDINARY PHYSICIAN IN THE THIRD REICH

Alexander Mitscherlich, the official envoy of the West German Chamber of Physicians at the Doctors' Trial, noted that many more physicians were involved in medical crimes than the 23 Nuremberg defendants, who were only the tip of an iceberg. An anecdote by a physician I interviewed about her wartime experience helps to elucidate this observation. In 1943, as a medical student, she was conducting experiments on the functioning of the kidney in a Berlin laboratory. She was doing these experiments on herself and her fellow students. One day an air force physician, who was on leave from the African front and had stopped by her lab, exclaimed: "Are you crazy, doing those experiments on yourself? We have concentration camps for this!"[1]

Hermann Voss, professor of anatomy at Posen University in occupied Poland, conducted experiments on the content of the blood in the spleen. He received his "material" from the guillotine of the Posen Gestapo, which was very busy fighting the Polish resistance. In his diary, which he failed to destroy when the Russians arrived, he noted:

> Yesterday I looked at the mortuary morgue in the basement and the furnace in the crematorium. The furnace was originally intended to dispose of the remnants of the dissecting course for the students. Now it serves to incinerate executed Poles. Almost daily the gray limousine arrives with the gray men, the SS-men from the Gestapo, carrying material for the furnace. As it was not working yesterday we could look inside the furnace, where we could see the ashes of four Poles. How little remains from a human being after all organic material has been burnt! Looking into such a furnace makes me feel very calm and comfortable. The Poles recently have become increasingly impudent and thus our furnace is very busy. How nice it would be to chase the whole population through such furnaces! Then the German people finally would get some rest in the East. . . . Today I wrote to Prof. Schoen in Göttingen and asked him to remember me when the chair for anatomy at the university becomes vacant.[2]

Voss was an average physician, not an ardent Nazi. He became one of the most prestigious professors of anatomy after the war and held the chair of anatomy at the University of Jena, East Germany. Virtually every medical student in both Germanies learned anatomy from his handy little textbook, the "Voss-Herrlinger book."

The Posen diaries of Voss give an unusual insight into the inner life of a rather average perpetrator. They are based on documents written at the time, uncensored and unfalsified by the need for excuses and for some kind of postwar identity. To a certain extent, they resemble the autobiography of the commander of Auschwitz, Rudolf Höß, written after his arrest by the Allies. His whining and philistine language bore the stamp of the typical culprit: the German sentimentality of the mass murderer, who emphasizes his own suffering in the face of the mountain of corpses he himself produces. The autobiography of Rudolf Höß gave support to the theory of the "banality of evil." Remarkably, this notion supported the dispersion of a sense of threat from the continued presence of these men among the population in Germany. The idea quickly became the common currency of the task of mastering the past, utterly contrary to Hanna Arendt's intent. The concept, intended as a rhetorical spur to focus attention on the inconceivable, merely made it tangible, so that it could be pushed aside. Immediately the actual perpetrator Höß managed to disappear behind the image of the culprit Höß. He was perfectly willing to admit to mass murder, but he did not mention the removal of three carloads of valuables from Auschwitz. This silence concerning the evidence of baser motives was accepted without question. Amazingly, it seemed easier to deal with a profile of the perpetrator that remained unblemished by any trace of sadism or greed.

The diaries of Voss, however, reveal such baser motives as envy, greed, careerism and mutual elbowing, malicious joy, and contempt for the subhumans at his disposal. They exhibit a peculiar coexistence of the enjoyments of everyday life, tender feelings for flowers and loved ones — and the routine of selecting and killing. One might expect that petit bourgeois intimacy and human destruction would somehow be linked in these private documents, but somehow, seeing the mixture of these two elements in their particularity overwhelms one with a sense of shock. Voss's diary is a mixture of whining over his unsatisfying career, pleasure in nature, and greed for the marginal profits of the great war, for the "special distributions."

The conquest of the East brought him a professorship at the university in Posen. Even if his drive for advancement couldn't be stilled by this position, the anatomical institute of the *Reichsuniversität* Posen represented one object of his desire: the crematorium in the service of the Gestapo. The oven was his social utopia. These quotes of an average doctor, who did not stand at the ramp in Auschwitz, demonstrate to what extent the officially organized murders were supported by the anticipatory consent of the people, including the intelligentsia. The German intelligentsia lent a vocabulary to the hatred of the little people and rationalized the will for annihilation to the point where it could become realized. It is, in fact, a singular accomplishment of the German intelligentsia that the crematoria could be promoted as a solution for social ills. Voss's diary is important, above all, because it shows that it was not only unrestrained desire for knowledge that energized the fury of destruction, but simple hate.[3]

One of the leading German surgeons, Ferdinand Sauerbruch, was on the Research Review Committee of the *Reichsforschungsrat* (the Reich Research Council) that approved the grants for Mengele's twin studies in Auschwitz.[4] The prosecutor in the Doctors' Trial named Sauerbruch and other leading German medical professors as accessories to medical crimes because they

had participated in a conference on the extremely cruel and fatal sulfonamide experiments in the Ravensbrück concentration camp. In that conference, the results of the experiments were openly discussed among special-
ists, without anybody questioning their ethics.[5]

Another high-ranking surgeon, Erwin Gohrbandt, director of Surgery III
of the University Clinic of Berlin and chief medical advisor for aeronautical
medicine at the Luftwaffe's sanitary services division, participated in a secret 1942 conference on the results of the fatal freezing experiments at
Dachau. Later he reported on these results in the leading surgical journal,
Zentralblatt für Chirurgie.[6] By participating in the scientific discourse on
these experiments in a value-free manner, or by approving of grants for these
experiments or publishing the results under their names in prestigious medical journals, Sauerbruch and Gohrbandt gave them the appearance of legiti-
macy.

Gastroenterologist Kurt Gutzeit, professor of medicine at the University
of Breslau, directed hepatitis experiments on Jewish children from Auschwitz. He wanted to identify the carrier of hepatitis by artificially infecting
these children with serum from hepatitis patients. When his assistant, Dr.
Arnold Dohmen, tried to avoid the human experiments by doing animal
experiments, Gutzeit threatened to wake him up from his "animal-experi-
ment lethargy." Finally, Dohmen infected 11 Jewish children and carried out
liver punctures on them, but with no satisfying results. Further "massive"
artificial infections, which Gutzeit demanded, were never carried out because of Germany's defeat.[7]

Heinrich Berning, associate professor at Hamburg University, carried out
famine experiments on Soviet prisoners of war to investigate the nature of
famine disease. While the prisoners starved to death, he observed their body
functions, such as the ceasing of libido, dizziness, headache, edema, and
swelling of the lower abdomen. "The changes in the gastrointestinal tract,
that we find in the autopsies, are particularly interesting," he wrote in a
secret preliminary report. He published a sanitized version of his results in a
monograph after the war.[8]

Neuropathologist Julius Hallervorden from the Kaiser Wilhelm Institute
for Brain Research in Berlin-Buch, together with his chief, Hugo Spatz, is
known in the medical world as the discoverer of the Hallervorden-Spatz
disease, a rare congenital brain disease. In the early 1940s, he ordered hundreds of brains of the victims of euthanasia from the killing hospital in
Brandenburg-Görden for his neuropathological studies. In 1945 an American interrogator asked him about his research and quoted Hallervorden's
excuses in his report:

> I heard that they were going to do that, and so I went up to them and told them
> "Look here now, boys, if you are going to kill all these people, at least take the
> brains but so that the material could be utilized." They asked me: "How many can
> you examine?" and so I told them an unlimited number—"the more the better." I
> gave them fixatives, jars and boxes and instructions for removing and fixing the

brains and then they came bringing them like the delivery van from the furniture company. There was wonderful material among these brains, beautiful mental defectives, malformations and early infantile disease. I accepted these brains of course. Where they came from and how they came to me, was really none of my business.[9]

Hallervorden's statement shows that he was so preoccupied with his scientific curiosity that he accepted the killing of patients as normal.

Robert Ritter, a psychiatrist who was trained at the Psychiatric Clinic of the University of Tübingen, worked on the racial identification and genealogy of the Gypsies and the *Asozialen* (antisocials). In 1938, when he became director of the Research Institute of the Reich Health Office for Race Hygiene and Criminal Biology, he systematically searched for and examined all Gypsies living within the borders of the Reich (after 1939 he included those in the occupied territories). He discovered that most Gypsies were not racially pure, but rather half-breeds. He considered these half-breeds, who, according to him, had intermarried with the "antisocial and criminal German subproletariat," more dangerous than pure Gypsies. The half-Gypsies, as he saw it, were a primitive, intellectually underdeveloped species that neither education nor punishment could mold into tidy, settled citizens. They would inevitably cost the state tremendous sums for welfare. Ritter proposed that they be incarcerated in forced labor camps and prevented from procreating. In a proposal to the SS chief, Himmler, he suggested that the pure Gypsies, on the other hand, be assigned to reservations, where their exotic customs and culture could be preserved for anthropological science. Ritter presented his first report in 1941 and announced that 30,000 Gypsies had been registered, among them 19,000 within the borders of the Reich and 11,000 in the occupied territories. During a conference of the *Reichssicherheitshauptamt* in 1941, SS leaders discussed various means of exterminating the Gypsies. One proposal was to drown them in the Mediterranean. Ritter, who took part in this conference, managed to persuade the SS leaders to postpone the killing for another year until his racial studies were finished and the racially pure Gypsies had been separated from the mass of the half-breeds. Himmler ordered the deportation of the majority of the Gypsies to Auschwitz in December 1942. Only nine Gypsy clans, who were considered racially pure, were exempt from the deportation. Ritter's contribution to the genocide of the Gypsies was essential. His medical expert opinions defining who was a Gypsy and who wasn't, and what kind of Gypsy one was, gave the selection and destruction of socially undesired elements a medical, scientific underpinning.[10]

The director of the Institute of Anatomy of Berlin University, Hermann Stieve, conducted experiments on female prisoners from the Plötzensee prison and the Ravensbrück concentration camp. He studied the female menstrual cycle under severe stress, that is, the irregular bleedings in women after they learned about their imminent execution. At autopsy he proved that the bleedings were not regular menstruations after ovulation but stress-induced bleeding. He published his results after the war as the honored leading specialist in gynecological anatomy at East Berlin's Humboldt University.[11]

None of the above-mentioned physicians was indicted at Nuremberg. They represent not the extremes, but rather the attitude, thinking, and daily routine of a large part of the average physician population. They were not fanatic Nazis or high-ranking SS physicians, but they profited from the unique opportunity to experiment on living humans, and they supported the Nazi utopian view of a society cleansed of everything sick, alien, and disturbing. These facts have been revealed only in the past 10 years and have stirred a debate among the German medical profession that was long overdue.

THE TOPICALITY OF NAZI MEDICINE

It is fear of medical technology, the uncertainty of how to handle it, and the erosion of traditional ethical standards that makes people look for historical lessons from the Nazi experience. (See chapter 14) Yet it is difficult to find an answer to present-day problems in historical analogies. Long before 1933, physicians and anthropologists had tried to prove that certain human beings were less worthy of living than others. In the nineteenth century, the theory of the inequality of the human races, of the differentiation of "superiors" and "inferiors," was an attack of the declining European gentry on the demands for equality, freedom, and brotherhood and the declaration of human rights during the French Revolution. It provided the ideological tools for a biological solution to the social question. Despite the fact that in the period of industrialization poverty, venereal disease, tuberculosis, and alcoholism spread in the slums of the big cities, their social causes were simply denied, and it was suggested that it was the individual's fault if he was poor and sick. Poverty was understood as a sign of degeneration and hereditary inferiority.

Leading psychiatrists and anthropologists translated ideological slogans into scientific categories and applied them as apparently objective medical diagnoses.[12] The new science was called *racial hygiene*. The Nazi seizure of power in 1933 provided the long-desired opportunity for racial hygiene to be applied in practice, to solve the economic and social crisis of German society by a radical biological cure. Yet racism was not the only source of the disaster. Alexander Mitscherlich, noted in his first-hand impressions from Nuremberg in 1947:

> Before such monstrous deeds and thoughts shape everyday routine and real life, the disaster must have originated from many sources. Only in the crossing of two currents could the doctor turn into a licensed killer and publicly employed torturer: at the point where his aggressive search for the truth met with the ideology of

the dictatorship. It is almost the same, if one sees a human being as a "case" or as a number tattooed on his arm. This is the double facelessness of a merciless epoch.[13]

The search for truth, the search for new notions, has motivated scientists and doctors for centuries. Without it there would be no progress, no modern diagnostic and therapeutic knowledge and technique. However, in nineteenth-century science, this search became more and more a search for objective truths. The search for truth in medicine turned into destruction. It abandoned its purpose of healing the sick individual, of alleviating his suffering, and abandoned the Hippocratic *nil nocere* when experimentation was done for its own sake, for "superior" aims.

What physician is not tempted by the enormous range of invasive diagnostic measures and fascinated by the chance to look into the most remote parts of the human organism? Today sheer curiosity, competition, and careerism among doctors, defensive medicine, the corporatization of medicine, and the disappearance of the classic elements of medicine, such as the art of listening to the patient and using one's senses, lead to an inflated application of machinery. They seduce the physician who is permanently confronted with the imperfect, unpredictable human being to escape into the apparently safe world of laboratory parameters and computer scans. In the Weimar Republic, numerous physicians complained about the decay of medicine into a purely diagnostic science.[14] Under the Nazis, it was as if an already unstable dam had broken. The abundant availability of human guinea pigs among people labeled as "inferior" or "subhuman" was exploited by doctors as a unique opportunity for scientific research. The chief managers of euthanasia did not simply kill their victims; they thoroughly investigated them before and afterward, hoping to find eventually the clue to the nature of mental disease.

Another source of the disaster was the tension between the physicians' fantasies of omnipotence and their factual impotence. Medicine is often like the works of Sisyphus, because it alone can do little to overcome the misery of many patients, nor can it change the often puzzling and stubborn human nature. When the young physician graduates from medical school and enters the rough reality of medical practice, he quickly feels the limitations of his professional skills and his own helplessness. He can change neither men nor society. The idealism of the helpless helper can turn into an aggressive attitude toward the sick and a search for radical and final prescriptions. The relapsing, incurable, and chronically ill patient mobilizes the helper's hidden fears of disease and death. If these emotions coincide with a loss of job security, a financial crisis of the health care system, and a fear of the future, ethical standards tend to erode very quickly. The propaganda for the sterilization of the "inferior" and the elimination of "unnecessary eaters" in Weimar Germany gained broad support only when the Great Depression of 1929 caused an acute shortage of funds in the health service. Growing unemployment after 1929 drove thousands of doctors into the ranks of the National Socialists Physicians' League.

In contemporary Germany, the official dramatic rhetoric about the "cost explosion" in health care and the continuous cuts in spending have produced new prophets of euthanasia. In a prepared television show, surgeon Julius Hackethal handed a cancer patient potassium cyanide and advocated active euthanasia.[15] A growing number of court cases are being reported in which nurses have intentionally killed old and chronically ill patients in nursing homes and intensive care units.[16] The *Journal of the American Medical Association* in 1988 published the anonymous report of a young physician on duty who gave a young cancer patient he did not know but had just come across during his night shift a fatal injection.[17] What did the editors have in mind when they published this report? The United States and Germany in 1991 are not pre-Nazi Germany, yet there is an economic crisis, unemployment, serious cuts in health care spending, and new talk about certain people being less qualified for full medical care than others. Could calls for a discontinuation of sophisticated medical care and life-prolonging measures for the elderly be the catalyst for an attack on the life of the elderly,[18] as much as Binding and Hoche's call for "the destruction of life unworthy of living" was an attack on the mentally ill and the handicapped in 1920 in Germany?[19]

HISTORIOGRAPHY AND POLITICS

As Mitscherlich and Mielke noted in 1947, "only the secret consent of the practice of science and politics can explain why the names of high-ranking scientists are constantly dropped during this trial, of men, who perhaps did not right off commit any crime but took advantage of the cruel fate of defenseless individuals."[20] Mitscherlich and Mielke had the courage to break the taboo of their profession by publishing trial documents, which charged Ferdinand Sauerbruch, Germany's leading surgeon, and Wolfgang Heubner, director of the Pharmacological Institute of Berlin University, with being accessories to medical crimes by participating in a conference on the extremely cruel and partly fatal sulfonamide experiments in Ravensbrück.[21] Mitscherlich had to pay a high price for it. Sauerbruch and Heubner sued him and forced him to remove this paragraph from the trial report. At the same time, the leading physiologist and specialist of aviation medicine in Göttingen, Friedrich Rein, accused Mitscherlich of irresponsibly attacking the basis of scientific research and dishonoring the German medical profession.[22]

Ten thousand copies of the final version of Mitscherlich's documentation of the Nuremberg Doctors' Trial[23] were printed in 1949 exclusively for the members of the West German Chambers of Physicians. Yet the book did not become known to the public. There were no reviews, no letters to the editor. "It was as if the book had never been written," Mitscherlich recalled. It is as if the 10,000 copies disappeared in the basement of the West German Chambers of Physicians without a single German doctor ever having read the book. However, the World Medical Association received a copy and took it as proof that the German medical profession had distanced itself from the medical crimes committed under the Nazis and thus was qualified for renewed membership.[24] Mitscherlich, who had helped to save the international reputation of the German medical profession, was subjected to a campaign of slander by his colleagues, who labeled him a traitor to his country and succeeded in hurting his career. In 1956 the medical faculty of Frankfurt University refused to give him the chair of an institute of psychoanalysis and psychosomatic medicine that the state government had offered him. In his autobiography, Mitscherlich bitterly notes that he had virtually pulled the chestnuts out of the fire for his profession but had been stabbed in the back for it.[25]

In the following three decades after the repression of Mitscherlich's documentation, there was a loud silence. Very little was published, and it got little public attention.[26] In 1960 there was some news coverage of the leading protagonist of the killing of handicapped children in the Third Reich, Werner Catel, who was forced to resign as director of the pediatric hospital of Kiel University.[27] In 1959 the former professor of psychiatry of Würzburg University and chief manager of euthanasia, Werner Heyde, was arrested. For 15 years he had been practicing medicine in a small town in northern Germany under a false name, protected by the local medical establishment, who knew his identity. Heyde committed suicide in prison and thus evaded trial.[28] The East German lawyer Friedrich Karl Kaul, who was an observer of many trials of Nazi criminals in West Germany, published a book on the cover-up of Heyde, as well as a book on physicians in Auschwitz, some of whom went on trial in Frankfurt in the mid-1960s.[29] But in those days, with the cold war at its height, anything that came from an East German source was considered obscure or at least not worth listening to. At least as a result of those events, Mitscherlich's documentation was reedited.[30]

During the student rebellion of the late 1960s, some facts were revealed about the Nazi past of prominent members of medical schools. In 1968 the director of the National Cancer Institute in Heidelberg, Karl Heinrich Bauer, faced a sit-in by medical students confronting him with his involvement in compulsory sterilization during the Third Reich. A hand-made document was published but did not become known beyond the Heidelberg academic community. The whole medical faculty backed Bauer and obstructed the medical career of the author of the document.[31]

The history of medicine community at German medical schools, with few exceptions, produced the apologetic literature on the profession's past that its leaders were asking for. Hans Schadewaldt, the last director of the Institute of the History of Medicine in Düsseldorf, in a 1969 essay on the 75-year history of the largest physician lobby organization, *Hartmannbund*, denied that its pre-1933 leaders had actively participated in the Nazi seizure of power.[32] Until recently, Schadewaldt was the official historian of the German

Federal Chamber of Physicians. Another influential figure in the postwar German history of medicine was Paul Diepgen, who as director of the prestigious Berlin Institute during the Third Reich had created a list of Jewish authors who were no longer to be cited.[33] In the 1947 and 1953 editions of his popular textbook *Die Heilkunde und der ärztliche Beruf* he eliminated all the Nazi phraseology that the 1938 edition had carried.[34] Another example of the zeitgeist is the 1972 *Festschrift* brochure on the 100th anniversary of the renowned Moabit Hospital in Berlin, in which Berlin medical historian Manfred Stürzbecher gave an industrious and detailed account of the admission figures of patients, the hospital budgets, the construction of hospital buildings, and the changing patient menus of the past 100 years, while skipping almost entirely the events between 1933 and 1945, when the hospital's predominantly Jewish physicians were persecuted and an underground resistance group of physicians was arrested and some of its members killed.[35] It is the typical blank spot that one finds in most postwar German *Festschriften* and biographies.

Another factor that impeded attempts to deal openly with the profession's past was that, until the end of the 1970s, many leading positions in the professional organizations and university chairs were held by physicians who had been active members of the Nazi Party or its affiliated organizations, the SA and the SS. In 1983, the president of the West Berlin Chamber of Physicians was surgeon Wilhelm Heim, who had been a member of the SA stormtrooper squad that was involved in the purge of Jewish physicians at the *Urbankrankenhaus* in Berlin in 1933.[36] Important data on these physicians exist in the archives of the U.S.-administered Berlin Document Center, which until recently was almost inaccessible to German researchers. Equally significant are the files of the *Kassenärztliche Vereinigung Deutschlands*, the federation of panel doctors, which took away the licenses of Jewish doctors after 1933. These files were discovered in the late 1970s in the archives of the *Kassenärztliche Bundesvereinigung* Berlin office, the West German panel doctors federation, by the Canadian historian Michael Kater. Kater was farsighted enough to copy most of the material and move it to the archives of York University in Ontario, Canada, because when researchers asked for the files a couple of years later, they had mysteriously disappeared. After repeated requests, Kater in 1986 got an official letter from the *Kassenärztliche Bundesvereinigung* headquarters in Köln saying that "unfortunately" the papers had now been "destroyed."[37]

In the late 1970s and early 1980s, starting with the catalyzing effect of the American television series *Holocaust*, the political climate changed. The old Nazi generation was retiring or had already died. Suddenly archives were available that had not been accessible before. A fever of remembrance by grass-root historians broke out, culminating in the 50th anniversary of the Nazi seizure of power in 1983 and the 50th anniversary of the *Kristallnacht* pogrom in 1988. Politicians, professional organizations, and village or city governments suddenly discovered their former Jewish "fellow citizens," and invited and honored them. As Raoul Hilberg noted 28 years ago in a sarcastic comment on the reception of Anne Frank's diary in Germany, the Germans tend to praise and deify their former victims with an ardor that seems uncanny.[38]

Apart from all the official memorial ceremonies, the movement of grass-root historians has persistently dug out document after document about what happened between 1933 and 1945. They continued where the Nuremberg trials and the postwar German trials of perpetrators had stopped or remained fragmentary. The evidence they provided about the involvement of almost every public institution, every professional organization, about the forgotten victims — Gypsies, Communists, homosexuals, sterilization victims, deserters, and conscientious objectors — who never got compensation, pervaded the consciousness of a broader public and has to a certain extent influenced the official rhetoric since that time. It is this new consciousness that so far has prevented the attempt of conservative historians like Ernst Nolte to quietly imprint their revisionist version of history outside any public debate on the concept of a planned National Museum of History in Berlin.

THE TURN OF THE TIDE

In the historiography of Nazi medicine, the turn of the tide occurred during a national conference of physicians and health workers called the *Gesundheitstag* in West Berlin in May 1980. It was a deliberate counterconference to the simultaneous annual meeting of the *Deutsche Ärztetag*, the physicians' parliament, whose host was the above-mentioned former SA member Wilhelm Heim. As an attempt to recapture destroyed alternative models of health care from the Weimar period, the organizers of the *Gesundheitstag* had invited five Jewish refugee physicians from abroad, most of them former members of the Socialist Doctors' Association (*Verein Sozialistischer Ärzte*). "Medicine Under National Socialism. Repressed Past — Unbroken Tradition?" was the title of the conference, which for the first time presented the work of a small group of outsiders.[39] Among them was the investigative reporter Günther Schwarberg, who had written a book on the fatal experiments on tuberculous children in Hamburg;[40] the Bremen law professor Stephan Leibfried and the Kassel sociologist Florian Tennstedt, who had documented the purge of Jewish and socialist doctors from the health insurance panels;[41] the historian Walter Wuttke-Groneberg, who had published a voluminous collection of documents on Nazi health policy;[42] and the Hamburg family physician Karl Heinz Roth, who had studied family planning and population control in the Third Reich.[43] From the institutes of the history of medicine, two nonconformists had the courage to attend the conference. Fridolf Kudlien from Kiel University gave a paper on anti-Nazi resistance among physicians, and Gerhard Baader of Berlin University spoke about the history of social Darwinism.[44]

The conference sparked further research. A social worker for the handicapped, Ernst Klee, came out with a profound study of euthanasia based on material from the archives of mental hospitals run by the Innere Mission, the charitable organization of the Lutheran church.[45] Walter-Wuttke Groneberg and his associates created an exhibit on Nazi medicine, which was shown throughout West Germany, that focused on the role of psychiatrists, on the role of occupational health care, and on the preference of early Nazi health policy for holistic medicine and natural healing as opposed to decadent "Jewish" scientific medicine.[46] Benno Müller-Hill, a geneticist from Cologne University, revealed the involvement of leading German geneticists and anthropologists in the selection of Jews, Gypsies, and the mentally ill and retarded for sterilization and genocide. Among them he focused on the director of the prestigious Kaiser Wilhelm Institute for Anthropology, menschliche Erblehre und Eugenik, Otmar von Verschuer, who directed Mengele's research on twins in Auschwitz.[47] To this day, Verschuer's twin studies are still cited by many of the world's leading geneticists.[48] The Berlin historian Gisela Bock published a profound study on compulsory sterilization, in which she suggests that sterilization was directed mainly against women, who were considered inferior to men.[49]

Other classic works that were published after the *Gesundheitstag* include Götz Aly and Karl-Heinz Roth's analysis of compulsory registration of the German population, which was implemented in 1938 and provided the technical assumptions for the selection of racial and hereditary "superiors" and "inferiors."[50] Michael Kater studied the National Socialist Physicians' League, documenting the high percentage of physicians in Nazi organizations and the power struggle within the Nazi health administration.[51] Georg Lilienthal studied the *Lebensborn*, an SS-run foundation that established maternity homes for unmarried mothers and orphanages to raise racially selected children.[52] Geoffrey Cocks and Regine Lockot published a history of psychoanalysis and psychotherapy in Nazi Germany,[53] and Angelika Ebbinghaus and associates studied the Nazi model for a "modernized" health care system in the city of Hamburg.[54] There were also many other local studies.[55]

To coordinate and fund this new wave of research, which in general was not welcomed and sometimes was even obstructed by the academic community, Karl Heinz Roth, Götz Aly, and others in 1983 founded the *Verein zur Erforschung der nationalsozialistischen Gesundheitsund Sozialpolitik* (Association for Research on Nazi Health and Social Policy). The *Verein* received private contributions, and some of its members were sponsored by the foundation Hamburger Institut für Sozialforschung. In 1985 it came out with a periodical, *Beiträge zur nationalsozialistischen Gesundheits—und Sozialpolitik*, of which eight volumes have since been published.[56]

The impact of these numerous publications over the past 10 years has been powerful enough to finally force the German Federal Chamber of Physicians to change its attitude. On the 50th anniversary of the *Machtergreifung*, the Nazi seizure of power, the *Deutsche Ärzteblatt* (the equivalent of the *Journal of the American Medical Association*) still maintained in an editorial that "the new masters had appeared overnight" and seized control of the reluctant professional organizations, denying the fact that the leaders of these organizations had enthusiastically supported the new regime.[57] When the German pediatrician and peace activist Hartmut Hanauske-Abel published an article in *Lancet* in 1986 about the medical profession's continuing denial of the truth,[58] the chairman of the Federal Chamber of Physicians, Karsten Vilmar, accused him of distorting facts and slandering the profession.[59] Hanauske-Abel consequently lost his position as emergency physician at the panel (insurance) doctors association in Mainz for political reasons. His case and Vilmar's backward attitude were covered by the leading German newspapers as a scandal. In May 1989, the Berlin Chamber of Physicians, which was now controlled by the organizers of the 1980 *Gesundheitstag*, used the opportunity of hosting the 1989 annual meeting of the *Deutsche Ärztetag* to persuade Vilmar to put medicine under the Nazis on the agenda. Against considerable resistance from some state physicians' chambers, an exhibit was created, which was officially opened at the annual session in May 1989 in Berlin,[60] "The Value of the Human Being," created by the author and Götz Aly. Simultaneously, an international scientific symposium under the umbrella of the Federal Chamber of Physicians was organized and a series of articles was published on medicine under the Nazis in the *Deutsche Ärzteblatt*.[61] At the opening of the exhibit, Richard Toellner, medical historian at the University of Münster, stated in a widely noted speech that the majority of physicians had actively or passively participated in medical crimes and that the burden of the past had to be faced and no longer repressed:

> The whole spectrum of normal representatives of the medical profession was involved and they all knew what they did. . . . A medical profession, who accepts mass murder of sick people as a normality, and to a large degree explicitly approves of it as a necessary, justified act for the sake of the community, has failed and betrayed its mission. Such a medical profession as a whole has become morally guilty, no matter how many members of the profession directly or indirectly participated in the killing of sick people in a legal sense.

This clear statement was printed in the *Deutsche Ärzteblatt* and must be seen as a new interpretation of history, from which the Federal Chamber of Physicians can no longer retreat.[62] Does that mean that the German medical profession has finally shown the remorse Mitscherlich asked for in vain 42 years ago? The attitude of the official representatives of the profession remains contradictory. The 1989 *Deutsche Ärztetag* in Berlin certainly triggered a debate within the profession that was unthinkable before. The articles in the *Deutsche Ärzteblatt* provoked angry reactions from a number of readers; some of the letters to the editor were full of anti-Semitic and German chauvinist resentment.[63] On the one hand, some of the presidents of state physicians' chambers, such as the president of the *Ärztekammer Nordrhein*, Horst Bourmer, and the president of the *Ärztekammer Bremen*, Karsten Vilmar (who is also the president of the Federal Chamber of Physicians), have honored their former persecuted Jewish members in memorial ceremonies and apologized for the deeds of Nazi colleagues. On the other hand, Karsten Vilmar recently challenged Professor Toellner's notions by stating that the majority of German physicians had worked altruistically for their patients and had never been involved in or approved of any atrocities. He also repeated the official legend that as early as 1949 the West German Chamber of Physicians had confronted the past by publishing Mitscherlich's report of the Nuremberg Doctors' Trial.[64]

Meanwhile, German doctors are facing growing concern from abroad on the issue of Nazi medicine. At the 1986 meeting of the American College of Neuropsychopharmacology, a German scientist was questioned about the origin of the historical brain specimens, dating from the early 1940s, that he had used for his research and had presented at the meeting. It turned out that they originated from victims of euthanasia.[65] Physicians in Israel and the United States have expressed concern about the use of anatomical specimens from Nazi victims by German medical schools for teaching purposes. The pressure from abroad finally forced several universities and the prestigious Max Planck Society for Brain Research to remove all specimen of Nazi victims from their collections and bury them.[66] The speech given by the director of the Institute for Brain Research of the University of Tübingen, Prof. Jürgen Peiffer, at the burial in Tübingen shows how the debate of the past 10 years has stimulated leading representatives of academic medicine to confront the past of their own profession. Peiffer, who served as a soldier in World War II, confessed in his speech that he admired and respected the grand old man of German neuropathology, Julius Hallervorden, as a friendly colleague and dedicated teacher. He then tried to present a balanced judgment of Hallervorden's guilt: Although Hallervorden may have had doubts about the legality of his actions, he was so dazzled by scientific curiosity and ambition that he was not aware of serving as a cog in an inhumane machinery of extermination. The zeal of scientists like Hallervorden, Peiffer suggested, thus morally legitimized the crimes of the actual "death doctors."[67] Peiffer was stimulated by Götz Aly's research to initiate a controversial debate on Hallervorden[68] in the German Neuropathological Society and now works on a detailed history of the criminal involvement of a number of German neuropathologists in the Third Reich.

This process of dethronement has affected two other leading scientists who are still alive. One is Hans Harmsen, a leading racial hygienist during the Third Reich and a supporter of compulsory sterilization of patients in the welfare institutions of the Protestant church. After the war he was co-founder of the family planning organization Pro Familia and of the International Planned Parenthood Foundation. He was removed as honorary president of Pro Familia.[69] The second scientist affected was Siegfried Koller, a leading medical statistician during the Third Reich and the author of a study on the hereditary inferiority of "antisocials" and "deviants," whose elimination he had propounded. Koller became the director of the Institute for

Medical Statistics of Mainz University after the war. The majority of the members of the German branch of the International Biometric Society, in their annual conference on March 15, 1990, declared that they no longer regarded Koller as an honorary member of the society because of his role in the Nazi period.[70]

The system of silence, lies, half-truths, excuses, and angry denials of the last four decades is in retreat. The open debate about the Nazi past has raised the consciousness of many German doctors and of parts of the German public toward contemporary medical abuses. It has shaken the German doctors' self-image of infallibility, of a profession that stands above political and social forces and that presumably has always had a clean shirt and has acted out of noble, altruistic motives.

NOTES

1. Interview with Ilse Bürgel in Berlin, July 12, 1983, cited from Christian Pross, "Das Krankenhaus Moabit 1920, 1933, 1945," in Christian Pross and Rolf Winau, ed., *Nicht mißhandeln* (Berlin: Edition Hentrich, 1984), p. 226.

2. Götz Aly, "Das Posener Tagebuch des Anatomen Hermann Voss," in *Biedermann und Schreibtischtäter, Beiträge zur nationalsozialistischen Gesundheits- und Sozialpolitik*, Bd. 4 (Berlin: Rotbuch-Verlag, 1987), pp. 43–44.

3. For a detailed excerpt of the Voss diaries see Götz Aly, note 2, pp. 15–66.

4. Berlin Document Center, Akte von Verschuer, cited in Benno Müller-Hill, *Tödliche Wissenschaften* (Reinbek: Rowohlt Taschenbuchverlag 1984), p. 72.

5. Alexander Mitscherlich and Fred Mielke, ed., *Das Diktat der Menschenverachtung* (Heidelberg: Verlag Lambert Schneider, 1947), pp. 83–84.

6. Erwin Gohrbandt, "Auskühlung," *Zentralblatt für Chirurgie*. 70 (1943): 1553–1557. The Gohrbandt case is described in detail in Pross, "Das Krankenhaus Moabit 1920, 1933, 1945, pp. 224–226.

7. Brigitte Leyendecker and Burghardt F. Klapp, "Deutsche Hepatitisforschung im Zweiten Weltkrieg," in Christian Pross, Götz Aly and Ärztekammer Berlin, ed., *Der Wert des Menschen, Medizin in Deutschland 1918-1945* (Berlin: Edition Hentrich, 1989), pp. 261–293.

8. Götz Aly, "Die Menschenversuche des Doktor Heinrich Berning," in Angelika Ebbinghaus et al., ed., *Heilen und Vernichten im Mustergau Hamburg* (Hamburg, Konkret Literatur Verlag, 1984), pp. 184–187.

9. Leo Alexander, *Neuropathology and Neurophysiology Including Electro-Encephalography in Wartime Germany*, CIOS Report, Item No. 24, File No. XXVII-I (London: His Majesty's Stationery Office, 1945); see also Götz Aly, "Der saubere und der schmutzige Fortschritt," in *Reform und Gewissen, Beiträge zur nationalsozialistischen Gesundheits und Sozialpolitik* Bd. 2 (Berlin: Rotbuch Verlag, 1985), pp. 64–71.

10. Reimar Gilsenbach, "Die Verfolgung der Sinti — Ein Weg, der nach Auschwitz führte," in *Feinderklärung und Prävention, Beiträge zur nationalsozialistischen Gesundheits- und Sozialpolitik*, Bd. 6 (Berlin: Rotbuch Verlag, 1988), S. 11–41; Donald Kenrick and Grattan Puxton, *Sinti und Roma, die Vernichtung eines Volkes im NS-Staat* (Göttingen: 1981), pp. 53–61.

11. Aly, "Das Posener Tagebuch," pp. 61–62.

12. For the history of the politics of eugenics in Germany, see Hedwig Conrad-Martius, *Utopien der Menschenzüchtung. Der Sozialdarwinismus und seine Folgen* (Munich: 1955); Gerhard Baader, "Die Medizin im Nationalsozialismus: Ihre Wurzeln und die erste Periode ihrer Realisierung 1933-1938," in Pross and Winau, *Nicht mißhandeln*, pp. 61–75; Anna Bergmann, Gabriele Czarnowski, and Annegret Ehmann, "Menschen als Objekte humangenetischer Forschung und Politik im 20. Jahrhundert. Zur Geschichte des Kaiser Wilhelm Instituts für Anthropologie, menschliche Erblehre und Eugenik in Berlin-Dahlem (1927-1945)," in *Der Wert des Menschen*, Christian Pross and Götz Aly, ed., *Herausgegeben von der Ärztekammer Berlin in Zusammenarbeit mit der Bundesärztekammer* (Berlin: Edition Hentrich, 1989), pp. 121–142; Sheila Faith Weiss, *Race Hygiene and National Efficiency. The Eugenics of Wilhelm Schallmeyer* (Berkeley: University of California Press, 1987).

13. Alexander Mitscherlich and Fred Mielke, ed., *Das Diktat der Menschenverachtung* (Heidelberg: Verlag Lambert Schneider, 1947), preface.

14. See Heinz-Peter Schmiedebach, "Zur Standesideologie in der Weimarer Republik am Beispiel Erwin Liek," in *Medizin in Deutschland 1918-1945*, Pross and Aly, *Herausgegeben von der Ärztekammer Berlin*, pp. 26–35; and: Susanne Hahn, "Revolution der Heilkunst — Ausweg aus der Krise? Julius Moses (1968-1942) zur Rolle der Medizin in der Gesundheitspolitik in der Weimarer Republik," *Der Wert des Menschen*, pp. 71–85.

15. Götz Aly, "Medizin gegen Unbrauchbare," in *Aussonderung und Tod, Beiträge zur nationalsozialistischen Gesundheits- und Sozialpolitik* (Berlin: Rotbuch Verlag, 1985), pp. 9–10.

16. The most recent one is the case of the "Vienna death nurses": Die Mordschwestern von Wien, "Ruhig, unauffällig, hilfsbereit," *Stern* Nr. 17 (April 20, 1989), pp. 32–39.

17. Anonymous, "It's Over, Debbie," 259 (1988): 272.

18. See e.g., Daniel Callahan, *Setting Limits. Medical Goals in an Aging Society* (New York: Simon and Schuster, 1987). See also the critical review of Callahan's book by Amitai Etzioni: "Spare the Old, Save the Young," *The Nation* (June 11, 1988), pp. 818–822, and the debate on Callahan's book "The Nazi Analogy in Bioethics," *Hastings Center Report* (August–September 1988): pp. 29–33.

19. Karl Binding and Alfred Hoche, *Die Freigabe der Vernichtung lebensunwerten Lebens. Ihr Maß und ihre Form* (Leipzig: F. Meiner, 1920).

20. Mitscherlich and Mielke, *Das Diktat*, preface.

21. Ibid., pp. 83–84.

22. Rein, Sauerbruch, and Heubner's campaign against Mitscherlich is documented in the *Göttingen Universitätszeitung* Nr. 14 (1947): 3–5; Nr. 17/18 (1947): 6–8; Nr. 3 (1948): 4–7; Nr. 10 (1948): 6–8.

23. Alexander Mitscherlich and Fred Mielke, *Wissenschaft ohne Menschlichkeit* (Heidelberg, 1949). The book was published in an incomplete translated version in the United States: *Doctors of Infamy* (New York: Henry Schuman, 1949).

24. Alexander Mitscherlich and Fred Mielke, *Medizin ohne Menschlichkeit* (Frankfurt: Fischer Verlag, 1978), p. 15.

25. Alexander Mitscherlich, *Ein Leben für die Psychoanalyse* (Frankfurt: Suhr-Kamp-Verlag, 1980), pp. 144–147, 157, 189–192.

26. In 1965 an apologetic book on Nazi euthanasia was published by the prominent psychiatrist Helmut Ehrhardt (Helmut Ehrhardt, *Euthanasie und die Vernichtung "lebensunwerten Lebens,"* Stuttgart: Ferdinand Enke Verlag, 1965). Ehrhardt

denied the true extent of the euthanasia program, did not name all the physicians involved in it, and overemphasized the resistance against the killing of patients by some psychiatrists. The same year, a report about the killings in the psychiatric state hospital Eglfing Haar near Munich was published by its postwar director, Gerhard Schmidt (*Selektion in der Heilanstalt 1939-1945*, Stuttgart: Evangelisches Verlagswerk, 1965).

27. Ulrich Schultz, "Dichtkunst, Heilkunst, Forschung, Der Kinderarzt Werner Catel," in *Reform und Gewissen, Euthanasie im Dienst des Fortschritts. Beiträge zur nationalsozialistischen Gesundheits- und Sozialpolitik*, Band 2 (Berlin: Rotbuch Verlag, 1985), p. 122.

28. Ernst Klee, *Was sie taten — Was sie wurden. Ärzte, Juristen und andere Beteiligte am Kranken- oder Judenmord* (Frankfurt: Fischer Taschenbuchverlag, 1986), pp. 19–29.

29. Friedrich Karl Kaul, *Dr. Sawade macht Karriere. Der Fall des Euthanasie-Arztes Dr. Heyde* (Frankfurt: Röderberg Verlag, 1971); Kaul, *Ärzte in Auschwitz* (Berlin: GDR: VEB Verlag Volk und Gesundheit, 1968).

30. Of the first new edition under the title *Medizin ohne Menschliehkeit* (op. cit.), 50,000 copies were printed in 1960 and another 25,000 in 1962.

31. *Dokumentation des Arbeitskreises Medizin und Verbrechen, Arbeit, Aktionen, Analysen zum Thema Zwangssterilisation im 3. Reich, Kritik heutiger Medizin* Kritische, Universit of Heidelberg, July 1968) (typewritten brochure in author's possession). The main initiator and author of the brochure, Ernst Scheurlen, a young internist, could not continue his career at the Department of Medicine at the University of Heidelberg. In 1936 Bauer had published the standard textbook on the sterilization of males under the Nazi sterilization law, in which he propagated the principles of Nazi racial hygiene concerning the "hereditary inferior" (Karl Heinrich Bauer and Felix von Mikulicz-Radecki, *Die Praxis der Sterilisierungsoperationen*, Leipzig: 1936). Bauer, who to this day is falsely regarded as an anti-Nazi, had been made the first postwar president of Heidelberg University by the American military government.

32. Hans Schadewaldt, *75 Jahre Hartmannbund: Ein Kapitel deutscher Sozialpolitik* (Bonn-Bad: Godesberg, 1975, p. 79). A detailed correction of Schadewaldt's apology is Michael Hubenstorf, "Deutsche Landärzte an die Front!" — Ärztekammer Standespolitik zwischen Liberalismus und Nationalsozialismus," in *Der Wert des Menschen*, 1989, pp. 200–223.

33. Werner Leibbrand reports this in his autobiography: "Fridolf Kudlien, Werner Leibbrand als Zeitzeuge: Ein ärztlicher Gegner des Nationalsozialismus im Dritten Reich," *Medizinhistorisches Journal* 21 (1986): 344.

34. A summary of the Diepgen story is William Coleman, "The Physician in Nazi Germany," *Bulletin of the History of Medicine* 60 (1986): 238–240. A detailed study of Paul Diepgen's role in the Third Reich will be published by the Institute of the History of Medicine at Humboldt University in Berlin.

35. Manfred Stürzbecher, "Aus der Geschichte des Städtischen Krankenhauses Moabit," in *1872-1972 Städtisches Krankenhaus Moabit, Festschrift zum 100jährigen Bestehen. Herausgegeben von Bezirksamt Tiergarten von Berlin* (Berlin: Abteilung Gesundheitswesen, 1972), pp. 13–98. For comparison, see Pross, "Das Krankenhaus Moabit 1920, 1933, 1945," pp. 7–10, 109–261.

36. Michael Kater, "The Burden of the Past: Problems of a Modern Historiography of Physicians and Medicine in Nazi Germany," *German Studies Review* 10 (1987): 31–56.

37. Ibid., 40.

38. Raoul Hilberg, *Die Vernichtung der europäischen Juden, Die Gesamtgeschichte des Holocaust* (Berlin: Olle und Wolter, 1982), p. 802.

39. The proceedings of the Gesundheitstag 1980 were published in Gerhard Baader and Ulrich Schultz, ed., *Medizin und Nationalsozialismus, Tabuisierte Vergangenheit — ungebrochene Tradition?* (Berlin: Verlagsgesellschaft Gesundheit, 1980).

40. Günther Schwarberg, "Der SS-Arzt und die Kinder," *Stern* Magazin im Verlag Gruner und Jahr, Hamburg, 1979.

41. Stephan Liebfried and Florian Tennstedt, *Berufsverbote und Sozialpolitik 1933, Die Auswirkungen der nationalsozialistischen Machtergreifung auf die Krankenkassenverwaltung und die Kassenärzte* (University of Bremen: Arbeitspapiere des Forschungsschwerpunktes Reproduktionsrisiken, soziale Bewegungen und Sozialpolitik Nr. 2, 1979).

42. Walter Wuttke-Groneberg, *Medizin im Nationalsozialismus, Ein Arbeitsbuch* (Tübingen: Schwäbische Verlagsanstalt, 1980).

43. See note 39.

44. Ibid.

45. Ernst Klee, *"Euthanasie" im NS-Staat, Die "Vernichtung lebensunwerten Lebens"* (Frankfurt: Fischer Verlag, 1983).

46. Projektgruppe "Volk und Gesundheit", Volk und Gesundheit, Heilen und Vernichten im Nationalsozialismus, Tübinger Vereinigung für Volkskunde e.V. Tübingen 1982; see also Walter Wuttke-Groneberg's paper on the 1980 Gesundheitstag: "Von Heidelberg nach Dachau. 'Vernichtungslehre' und Naturwissenschaftskritik in der nationalsozialistischen Medizin." See note 39, pp. 113–138.

47. Müller-Hill, *Tödliche Wissenschaft*. The book is now available in English under the title *Murderous Science* (Oxford: Oxford University Press, 1988).

48. See, for example, Victor McKusick, "Medical Genetics," in A. McGhee Harvey et al., *The Principles and Practice of Medicine*, 21st ed. (Norwalk, Conn.: Appleton-Century Crofts, 1984), p. 433.

49. Gisela Bock, *Zwangssterilisation im Nationalsozialismus* (Opladen: Westdeutscher Verlag, 1986).

50. Götz Aly and Karl-Heinz Roth, *Die restlose Erfassung, Volkszählen, Identifizieren, Aussondern im Nationalsozialismus* (Berlin: Rotbuch-Verlag, 1984).

51. See the following works by Michael H. Kater: "Hitlerjugend und Schule im Dritten Reich," *Historische Zeitschrift* 228 (1981): 572–623; *The Nazi Party: A Social Profile of Members and Leaders, 1919-1945* (Cambridge, Mass.: Harvard University Press, 1983), p. 112; "Hitler's Early Doctors: Nazi Physicians in Predepression Germany," *The Journal of Modern History* 59 (1987): 25–52; "The Nazi Physicians' League of 1929: Causes and Consequences," in Thomas Childers, ed., *The Formation of the Nazi Constituency 1919-1933* (London: Croom Helm, 1986), pp. 147–181; "Doctor Leonardo Conti and His Nemesis: The Failure of Centralized Medicine in the Third Reich," *Central European History* 18 (1985): 299–325; *Doctors Under Hitler* (Chapel Hill: University of North Caroline Press, 1989).

52. Georg Lilienthal, *Der "Lebensborn e.V."* (Stuttgart: Gustav Fischer Verlag, 1985).

53. Geoffrey Cocks, *Psychotherapy in the Third Reich* (New York: Oxford University Press, 1985); Regine Lockot, *Erinnern und Durcharbeiten, Zur Geschichte der Psychoanalyse und Psychotherapie im Nationalsozialismus* (Frankfurt: Fischer Taschenbuch Verlag, Frankfurt 1985).

54. Angelika Ebbinghaus, Heidrun Kaupen-Haas, and Karl Heinz Roth, *Heilen und Vernichten im Mustergau Hamburg* (Hamburg: Konkret Literatur Verlag, 1984).

55. To mention only a few examples: Pross, "Das Krankenhaus Moabit 1920, 1933, 1945"; Arbeitsgruppe zur Erforschung der Karl-Bonhoeffer-Nervenklinik, ed., *Totgeschwiegen 1933-1945, Die Geschichte der Karl-Bonhoeffer Nervenklinik* (Berlin: Edition Hentrich, 1988); Michael Wunder, Ingrid Genkel, and Harald Henner, *Auf dieser schiefen Ebene gibt es keine Halten mehr—Die Alsterdorfer Anstalten im Nationalsozialismus*, Kommissionsverlag (Hamburg: Agentur des Rauhen Hauses, 1987); Matthias Leipert, Rudolf Styrnal, and Winfried Schwarzer, *Verlegt nach unbekannt, Sterilisation und Euthanasie in Galkhausen 1933-1945* (Cologne: Rheinland-Verlag, 1987); Dagmar Hartung von Doetinchem, *Zerstörte Fortschritte— Zur Geschichte des Jüdischen Krankenhauses zu Berlin 1756-1861-1914-1989* (Berlin: Edition Hentrich, 1989).

56. *Beiträge zur nationalsozialistischen Gesundheits—und Sozialpolitik, Rotbuch Verlag Berlin*: Vol. 1, *Aussonderung und Todi* (1985); Vol. 2, *Reform und Gewissen* (1985); Vol. 3, *Herrenmensch und Arbeitsvölker* (1986); Vol. 4, *Biedermann und Schreibtischtäter* (1986); Vol. 5, *Sozialpolitik und Judenvernichtung* (1987); Vol. 6, *Feinderklärung und Prävention* (1988); Vol. 7, *Internationales Ärztliches Bulletin*, Reprint (1989); Vol. 8, *Arbeitsmarkt und Sonderelsaß* (1990); Another series of books and a journal are published by the Hamburg branch of the Verein: *Schriften der Hamburger Stiftung für Sozialgeschichte des 20. Jahrhunderts*. Vol. 1, *Der Griff nach der Bevölkerungspolitik*; Vol. 6, *Die Träume der Genetik*, Greno Nördlingen 1987ff; 1989, *Zeitschrift für Sozialgeschichte*, des 20. und 21; *Jahrhunderts*, Vol. 1, 1986ff.

57. Norbert Jachertz, "Die neuen Herren kamen über Nacht," *Deutsches Ärzteblatt* (1983): pp. 23-26.

58. Hartmut Hanauske-Abel, From Nazi Holocaust to Nuclear Holocaust: A Lesson to Learn?" *Lancet* (1986): 271-273.

59. "Die 'Vergangenheitsbewältigung' darf nicht kollektiv die Ärzte diffamieren, Interview mit Dr. Karsten Vilmar," *Deutsches Ärzteblatt* (1987): pp. 767-779.

60. An exhibit catalogue was published containing an anthology of scientific contributions: *Der Wert des Menschen*. See note 7.

61. The series of articles in the *Deutsche Ärzteblatt* were published as an anthology: Johanna Bleker and Norbert Jachertz, ed., *Medizin im Dritten Reich* (Cologne: Deutscher Ärzteverlag, 1989).

62. Richard Toellner, "Arzte im Dritten Reich, Wortlaut des Vortrages, gehalten auf der 1. Plenarsitzung des 92. Deutschen Ärztetages in Berlin," *Deutsches Ärzteblatt* (August 17, 1989), pp. 1427-1433.

63. See letters to the editor in *Deutsches Ärzteblatt* Heft 19, 1988ff.

64. "Rolle der Medizin bleibt umstritten," in *Süddeutsche Zeitung* (October 13, 1989).

65. *Archives of General Psychiatry* 45 (1988): 774-776.

66. William E. Seidelman, "In Memoriam: Medicine's Confrontation with Evil," *Hastings Center Report* (November–December 1989): 5-6. Meanwhile the University of Heidelberg has buried all anatomical specimens of Nazi victims. The University of Tübingen buried their specimens on July 8, 1990, in an official memorial ceremony. W. E. Seidelman, professor of family medicine at McMaster University in Hamilton, Ontario, and Arthur Caplan, professor at the Center for Bioethics at the University of Minnesota, both called for an international commemoration at the burial of the Hallervorden brain specimen. This call was ignored by the Max Planck Insti-

tute, which buried the brain specimens from the Hallervorden collection in an unspectacular closed ceremony in Munich on May 25, 1990 and in Frankfurt on December 21, 1990. See J. Peiffer, "Neuropathology in the Third Reich: Memorial to Those Victims of National-Socialist Atrocities in Germany Who Were Used by Medical Science," *Brain Pathology* 1 (1991): 125–131.

67. Jürgen Peiffer, "Gedenkrede aus Anlass der Aufstellung eines Steines auf dem Gräberfeld X zum Gedenken an die Opfer nationalsozialistischer Gewalt und deren Nutzung durch die medizinische Wissenschaft." The speech was published in English as "Neuropathology in the Third Reich: Memorial to those victims of National Socialist atrocities in Germany who were used by Medical Sciences," *Brain Pathology* 1 (1991): 125–131.

68. Götz Aly discovered the Hallvorden collection in the Max Planck Institute for Brain Research in Frankfurt in the early 1980s and published his findings in 1985 (see note 9.)

69. Harmsen's Nazi past was revealed by Heidrun Kaupen Haas: "Eine deutsche Biographie—der Bevölkerungspolitiker Hans Harmsen," in Angelika Ebbinghaus et al., ed., *Heilen und Vernichten im Mustergau Hamburg* (Hamburg: Konkret Literatur Verlag, 1984), pp. 41–44.

70. Koller's role in the Third Reich was exposed by Götz Aly and Karl Heinz Roth in their monograph *Die restlose Erfassung, Volkszählen, Indentifizieren, Aussondern im Nationalsozialismus* (Berlin: Rotbuch Verlag, 1984). The vote of the German branch of the International Biometric Society concerning Koller is documented in a letter to the members dating from February 1990. I am grateful to Rolf Lorenz, Tübingen, who made this letter available to me.

4

The Mengele Twins and Human Experimentation: A Personal Account

EVA MOZES-KOR

To look back at my childhood is to remember my experiences as a human guinea pig in the Birkenau laboratory of Dr. Josef Mengele. To recount such painful memories is to relive the horrors of human experimentation, where people were used as merely objects or means to a scientific end. I envision the chimneys, the smell of burning flesh, the medical injections, the endless blood taking, the tests, the dead bodies all around us, the hunger, and the rats. Nothing that is close to human existence existed in that place.

THE LABORATORY

It was early spring in 1944. I don't know the exact date. It was likely the beginning of April. We had traveled from our small village of Portz in Transylvania, not knowing where we were going or what fate lay ahead. Our cattle car train came to a sudden stop. I could hear a lot of German voices yelling orders outside. Inside I could smell the stench of the cramped bodies. We were packed like sardines. I could see a small patch of gray sky through the barbed wires. My father, Alexander Mozes, gathered the family around him. My mother was 38 years old, my oldest sister Edit was 14, my middle sister Aliz was 12 and we, the twins, Miriam and Eva, were 9. We listened quietly as my father spoke: "Promise me that if any of you survive this terrible war, you will go to your uncle Aaron Mozes in Palestine, where Jews can live in peace and freedom." I did not really understand what my father meant by those words, but I sensed that the situation was grave because he had never spoken to us that way before. We cried, and with tears in our eyes promised him that we would do as he said. My father was a very religious man; he was 44 years old at the time we were deported. His faith in God was the guiding force in his life, and with all that had happened to us, he had turned even closer to God.

My thoughts were interrupted by the sound of the cattle car door as it swung open. "*Schnell, schnell.*" The SS soldiers were ordering everybody out. As soon as we stepped out onto the cement platform, my mother grabbed my twin sister and me by the hand, hoping somehow to protect us. Everything was moving very fast. I suddenly realized that my father and my two older sisters, Edit and Aliz, were gone. I never saw them again. I think the whole thing took 10 minutes; they were lost in the crowd as Miriam and I clutched my mother's hand. The SS soldiers walked by, shouting louder. Suddenly, they stopped my mother and looked at my twin sister and me, because we were dressed alike and looked very much alike. "Are they twins?" one soldier asked my mother. My poor mother was bewildered. What was this place? she must have thought. What was happening here? What were the rules? What was a good answer and what was bad? She asked the SS soldier if being a twin was good. The guard nodded his head. My mother said very hesitantly, "Yes, they are." Without any further explanation, the officer grabbed Miriam and me, and another SS soldier grabbed my mother and pulled her in the opposite direction. We screamed and pleaded as we were separated. I remember looking back and seeing my mother's arm stretched in despair as she was being pulled away. I never even said goodbye to her. I did not know that was the last time we would see our mother.

Miriam and I joined a group of about 10 or 12 sets of twins. We waited for a long time at the edge of the railroad ramp. They seemed to be waiting for everybody to be detrained and all the twins to be gathered. I looked around the camp. Everything appeared dark, gray, and lifeless. Near the train, as the victims were being separated into two distinct groups, there stood one SS officer dressed in a neatly pressed uniform. He looked very sharp in his beautiful gleaming boots. It appeared to me that he was in charge. The officer doing the selection was Dr. Josef Mengele.

Our group was led to a huge building near a very tall barbed-wire fence. I had never seen a fence like this before. The building looked like a big gymnasium that was divided in two; one half was occupied by bleachers and the other half by many shower heads. We were ordered to undress, and our clothes were taken away. I felt numb, paralyzed in body and mind. It seemed like a nightmare that would be over as soon as I opened my eyes. All the twins were given short haircuts. Miriam and I had arrived at the camp with long braids and ribbons in our hair. The barber explained to us that the twins were privileged; therefore, we could have short hair instead of having our heads shaved. Our clothes were returned with a big red cross painted on the back. This identified the twins as part of medical experiments. We were lined up for registration and tattooing. Four people, two SS soldiers and two women prisoners, restrained me while they heated a pen-like gadget over an open flame, dipped it in ink, and forced it into my left arm, burning into my flesh, dot by dot, the number A-7063.

Early in the evening we were taken to a barrack in camp A, the women's camp. I could see groups of prisoners returning from work. They looked like walking skeletons. One poor victim stepped out of line, trying to talk to us. She said, "Children, children, where did you come from?" She was killed on the spot. The SS guards were everywhere. They marched us to every activity: to the lab, to the showers, to Auschwitz, and to the other experiments. Our interactions with the other prisoners was extremely limited, as the twin experiments were top secret.

In the barracks we met many other twin children. After our evening meal of a two-inch slice of black bread and a brownish liquid, two Hungarian twins briefed us about the camp. They explained that this camp was called Birkenau. Auschwitz, they said, had one gas chamber and one crematorium, while Birkenau had four gas chambers and four crematoriums. "We don't understand these words — *gas chambers, crematorium*," Miriam and I interrupted. They took us to the back door, where we looked toward the northern sky, to see a giant smoking chimney towering above the camps. I could see glowing flames rising high above the structure. I asked, "What are they burning so late at night?" "The Germans are burning people in the ovens. They want to kill all the Jews, and after every transport, the chimney burns day and night." "Burning people? That's crazy. Why would they want to burn people?" I asked. "Did you see the two groups of people on the railroad platform this morning?" they asked. "They are probably burning them right now. Only those who can work stay alive, and only as long as they are strong enough to work. The weak, the sick, the old, and the children all end up in the gas chambers and in the flames." "But," I said, "we are children too, and we are alive. Why don't they kill us?" It seemed to me a very good question. "They will someday, but right now, they want us alive because we are twins and they use us in experiments conducted by Dr. Josef Mengele," they replied. "You will meet him tomorrow; he comes in every morning after roll call."

THE EXPERIMENTS

No one ever attempted to explain anything to us. No one explained why we were in Mengele's "laboratory," what was going to be done to us, or what would be our ultimate destiny. There was never an attempt to minimize our risks. In fact, we were there for one reason: to be used as experimental objects and then to be killed. Mengele had two types of research programs. One set of experiments dealt with genetics and the other with germ warfare. In the germ experiments, Mengele would inject one twin with the germ.

Then, if and when that twin died, he would kill the other twin in order to compare the organs at autopsy.

In June or July, about 3 months after my arrival, I was injected with some kind of deadly germ. After a visit to Dr. Mengele's lab, I became ill with a very high fever. I was desperately afraid of revealing this fact because it was well known that the illness would result in my being separated from Miriam and sent to the hospital. We knew that many children became sick, were taken to the hospital, and never came back. On the next visit to the lab my fever was measured, and I was sent to the hospital.

The hospital was a camp filled with some 15 to 25 barracks for the sick. I was placed in a barrack filled with moving and screaming skeletons. I called the ward the "barrack of the living dead." I was told by the other children that we were not given anything to eat here because people were brought here to await their turn for a place in the gas chambers. Twice a week, a truck would come to pick up the living dead. These sick people were thrown on the truck like sacks of potatoes. The screaming of these poor souls will stay with me forever.

The next day a team of five doctors, including Mengele, came to study my case. They looked at my fever chart and then Mengele said sarcastically, "She is so young. Too bad. She has only two weeks to live."

The doctors never examined me and never ran any tests; they only looked at the fever chart. I was between life and death for 2 weeks. It was then that I made a silent pledge: "I will do everything in my power to prove Mengele wrong, and to survive and be reunited with my sister Miriam." During the first 2 weeks I was unconscious most of the time, but I do remember waking up on the barrack floor while trying to crawl to the other end of the barrack to a water faucet. I was given no food, no medication, and no water.

Then I realized that my temperature had to be normal before I would be reunited with Miriam. I understood that I had to convince Mengele and the other doctors who were monitoring my disease that I was getting well. I accomplished this by manipulating the thermometers so that it appeared that my fever had gradually disappeared. It took me 3 weeks to allow my temperature to be read as normal. Three weeks later, I was released and reunited with Miriam.

Upon my return, Miriam told me that during the first 2 weeks of my hospitalization, someone had stayed with her continually. She was not told of my condition, but it was clear that had I died in the hospital, Miriam would have been taken immediately to Mengele's lab to be killed. After the 2 weeks, when it appeared that I would not die, Miriam was no longer under surveillance at all times. Instead, she was taken back to the lab, together with all the other twins, and was injected with something. When I got back from the hospital, Miriam was very ill.

The daily routine for Mengele's twins was regimented. We awoke every morning at 5 A.M. and helped the younger twins to dress. In our barracks there were twins from 1 1/2 to 13 years of age. By 6 A.M. all of us were standing for roll call outdoors, whether it was winter or summer, rain or snow. Everybody had to be accounted for as either dead or alive. The bodies of dead children were brought out and counted as well. Mengele became very angry when a child died in bed because of the conditions in the camp. These deaths meant the loss of valuable guinea pigs for his medical experiments.

After Mengele's visit, we received some food and then were taken to the labs for tests. We were examined, measured, and given X-rays. Three times a week we were taken to the blood lab. There, blood was taken from my left arm, and three or more shots were injected into my right arm. Afterward, we were usually taken back to the barracks. On one occasion, while in the waiting area of the lab, I observed one twin faint. She was being tested to see how much blood could be taken before death occurred. These experiments were felt to have a practical application on the battlefield.

Three times a week we were marched from Birkenau to Auschwitz, where we would go to Barrack 10. We were assembled, naked, in an enormous room. There 10 or 12 doctors would study us. They measured parts of the body: the size of the mouth, the shape of the bones of the face and skull, and the colors of eyes and hair. We were compared to a chart in addition to each set of twins. Our bodies were marked with different color codes, and each doctor walked around us, continually taking notes. The "specimens" were photographed and catalogued. There was no way to protest and stay alive.

One of the twins, who was 19 years old, told of experiments involving a set of teenage boys and a set of teenage girls. Cross-transfusions were carried out in an attempt to "make boys into girls and girls into boys." Some of the boys were castrated. Transfusion reactions were similarly studied in the adolescent twins.

In the area of genetics, Mengele collected dwarfs, giants, hunchbacks, and people with abnormalities and defects. He studied genetic traits in the hope of "purifying" the "Aryan superrace." He closely monitored eye and hair color.

A set of Gypsy twins was brought back from Mengele's lab after they were sewn back to back. Mengele had attempted to create a Siamese twin by connecting blood vessels and organs. The twins screamed day and night until gangrene set in, and after 3 days they died. Mengele also attempted to connect the urinary tract of a 7-year-old girl to her own colon. Many experiments were performed on the male and female genitals.

LIBERATION

In early November 1944 all the Gypsies were exterminated, and we were transferred to their camp, which was next to the gas chambers and crematorium. After we were transferred to the Gypsy camp, the experiments became less routine. We were still taken to the lab, but not as frequently. It was clear that something was happening. It was a midnight in January, 1945. We were awakened by the unbearable heat coming from the roof of the barracks. I looked outside; the whole sky was red with flames. The SS had blown up the gas chambers and crematoriums. The SS guards stood outside with their machine guns and ordered us to march.

On a snowy day, January 27, 1945, just 4 days before my 10th birthday, Auschwitz was liberated. I thought that once we were free, we would be able to go home. Of course, that was not the case. We were held in refugee camps until September 1945. We were then transferred from one camp to another.

I eventually made it back to my home city. Our home had been looted and ransacked. I found a crumpled photograph—the last photograph I have of my family. The picture was taken in the fall of 1943.

In 1948, Miriam and I applied for a visa to emigrate to the newly formed country of Israel. After 2 years, we were finally granted our request, and in 1950 we settled in Israel. In 1960, I married an American tourist and came to live in the United States. My son Alex was born in 1961 and my daughter Rina in 1963. I have tried to obtain copies of the medical experimentation records from the U.S. Government. My sister Miriam suffers from renal disease, and I have donated my left kidney to her. To this day, we do not know what substances were injected into us when we served as Mengele's guinea pigs.

CONCLUSION

I hope that what was done to me will never again happen to another human being. This is the reason I have told my painful story. Those who do research must be compelled to obey international law. Scientists should continue to do research. But if a human being is ever used in the experiments, the scientists must make a moral commitment never to violate a person's human rights and human dignity. The scientist must respect the wishes of the subjects. Every time scientists are involved in human experimentation, they should try to put themselves in the place of the subject and see how they would feel. The scientists of the world must remember that the research is being done for the sake of mankind and not for the sake of science; scientists must never detach themselves from the humans they serve. I hope with all my heart that our sad stories will in some special way impel the international community to devise laws and rules to govern human experimentation.

The dignity of all human beings must be respected, preserved, and protected at all costs; life without dignity is mere existence. I experienced such loss of dignity every day as a guinea pig in Dr. Mengele's laboratory. Forty-five years later, I still feel deep pain and anger for the way I was treated by the doctors. These same doctors had taken an oath to help and to save human life.[1]

NOTES

1. For further discussion of Josef Mengele and the twin experiments see M. Nyiszli, *Auschwitz: An Eyewitness Account of Mengele's Infamous Death Camp* (New York: Seaver Books, 1986), and G. L. Posner and J. Ware, *Mengele: The Complete Story* (New York: McGraw-Hill, 1986). See also P. Aziz, *Doctors of Death*, Vol. 2, *Joseph Mengele, The Evil Doctor* (Geneva: Ferni Publishing, 1976), and C. Bernadac, *Devil's Doctors: Medical Experiments on Human Subjects in the Concentration Camps* (Geneva: Ferni Publishing, 1978), L. M. Lagnado and S. C. Dekel, *Children of the Flames: Dr. Josef Mengele and the Untold Story of the Twins of Auschwitz* (New York: William Morrow, 1991), A. Haas, *The Doctor and the Damned* (London: Granada, 1985); The International Auschwitz Committee on Nazi Medicine: *Doctors, Victims and Medicine in Auschwitz* (New York: Fertig Publishing, 1986); and R. J. Lifton, *The Nazi Doctors: Medical Killing and the Psychology of Genocide* (New York: Basic Books, 1986).

II

THE DOCTORS' TRIAL AND THE NUREMBERG CODE

This part contains the primary source documents from the Doctors' Trial; a summary of the aftermath of the trial; a discussion of the origin of the Nuremberg Code; and photographs of the judges, the courtroom, counsel, defendants, and exhibits.

Brigadier General Telford Taylor was the chief counsel for the trials of war criminals before the Nuremberg military tribunal from October 1946 to April 1949. Although James M. McHaney was the chief prosecutor for Tribunal No. I, Case 1, the Doctors' Trial, Taylor delivered the opening statement for the prosecution. In a 1990 discussion with the editors about the significance of the medical trials and the Nuremberg Code, Taylor suggested that his opening statement was more important than present-day personal reminiscence. Although rather reluctantly, we ultimately agreed. The opening statement appears almost in its entirety in Chapter 5.

We have not included the formal indictment because this material is contained in the final judgment. The judgment itself is reprinted almost in its entirety in Chapter 6. The concluding section of the judgment contains a discussion of the permissibility of medical experiments and the ten point Nuremberg Code.

Mitscherlich and Mielke were the official German court observers of the tribunal. Following the trial, they wrote a landmark account of the Doctors' Trial and published their observations in a book entitled *Doctors of Infamy*. We have included the epilogue to their book, which summarizes the verdicts and sentencing of the Nazi defendants.

The final chapter in this part of the book, Chapter 7, was written by one of the editors, Michael Grodin. It traces the history of codes of medical ethics and human experimentation. The sources of the various points in the Nuremberg Code are discussed in detail, and the context of the code is illuminated.

The twenty-three defendants at the trial (as described in the indictment) were:

Karl Brandt — Personal physician to Adolf Hitler; Gruppenfuehrer in the SS and Generalleutnant (Major General) in the Waffen SS; Reich Commissioner for Health and Sanitation (Reichskommissar fuer Sanitaets — und Gesundheitswesen); and member of the Reich Research Council (Reichsforschungsrat).

Siegfried Handloser — Generaloberstabsarzt (Lieutenant General, Medical Service); Medical Inspector of the Army (Heeressanitaetsinspekteur); and Chief of the Medical Services of the Armed Forces (Chef des Wehrmachtsanitaetswesens).

Paul Rostock — Chief Surgeon of the Surgical Clinic in Berlin; Surgical Adviser to the Army; and Chief of the Office for Medical Science and Research (Amtschef der Dienststelle Medizinische Wissenschaft und Forschung) under the defendant Karl Brandt, Reich Commissioner for Health and Sanitation.

Oskar Schroeder — Generaloberstabsarzt (Lieutenant General Medical Service); Chief of Staff of the Inspectorate of the Medical Service of the Luftwaffe (Chef des Stabes, Inspekteur des Luftwaffe-Sanitaetswesens); and Chief of the Medical Service of the Luftwaffe (Chef des Sanitaetswesens der Luftwaffe).

Karl Genzken — Gruppenfuehrer in the SS and Generalleutnant (Major General) in the Waffen SS; and Chief of the Medical Department of the Waffen SS (Chef des Sanitaetsamts der Waffen SS).

Karl Gebhardt — Gruppenfuehrer in the SS and Generalleutnant (Major General) in the Waffen SS; personal physician to Reichsfuehrer SS Himmler; Chief Surgeon of the Staff of the Reich Physician SS and Police (Oberster Kliniker, Reichsarzt SS und Polizei); and President of the German Red Cross.

Kurt Blome — Deputy [of the] Reich Health Leader (Reichsgesundheitsfuehrer); and Plenipotentiary for Cancer Research in the Reich Research Council.

Rudolf Brandt — Standartenfuehrer (Colonel) in the Allgemeine SS; Personal Administrative Officer to Reichsfuehrer SS Himmler (Persoenlicher Referent von Himmler); and Ministerial Counsellor and Chief of the Ministerial Office in the Reich Ministry of the Interior.

Joachim Mrugowsky — Oberfuehrer (Senior Colonel) in the Waffen SS; Chief Hygienist of the Reich Physician SS and Police (Oberster Hygieniker, Reichsarzt SS and Polizei); and Chief of the Hygienic Institute of the Waffen SS (Chef des Hygienischen Institutes der Waffen SS).

Helmut Poppendick — Oberfuehrer (Senior Colonel) in the SS; and Chief of the Personal Staff of the Reich Physician SS and Police (Chef des persoenlichen Stabes des Reichsarztes SS und Polizei).

Wolfram Sievers — Standartenfuehrer (Colonel) in the SS; Reich Manager of the "Ahnenerbe" Society and Director of its Institute for Military Scientific Research (Institut fuer Wehrwissenschaftliche Zweckforschung); and Deputy Chairman of the Managing Board of Directors of the Reich Research Council.

Gerhard Rose — Generalarzt of the Luftwaffe (Brigadier General, Medical Service of the Air Force); Vice President, Chief of the Department for Tropical Medicine, and Professor of the Robert Koch

Institute; and Hygienic Adviser for Tropical Medicine to the Chief of the Medical Service of the Luftwaffe.

Siegfried Ruff — Director of the Department for Aviation Medicine at the German Experimental Institute for Aviation (Deutsche Versuchsanstalt fuer Luftfahrt).

Hans Wolfgang Romberg — Doctor on the Staff of the Department for Aviation Medicine at the German Experimental Institute for Aviation.

Viktor Brack — Oberfuehrer (Senior Colonel) in the SS and Sturmbannfuehrer (Major) in the Waffen SS; and Chief Administrative Officer in the Chancellery of the Fuehrer of the NSDAP (Oberdienstleiter, Kanzlei des Fuehrers der NSDAP).

Hermann Becker-Freyseng — Stabsarzt in the Luftwaffe (Captain, Medical Service of the Air Force); and Chief of the Department for Aviation Medicine of the Chief of the Medical Service of the Luftwaffe.

Georg August Weltz — Oberfeldarzt in the Luftwaffe (Lieutenant Colonel, Medical Service of the Air Force); and Chief of the Institute for Aviation Medicine in Munich (Institut fuer Luftfahrtmedizin).

Konrad Schaefer — Doctor of the Staff of the Institute for Aviation Medicine in Berlin.

Waldemar Hoven — Hauptsturmfuehrer (Captain) in the Waffen SS; and Chief Doctor of the Buchenwald Concentration Camp.

Wilhelm Beiglboeck — Consulting Physician to the Luftwaffe.

Adolf Pokorny — Physician, Specialist in Skin and Venereal Diseases.

Herta Oberheuser — Physician at the Ravensbrueck Concentration Camp; and Assistant Physician to the defendant Gebhardt at the Hospital at Hohenlychen.

Fritz Fischer — Sturmbannfuehrer (Major) in the Waffen SS; and Assistant Physician to the defendant Gebhardt at the Hospital at Hohenlychen.

5

Opening Statement of the Prosecution December 9, 1946

TELFORD TAYLOR

[Editors' Note: This historical document is reproduced as written. Spelling errors are silently corrected.]

The defendants in this case are charged with murders, tortures, and other atrocities committed in the name of medical science. The victims of these crimes are numbered in the hundreds of thousands. A handful only are still alive; a few of the survivors will appear in this courtroom. But most of these miserable victims were slaughtered outright or died in the course of the tortures to which they were subjected.

For the most part they are nameless dead. To their murderers, these wretched people were not individuals at all. They came in wholesale lots and were treated worse than animals. They were 200 Jews in good physical condition, 50 Gypsies, 500 tubercular Poles, or 1,000 Russians. The victims of these crimes are numbered among the anonymous millions who met death at the hands of the Nazis and whose fate is a hideous blot on the page of modern history.

The charges against these defendants are brought in the name of the United States of America. They are being tried by a court of American judges. The responsibilities thus imposed upon the representatives of the United States, prosecutors and judges alike, are grave and unusual. It is owed, not only to the victims and to the parents and children of the victims, that just punishment be imposed on the guilty, but also to the defendants that they be accorded a fair hearing and decision. Such responsibilities are the ordinary burden of any tribunal. Far wider are the duties which we must fulfill here.

These larger obligations run to the peoples and races on whom the scourge of these crimes was laid. The mere punishment of the defendants, or even of thousands of others equally guilty, can never redress the terrible injuries which the Nazis visited on these unfortunate peoples. For them it is far more important that these incredible events be established by clear and public proof, so that no one can ever doubt that they were fact and not fable; and that this court, as the agent of the United States and as the voice of humanity, stamp these acts, and the ideas which engendered them, as barbarous and criminal.

We have still other responsibilities here. The defendants in the dock are charged with murder, but this is no mere murder trial. We cannot rest content when we have shown that crimes were committed and that certain persons committed them. To kill, to maim, and to torture is criminal under all modern systems of law. These defendants did not kill in hot blood, nor for personal enrichment. Some of them may be sadists who killed and tortured for sport, but they are not all perverts. They are not ignorant men. Most of them are trained physicians and some of them are distinguished scientists. Yet these defendants, all of whom were fully able to comprehend the nature of their acts, and most of whom were exceptionally qualified to form a moral and professional judgment in this respect, are responsible for wholesale murder and unspeakably cruel tortures.

It is our deep obligation to all peoples of the world to show why and how these things happened. It is incumbent upon us to set forth with conspicuous clarity the ideas and motives which moved these defendants to treat their fellow men as less than beasts. The perverse thoughts and distorted concepts which brought about these savageries are not dead. They cannot be killed by force of arms. They must not become a spreading cancer in the breast of humanity. They must be cut out and exposed, for the reason so well stated by Mr. Justice Jackson in this courtroom a year ago. "The wrongs which we seek to condemn and punish have been so calculated, so malignant, and so devastating, that civilization cannot tolerate their being ignored because it cannot survive their being repeated."

To the German people we owe a special responsibility in these proceedings. Under the leadership of the Nazis and their war lords, the German nation spread death and devastation throughout Europe. This the Germans now know. So, too, do they know the consequences to Germany: defeat, ruin, prostration, and utter demoralization. Most German children will never, as long as they live, see an undamaged German city.

To what cause will these children ascribe the defeat of the German nation and the devastation that surrounds them? Will they attribute it to the overwhelming weight of numbers and resources that was eventually leagued against them? Will they point to the ingenuity of enemy scientists? Will they perhaps blame their plight on strategic and military blunders by their generals?

If the Germans embrace those reasons as the true cause of their disaster, it will be a sad and fatal thing for Germany and for the world. Men who have never seen a German city intact will be callous about flattening English or American or Russian cities. They may not even realize that they are destroying anything worthwhile, for lack of a normal sense of values. To reestablish the greatness of Germany they are likely to pin their faith on improved military techniques. Such views will lead the Germans straight into the arms of the Prussian militarists to whom defeat is only a glorious opportunity to start a new war game. "Next time it will be different." We know all too well what that will mean.

This case, and others which will be tried in this building, offer a signal opportunity to lay before the German people the true cause of their present misery. The walls and towers and churches of Nuernberg were, indeed, reduced to rubble by Allied bombs, but in a deeper sense Nuernberg had been destroyed a decade earlier, when it became the seat of the annual Nazi Party rallies, a focal point for the moral disintegration in Germany, and the private domain of Julius Streicher. The insane and malignant doctrines that Nuernberg spewed forth account alike for the crimes of these defendants and for the terrible fate of Germany under the Third Reich.

A nation which deliberately infects itself with poison will inevitably sicken and die. These defendants and others turned Germany into an infernal combination of a lunatic asylum and a charnel house. Neither science, nor industry, nor the arts could flourish in such a foul medium. The country could not live at peace and was fatally handicapped for war. I do not think the German people have as yet any conception of how deeply the criminal folly that was Nazism bit into every phase of German life, or of how utterly ravaging the consequences were. It will be our task to make these things clear.

These are the high purposes which justify the establishment of extraordinary courts to hear and determine this case and others of comparable importance. That murder should be punished goes without the saying, but the full performance of our task requires more than the just sentencing of these defendants. Their crimes were the inevitable result of the sinister doctrines which they espoused, and these same doctrines sealed the fate of Germany, shattered Europe, and left the world in ferment. Wherever those doctrines may emerge and prevail, the same terrible consequences will follow. That is why a bold and lucid consummation of these proceedings is of vital importance to all nations. That is why the United States has constituted this Tribunal.

I pass now to the facts of the case in hand. There are 23 defendants in the box. All but three of them — Rudolf Brandt, Sievers, and Brack — are doctors. Of the 20 doctors, all but one — Pokorny — held positions in the medical services of the Third Reich. To understand this case, it is necessary to understand the general structure of these state medical services, and how these services fitted into the over-all organization of the Nazi State. [The material on the organization of the military medical personnel, and where the individual defendants fit into it, has been deleted.]

CRIMES COMMITTED IN THE GUISE OF SCIENTIFIC RESEARCH

I turn now to the main part of the indictment and will outline at this point the prosecution's case relating to those crimes alleged to have been committed in the name of medical or scientific research. The charges with respect to "euthanasia" and the slaughter of tubercular Poles obviously have no relation to research or experimentation and will be dealt with later. What I will cover now comprehends all the experiments charged as war crimes in paragraph 6 and as crimes against humanity in paragraph 11 of the indictment, and the murders committed for the so-called anthropological purposes which are charged as war crimes in paragraph 7 and as crimes against humanity in paragraph 12 of the indictment.

Before taking up these experiments one by one, let us look at them as a whole. Are they a heterogeneous list of horrors, or is there a common denominator for the whole group?

A sort of rough pattern is apparent on the face of the indictment. Experiments concerning high altitude, the effect of cold, and the potability of processed sea water have an obvious relation to aeronautical and naval combat and rescue problems. The mustard gas and phosphorus burn experiments, as well as those relating to the healing value of sulfanilamide for wounds, can be related to air-raid and battlefield medical problems. It is well known that malaria, epidemic jaundice, and typhus were among the principal diseases which had to be combated by the German Armed Forces and by German authorities in occupied territories. To some degree, the therapeutic pattern outlined above is undoubtedly a valid one, and explains why the Wehrmacht, and especially the German Air Force, participated in these experiments. Fanatically bent upon conquest, utterly ruthless as to the means or instruments to be used in achieving victory, and callous to the sufferings of people whom they regarded as inferior, the German militarists were willing to gather whatever scientific fruit these experiments might yield.

But our proof will show that a quite different and even more sinister objective runs like a red thread through these hideous researches. We will show that in some instances the true object of these experiments was not how to rescue or to cure, but how to destroy and kill. The sterilization experiments were, it is clear, purely destructive in purpose. The prisoners at Buchenwald who were shot with poisoned bullets were not guinea pigs to test an antidote for the poison; their murderers really wanted to know how quickly the poison would kill. This destructive objective is not superficially as apparent in the other experiments, but we will show that it was often there.

Mankind has not heretofore felt the need of a word to denominate the science of how to kill prisoners most rapidly and subjugated people in large numbers. This case and these defendants have created this gruesome question for the lexicographer. For the moment we will christen this macabre science *thanatology*, the science of producing death. The thanatological knowledge, derived in part from these experiments, supplied the techniques for genocide, a policy of the Third Reich, exemplified in the "euthanasia" program and in the widespread slaughter of Jews, Gypsies, Poles, and Russians. This policy of mass extermination could not have been so effectively carried out without the active participation of German medical scientists.

I will now take up the experiments themselves. Two or three of them I will describe more fully, but most of them will be treated in summary fashion, as Mr. McHaney will be presenting detailed proof of each of them.

High-Altitude Experiments

The experiments known as *high-altitude* or *low-pressure* experiments were carried out at the Dachau concentration camp in 1942. According to the proof, the original proposal that such experiments be carried out on human beings originated in the spring of 1941 with a Dr. Sigmund Rascher. Rascher was at that time a captain in the Medical Service of the German Air Force, and also held officer rank in the SS. He is believed now to be dead.

The origin of the idea is revealed in a letter which Rascher wrote to Himmler in May 1941 at which time Rascher was taking a course in aviation medicine at a German Air Force headquarters in Munich. According to the letter, this course included researches into high-altitude flying and "considerable regret was expressed at the fact that no tests with human material had yet been possible for us, as such experiments are very dangerous and nobody volunteers for them."

Rascher, in this letter, went on to ask Himmler to put human subjects at his disposal and baldly stated that the experiments might result in death to the subjects but that the tests theretofore made with monkeys had not been satisfactory. Rascher's letter was answered by Himmler's adjutant, the defendant, Rudolf Brandt, who informed Rascher that "prisoners will, of course, gladly be made available for high-flight researches."

Subsequently, Rascher wrote directly to Rudolf Brandt, asking for permission to carry out the experiments at the Dachau concentration camp, and he mentioned that the German Air Force had provided "a movable pressure chamber" in which the experiments might be made. Plans for carrying out the experiments were developed at a conference late in 1941, or early in 1942, attended by Dr. Rascher and by the defendants Weltz, Romberg, and Ruff, all of whom were members of the German Air Force Medical Service. The tests themselves were carried out in the spring and summer of 1942, using the pressure chamber which the German Air Force had provided. The victims were locked in the low-pressure chamber, which was an airtight ball-like compartment, and then the pressure in the chamber was altered to simulate the atmospheric conditions prevailing at extremely high altitudes. The pressure in the chamber could be varied with great rapidity, which permitted the defendants to duplicate the atmospheric conditions which an aviator might encounter in falling great distances through space without a parachute and without oxygen.

The reports, conclusions, and comments on these experiments, which were introduced here and carefully recorded, demonstrate complete disregard for human life and callousness to suffering and pain. These documents reveal at one and the same time the medical results of the experiments and the degradation of the physicians who performed them. The first report by Rascher was made in April 1942 and contains a description of the effect of the low-pressure chamber on a 37-year-old Jew. I quote:

> The third experiment of this type took such an extraordinary course that I called an SS physician of the camp as witness, since I had worked on these experiments all by myself. It was a continuous experiment without oxygen at a height of 12 kilometers conducted on a 37-year-old Jew in good general condition. Breathing continued up to 30 minutes. After 4 minutes the experimental subject began to perspire, and wiggle his head; after 5 minutes cramps occurred; between 6 and 10 minutes breathing increased in speed and the experimental subject became unconscious; from 11 to 30 minutes breathing slowed down to three breaths per minute, finally stopping altogether.
> Severest cyanosis developed in between and foam appeared at the mouth.
> At 5 minute intervals electrocardiograms from three leads were written. After breathing had stopped [the] EKG [electrocardiogram] was continuously written until the action of the heart had come to a complete standstill. About 1/2 hour after breathing had stopped, dissection was started.

Rascher's report also contains the following record of the "autopsy":

> When the cavity of the chest was opened the pericardium was filled tightly (heart tamponade). Upon opening of the pericardium, 80 cc of clear yellowish liquid gushed forth. The moment the tamponade had stopped, the right auricle of the heart began to beat heavily, at first at the rate of 60 actions per minute, then progressively slower. Twenty minutes after the pericardium had been opened, the right auricle was opened by puncturing it. For about 15 minutes, a thin stream of blood spurted forth. Thereafter, clogging of the puncture wound in the auricle by coagulation of the blood and renewed acceleration of the action of the right auricle occurred.
> One hour after breathing had stopped, the spinal marrow was completely severed and the brain removed. Thereupon, the action of the auricle of the heart stopped for 40 seconds. It then renewed its action, coming to a complete standstill 8 minutes later. A heavy subarachnoid oedema was found in the brain. In the veins and arteries of the brain, a considerable quantity of air was discovered. Furthermore, the blood vessels in the heart and liver were enormously obstructed by embolism.

After seeing this report Himmler ironically ordered that if a subject should be brought back to life after enduring such an experiment, he should be "pardoned" to life imprisonment in a concentration camp. Rascher's reply to this letter, dated 20 October 1942, reveals that up to [that] time the victims of these experiments had all been Poles and Russians, that some of them had been condemned to death, and Rascher inquired whether Himmler's benign mercy extended to Poles and Russians. A teletyped reply from the defendant, Rudolf Brandt, confirmed Rascher's belief that Poles and Russians were beyond the pale and should be given no amnesty of any kind.

The utter brutality of the crimes committed in conducting this series of experiments is reflected in all the documents. A report written in May 1942 reflects that certain of these tests were carried out on persons described therein as "Jewish professional criminals." In fact, these Jews had been condemned for what the Nazis called *Rassenschande*, which literally means "racial shame." The crime consisted of marriage or intercourse between Aryans and non-Aryans. The murder and torture of these unfortunate Jews is eloquently reflected in the following report:

> Some of the experimental subjects died during a continued high altitude experiment; for instance, after one-half hour at a height of 12 kilometers. After the skull had been opened under water, an ample amount of air embolism was found in the brain vessels and, in part, free air in the brain ventricles.
>
> In order to find out whether the severe psychic and physical effects, as mentioned [elsewhere] are due to the formation of embolism, the following was done: After relative recuperation from such a parachute descending test had taken place, however before regaining consciousness, some experiment subjects were kept under water until they died. When the skull and cavities of the breast and of the abdomen were opened under water, an enormous amount of air embolism was found in the vessels of the brain, the coronary vessels, and the vessels of the brain, the coronary vessels, and the vessels of the liver and the intestines.

The victims who did not die in the course of such experiments surely wished that they had. A long report written in July 1942 by Rascher, and by the defendants Ruff and Romberg, describes an experiment on a former delicatessen clerk, who was given an oxygen mask and raised in the chamber to an atmospheric elevation of over 47,000 feet, at which point the mask was removed and a parachute descent was simulated. The report describes the victim's reactions — "spasmodic convulsions," "agonal convulsive breathing," "clonic conclusions, groaning," "yells aloud," "convulses arms and legs," "grimaces, bites his tongue," "does not respond to speech," "gives the impression of someone who is completely out of his mind."

The evidence which we will produce will establish that the defendants Ruff and Romberg personally participated with Rascher in experiments resulting in death and torture; that the defendant Sievers watched the experiments for an entire day and made an oral report to Himmler on his observations; that the defendant Rudolf Brandt was the agent of Himmler in providing the human subjects for these experiments and in making many other facilities available to Rascher and rendering him general assistance; and that the defendant Weltz, in his official capacity, repeatedly insisted on supervision over and full responsibility and credit for the experiments. The higher authorities of both the German Air Force and the SS were fully informed concerning what was going on. . . .

Freezing Experiments

The deep interest of the German Air Force in capitalizing on the availability of inmates of concentration camps for experimental purposes is even more apparent in the case of the freezing experiments. These, too, were conducted at Dachau. They began immediately after the high-altitude experiments were completed and they continued until the spring of 1943. Here again, the defendant Weltz was directly in charge of the experiments, with Rascher as his assistant. . . .

The purpose of these experiments was to determine the most effective way of rewarming German aviators who were forced to parachute into the North Sea. The evidence will show that in the course of these experiments, the victims were forced to remain outdoors without clothing in freezing weather from 9 to 14 hours. In other cases, they were forced to remain in a tank of iced water for 3 hours at a time. The water experiments are described in a report by Rascher written in August 1942. I quote:

> Electrical measurements gave low temperature readings of 26.4° in the stomach and 26.5° in the rectum. Fatalities occurred only when the brain stem and the back of the head were also chilled. Autopsies of such fatal cases always revealed large amounts of free blood, up to 1/2 liter, in the cranial cavity. The heart invariably showed extreme dilation of the right chamber. As soon as the temperature in those experiments reached 28°, the experimental subjects died invariably, despite all attempts at resuscitation.

Other documents set forth that from time to time the temperature of the water would be lowered by 10° Centigrade and a quart of blood would be taken from an artery in the subject's throat for analysis. The organs of the victims who died were extracted and sent to the Pathological Institute at Munich.

Rewarming of the subjects was attempted by various means, most commonly and successfully in a very hot bath. In September, Himmler personally ordered that rewarming by the warmth of human bodies also be attempted, and the inhuman villains who conducted these experiments promptly produced four Gypsy women from the Ravensbrueck concentration camp. When the women had arrived, rewarming was attempted by placing the chilled victim between two naked women.

A voluminous report on the freezing experiments conducted in tanks of ice water, written in October 1942, contains the following:

> If the experimental subject were placed in the water under narcosis, one observed a certain arousing effect. The subject began to groan and made some defensive movements. In a few cases, a state of excitation developed. This was especially severe in the cooling of the head and neck. But never was a complete cessation of the narcosis observed. The defensive movements ceased after about 5 minutes. There followed a progressive rigor, which developed especially strongly in the arm musculature; the arms were strongly flexed and pressed to the body.

The rigor increased with the continuation of the cooling, now and then interrupted by tonic-clonic twitching. With still more marked sinking of the body temperature, it suddenly ceased. These cases ended fatally, without any successful results from resuscitation efforts.

Experiments without narcosis showed no essential differences in the course of cooling. Upon entry into the water, a severe cold shuddering appeared. The cooling of the neck and back of the head was felt as especially painful, but already after 5 to 10 minutes, a significant weakening of the pain sensation was observable. Rigor developed after this time in the same manner as under narcosis, likewise the tonic-clonic twitchings. At this point, speech became difficult because the rigor also affected the speech musculature.

Simultaneously with the rigor, a severe difficulty in breathing set in with or without narcosis. It was reported that, so to speak, an iron ring was placed about the chest. Objectively, already at the beginning of this breathing difficulty, a marked dilatation of the nostrils occurred. The expiration was prolonged and visibly difficult. This difficulty passed over into a rattling and snoring breathing.

During the winter of 1942 and 1943, experiments with "dry" cold were conducted. And Rascher reported on these in another letter to Himmler:

> Up to now, I have cooled off about 30 people stripped in the open air during nine to fourteen hours at 27° to 29°. After a time, corresponding to a trip of 1 hour, I put these subjects in a hot bath. Up to now, every single patient was completely warmed up within 1 hour at most, although some of them had their hands and feet frozen white.

The responsibility among the defendants for the freezing experiments is substantially the same as for the high-altitude tests. The results were, if anything, ever more widely known in German medical circles. In October 1942, a medical conference took place here in Nuernberg at the Deutscher Hof Hotel, at which one of the authors of the report from which I have just quoted spoke on the subject "Prevention and Treatment of Freezing," and the defendant Weltz spoke on the subject "Warming Up After Freezing to the Danger Point." Numerous documents which we will introduce show the widespread responsibility among the defendants, and in the highest quarters of the German Air Force, for these sickening crimes.

Malaria Experiments

Another series of experiments carried out at the Dachau concentration camp concerned immunization for and treatment of malaria. Over 1,200 inmates of practically every nationality were experimented upon. Many persons who participated in these experiments have already been tried before a general military court held at Dachau, and the findings of that court will be laid before this Tribunal. The malaria experiments were carried out under the general supervision of a Dr. Schilling, with whom the defendant Sievers and others in the box collaborated. The evidence will show that healthy persons were infected by mosquitoes or by injections from the glands of

mosquitoes. Catholic priests were among the subjects. The defendant Gebhardt kept Himmler informed of the progress of these experiments. Rose furnished Schilling with fly eggs for them, and others of the defendants participated in various ways which the evidence will demonstrate.

After the victims had been infected, they were variously treated with quinine, neosalvarsan, pyramidon, antipyrin, and several combinations of these drugs. Many deaths occurred from excessive doses of neosalvarsan and pyramidon. According to the findings of the Dachau court, malaria was the direct cause of 30 deaths, and 300 to 400 others died as the result of subsequent complications.

Mustard Gas Experiments

The experiments concerning mustard gas were conducted at Sachsenhausen, Natzweiler, and other concentration camps and extended over the entire period of the war. Wounds were deliberately inflicted on the victims, and the wounds were then infected with mustard gas. Other subjects were forced to inhale the gas or to take it internally in liquid form, and still others were injected with the gas. A report on these experiments written at the end of 1939 described certain cases in which wounds were inflicted on both arms of the human guinea pigs and then infected, and the report states: "The arms in most of the cases are badly swollen and pains are enormous."

The alleged purpose of these experiments was to discover an effective treatment for the burns caused by mustard gas. . . .

Ravensbrueck Experiments Concerning Sulfanilamide and Other Drugs; Bone, Muscle, and Nerve Regeneration and Bone Transplantation

The experiments conducted principally on the female inmates of Ravensbrueck concentration camp were perhaps the most barbaric of all. These concerned bone, muscle, and nerve regeneration and bone transplantation, and experiments with sulfanilamide and other drugs. They were carried out by the defendants Fischer and Oberheuser under the direction of the defendant Gebhardt.

In one set of experiments, incisions were made on the legs of several of the camp inmates for the purpose of simulating battle-caused infections. A bacterial culture, or fragments of wood shavings, or tiny pieces of glass were forced into the wound. After several days, the wounds were treated with sulfanilamide. Grawitz, the head of the SS Medical Service, visited Ravensbrueck and received a report on these experiments directly from the defendant Fischer. Grawitz thereupon directed that the wounds inflicted on the subjects should be even more severe so that conditions similar to those prevailing at the front lines would be more completely simulated.

Bullet wounds were simulated on the subjects by tying off the blood vessels at both ends of the incision. A gangrene-producing culture was then placed in the wounds. Severe infection resulted within 24 hours. Operations

were then performed on the infected areas, and the wounds were treated with sulfanilamide. In each of the many sulfanilamide experiments, some of the subjects were wounded and infected but were not given sulfanilamide, so as to compare their reactions with those who received treatment.

Bone transplantation from one person to another and the regeneration of nerves, muscles, and bones were also tried out on the women at Ravensbrueck. The defendant Gebhardt personally ordered that bone transplantation experiments be carried out, and in one case the scapula of an inmate at Ravensbrueck was removed and taken to Hohenlychen Hospital and there transplanted. We will show that the defendants did not even have any substantial scientific objective. These experiments were senseless, sadistic, and utterly savage. . . .

Other experiments in this category were conducted at Dachau to discover a method of bringing about coagulation of the blood. Concentration camp inmates were actually fired upon, or were injured in some other fashion in order to cause something similar to a battlefield wound. These wounds were then treated with a drug known as polygal in order to test its capacity to coagulate the blood. Several inmates were killed. Sulfanilamide was also administered to some and withheld from other inmates who had been infected with the pus from a phlegmon-diseased person. Blood poisoning generally ensued. After infection, the victims were left untreated for 3 or 4 days, after which various drugs were administered experimentally or experimental surgical operations were performed. Polish Catholic priests were used for these tests. Many died and others became invalids.

As a result of all of these senseless and barbaric experiments, the defendants are responsible for manifold murders and untold cruelty and torture.

Sea-Water Experiments

For the sea-water experiments we return to Dachau. They were conducted in 1944 at the behest of the German Air Force and the German Navy in order to develop a method of rendering sea water drinkable. Meetings to discuss this problem were held in May 1944, attended by representatives of the Luftwaffe, the Navy, and I. G. Farben. The defendants Becker-Freyseng and Schaefer were among the participants. It was agreed to conduct a series of experiments in which the subjects, fed only with shipwreck emergency rations, would be divided into four groups. One group would receive no water at all; the second would drink ordinary sea water; the third would drink sea water processed by the so-called "Berka" method, which concealed the taste but did not alter the saline content; the fourth would drink sea water treated so as to remove the salt.

Since it was expected that the subject would die, or at least suffer severe impairment of health, it was decided at the meeting in May 1944 that only persons furnished by Himmler could be used. Thereafter in June 1944 the defendant Schroeder set the program in motion by writing to Himmler, and I quote from his letter:

Earlier you made it possible for the Luftwaffe to settle urgent medical matters through experiments on human beings. Today I again stand before a decision which, after numerous experiments on animals and also on voluntary human subjects, demands final solution: The Luftwaffe has simultaneously developed two methods for making sea water drinkable. The one method, developed by a medical officer, removes the salt from the sea water and transforms it into real drinking water; the second method, suggested by an engineer, only removes the unpleasant taste from the sea water. The latter method, in contrast to the first, requires no critical raw material. From the medical point of view this method must be viewed critically, as the administration of concentrated salt solutions can produce severe symptoms of poisoning.

As the experiments on human beings could thus far only be carried out for a period of 4 days, and as practical demands require a remedy for those who are in distress at sea up to 12 days, appropriate experiments are necessary.

Required are 40 healthy test subjects, who must be available for 4 whole weeks. As it is known from previous experiments that necessary laboratories exist in the Dachau concentration camp, this camp would be very suitable.

Due to the enormous importance which a solution of this question has for soldiers of the Luftwaffe and Navy who have become shipwrecked, I would be greatly obliged to you, my dear Reich Minister, if you would decide to comply with my request.

Himmler passed this letter to Grawitz who consulted Gebhardt and other SS officials. A typical nauseating Nazi discussion of racial questions ensued. One SS man suggested using quarantined prisoners and Jews; another suggested Gypsies. Grawitz doubted that experiments on Gypsies would yield results that were scientifically applicable to Germans. Himmler finally directed that Gypsies be used, with three others as a check.

The tests were actually begun in July 1944. The defendant Beiglboeck supervised the experiments, in the course of which the Gypsy subjects underwent terrible suffering, became delirious or developed convulsions, and some died.

EPIDEMIC JAUNDICE

The epidemic jaundice experiments, which took place at Sachsenhausen and Natzweiler concentration camps, were instigated by the defendant Karl Brandt. A letter written in 1943 by Grawitz stresses the enormous military importance of developing an inoculation against epidemic jaundice, which had spread extensively in the Waffen SS and the German Army, particularly in southern Russia. In some companies, up to 60 percent casualties from epidemic jaundice had occurred. Grawitz further informed Himmler that, and I quote:

The General Commissioner of the Fuehrer, SS Brigadefuehrer Professor Dr. Brandt, has approached me with the request to help him obtain prisoners to be used in connection with his research on the causes of Epidemic Jaundice which has been furthered to a large degree by his efforts. . . . In order to enlarge our knowledge, so far based only on inoculation of animals with germs taken from human beings, it would not be necessary to reverse the procedure and inoculate human beings with germs cultivated in animals. Casualties [*Todesfaelle*] must be anticipated.

Grawitz also had been doing research on this problem with the assistance of a Dr. Dohmen, a medical officer attached to the Army Medical Inspectorate. Himmler made the following reply to the Grawitz letter:

I approve that eight criminals condemned in Auschwitz [eight Jews of the Polish Resistance Movement condemned to death] should be used for these experiments.

Other evidence will indicate that the scope of these experiments was subsequently enlarged and that murder, torture, and death resulted from them.

STERILIZATION EXPERIMENTS

In the sterilization experiments conducted by the defendants at Auschwitz, Ravensbrueck, and other concentration camps, the destructive nature of the Nazi medical program comes out most forcibly. The Nazi were searching for methods of extermination, both by murder and sterilization, of large population groups by the most scientific and least conspicuous means. They were developing a new branch of medical science which would give them the scientific tools for the planning and practice of genocide. The primary purpose was to discover an inexpensive, unobtrusive, and rapid method of sterilization which could be used to wipe out Russians, Poles, Jews, and other people. Surgical sterilization was thought to be too slow and expensive to be used on a mass scale. A method to bring about an unnoticed sterilization was thought desirable.

Medicinal sterilizations were therefore carried out. A Dr. Madaus had stated that caladium sequinum, a drug obtained from a North American plant, if taken orally or by injection, would bring about sterilization. In 1941 the defendant Pokorny called this to Himmler's attention, and suggested that it should be developed and used against Russian prisoners of war. I quote one paragraph from Pokorny's letter written at that time:

If, on the basis of this research, it were possible to produce a drug which, after a relatively short time, effects an imperceptible sterilization on human beings, then we would have a powerful new weapon at our disposal. The thought alone that the 3 million Bolsheviks, who are at present German prisoners, could be sterilized so that they could be used as laborers but be prevented from reproduction, opens the most far-reaching perspectives.

As a result of Pokorny's suggestion, experiments were conducted on concentration camp inmates to test the effectiveness of the drug. At the same time, efforts were made to grow the plant on a large scale in hothouses.

At the Auschwitz concentration camp sterilization experiments were also conducted on a large scale by a Dr. Karl Clauberg, who had developed a method of sterilizing women, based on the injection of an irritating solution. Several thousand Jews and Gypsies were sterilized at Auschwitz by this method.

Conversely, surgical operations were performed on sexually abnormal inmates at Buchenwald in order to determine whether their virility could be increased by the transplantation of glands. Out of 14 subjects of these experiments, at least 2 died.

The defendant Gebhardt also personally conducted sterilizations at Ravensbrueck by surgical operation. The defendant Viktor Brack, in March 1941, submitted to Himmler a report on the progress and state of X-ray sterilization experiments. Brack explained that it had been determined that sterilization with powerful X-rays could be accomplished and that castration would then result. The danger of this X-ray method lay in the fact that other parts of the body, if they were not protected with lead, were also seriously affected. In order to prevent the victims from realizing that they were being castrated, Brack made the following fantastic suggestion in his letter written in 1941 to Himmler, from which I quote:

> One way to carry out these experiments in practice would be to have those people who are to be treated line up before a counter. There they would be questioned and a form would be given them to be filled out, the whole process taking 2 or 3 minutes. The official attendant who sits behind the counter can operate the apparatus in such a manner that he works a switch which will start both tubes together (as the rays have to come from both sides). With one such installation with two tubes about 150 to 200 persons could be sterilized daily, while 20 installations would take care of 3,000 to 4,000 persons daily. In my opinion the number of daily deportations will not exceed this figure.

In this same report the defendants Brack related that, and I quote,

> the latest X-ray technique and research make it easily possible to carry out mass sterilization by means of X-rays. However, it appears to be impossible to take these measures without having those who were so treated finding out sooner or later that they definitely had been either sterilized or had been castrated by X-rays.

Another letter from Brack to Himmler, in June 1942, laid [out] the basis for X-ray experiments which were subsequently carried out at Auschwitz. The second paragraph of this letter forms a fitting conclusion to this account of Nazi depravity, and I quote:

Among 10 millions of Jews in Europe there are, I figure, at least 2 to 3 millions of men and women who are fit enough to work. Considering the extraordinary difficulties the labor problem presents us with, I hold the view that these 2 to 3 millions should be specially selected and preserved. This can, however, only be done if at the same time they are rendered incapable to propagate. About a year ago I reported to you that agents of mine have completed the experiments necessary for this purpose. I would like to recall these facts once more. Sterilization, as normally performed on persons with hereditary diseases, is here out of the question because it takes too long and is too expensive. Castration by X-rays, however, is not only relatively cheap but can also be performed on many thousands in the shortest time. I think that at this time it is already irrelevant whether the people in question become aware of having been castrated after some weeks or months, once they feel the effects.

TYPHUS (*FLECKFIEBER*) AND RELATED EXPERIMENTS

From December 1941 until near the end of the war, a large program of medical experimentation was carried out upon concentration camp inmates at Buchenwald and Natzweiler to investigate the value of various vaccines. This research involved a variety of diseases—typhus, yellow fever, smallpox, paratyphoid A and B, cholera, and diphtheria. A dozen or more of the defendants were involved in these experiments, which were characterized by the most cynical disregard of human life. Hundreds of persons died. The experiments concerning typhus—known in Germany as *Fleckfieber* or "spot fever," but is not to be confused with American spotted fever—were particularly appalling.

The typhus experiments at Natzweiler were conducted by Dr. Eugen Haagen, an officer in the Air Force Medical Service and a professor at the University of Strasbourg. In the fall of 1943, through the defendant Sievers, Haagen obtained 100 concentration camp prisoners for experiments with typhus vaccines. Two hundred more prisoners were furnished in the summer of 1944. These experiments caused many fatalities among the prisoners.

The general pattern of these typhus experiments was as follows. A group of concentration camp inmates, selected from the healthier ones who had some resistance to disease, were injected with an antityphus vaccine, the efficacy of which was to be tested. Thereafter, all the persons in the group would be infected with typhus. At the same time, other inmates who had not been vaccinated were also infected for purposes of comparison—these unvaccinated victims were called the "control" group. But perhaps the most wicked and murderous circumstance in this whole case is that still other inmates were deliberately infected with typhus with the sole purpose of keeping the typhus virus alive and generally available in the bloodstream of the inmates.

The typhus murders at Buchenwald were carried out in 1942 and 1943 under the direction of the defendants Genzken and Mrugowsky. Requests for the human guinea pigs were turned over to, and filled by, the defendant Hoven. The bulk of the actual work was done by an infamous physician known as Dr. Ding, who committed suicide after the war. But Dr. Ding's professional diary has survived.

The first entry in Ding's diary, for 29, December 1941, reveals that here again, the impetus for these murderous researches came from the Wehrmacht. This entry describes a conference sponsored by the defendant Handloser and Dr. Conti, respective heads of the military and civilian medical services of the Reich, which was also attended by the defendant Mrugowsky. Typhus had been making serious inroads on the German troops fighting in Russia. The account of this conference relates that, and I quote:

> Since tests on animals are not of sufficient value, tests on human beings must carried out.

Other entries in the Ding diary quoted below are typical of those made over a period of 3 years, and give some idea of the mortality among the victims:

> 10 Jan 42: Preliminary test B: Preliminary test to establish a sure means of infection: Much as in smallpox vaccination, 5 persons were infected with virus through 2 superficial and 2 deeper cuts in the upper arm. All of the humans used for this test fell ill with true typhus. Incubation period up to 6 days.
>
> 20 Feb 42: Chart of the case history of the preliminary tests to establish a sure means of infection were sent to Berlin. One death out of five sick.
>
> 17 Mar 42: Visit of Prof. Gildemeister and Prof. Rose [department head for tropical medicine of the Robert Koch Institute] at the experimental station. All persons experimented on fell sick with typhus, except two, who, the fact was established later, already had been sick with typhus during an epidemic at the police prison in Berlin.
>
> 9 Jan 43: By order of the surgeon general of the Waffen SS, SS Gruppenfuehrer and Major General of the Waffen SS, Dr. Genzken, the hitherto existing typhus research station at the concentration camp Buchenwald becomes the "Department for Typhus and Virus Research." The head of the department will be SS Sturmbannfuehrer Dr. Ding. During his absence, the station medical officer of the Waffen SS, Weimar, SS Hauptsturmfuehrer Hoven, will supervise the production of vaccines.
>
> 13 and 14 Apr 43: Unit of SS Sturmbannfeuhrer Dr. Ding ordered to I. G. Farbenindustrie A. G., Hoechst. Conference with Prof. Lautenschlaeger, Dr. Weber and Dr. Fussgaenger about experimental series "Acridine Granulate and Rutenol" in the concentration camp Buchenwald. Visit to Geheimrat Otto and Prof. Prigge in the institute for experimental therapeutics in Frankfurt-on-Main.
>
> 24 Apr 1943: Therapeutic experiments Acridine-Granulate (A-Gr2) and Rutenol (R-2) to carry out the therapeutic experiments Acridine Granulate and Rutenol, 30 persons (15 each) and 9 persons for control were infected by intravenous injection of 2 cc. each of fresh blood of a typhus sick person. All experimental persons got very serious typhus.
>
> 1 Jun 1943: Charts of case history completed. The experimental series was

concluded with 21 deaths; of these, 8 were in Buchenwald, 8 with Rutenol and 5 control.

7 Sep 1943: Chart and case history completed. The experimental series was concluded with 53 deaths.

8 Mar–18 Mar 1944: It is suggested by Colonel of the Air Corps, Prof. Rose, [that] the vaccine "Kopenhagen," produced from mouse liver by the National Serum Institute in Kopenhagen, be tested for its compatibility on humans. Twenty persons were vaccinated for immunization by intramuscular injection.

Ten persons were contemplated for control and comparison.

16 Apr 1944: The remaining experimental persons were infected on 16 April by subcutaneous injection of 1/20 cc. typhus sick fresh blood. The following fell sick: 17 persons immunized: 9 medium, 8 seriously. Nine persons from the control: 2 medium, 7 seriously.

13 Jun 1944: Chart and case history completed and sent to Berlin. Six deaths (3 "Kopenhagen") (3 control).

4 Nov 1944: Chart and case history completed. Twenty-four deaths.

Copies of each of Dr. Ding's official reports went to the defendants Mrugowsky and Poppendick, as well as to the I. G. Farben laboratories at Hoechst. Nowhere will the evidence in this case reveal a more wicked and murderous course of conduct by men who claimed to practice the healing art than in the entries of Dr. Ding's diary relating to the typhus experiments.

POISON EXPERIMENTS

Here again the defendants were studying how to kill, and the scene is Buchenwald. Poisons were administered to Russian prisoners of war in their food, and German doctors stood behind a curtain to watch the reactions of the prisoners. Some of the Russians died immediately, and the survivors were killed in order to permit autopsies.

The defendant Mrugowsky, in a letter written in September 1944, has provided us with a record of another experiment in which the victims were shot with poisoned bullets, and I quote:

In the presence of SS Sturmbannfuehrer Dr. Ding, Dr. Widmann and the undersigned, experiments with aconitine nitrate projectiles were conducted on 11 September 1944 on 5 persons who had been condemned to death. The projectiles in question were of a 7.64 mm. caliber, filled with crystallized poison. The experimental subjects, in a lying position, were each shot in the upper part of the left thigh. The thighs of two of them were cleanly shot through. Afterwards, no effect of the poison was to be observed. These two experimental subjects were therefore exempted. . . .

During the first hour of the experiment the pupils did not show any changes. After 78 minutes the pupils of all three showed a medium dilation, together with a retarded light reaction. Simultaneously, maximum respiration with heavy breathing inhalations set in. This subsided after a few minutes. The pupils contracted again and their reaction improved. After 65 minutes the patellar and achilles tendon reflexes of the poisoned subjects were negative. The abdominal reflexes of two of them were also negative. After approximately 90 minutes, one of the subjects again started breathing heavily; this was accompanied by an increasing motor unrest. Then the heavy breathing changed into a flat, accelerated respiration, accompanied by extreme nausea. One of the poisoned persons tried in vain to vomit. To do so he introduced four fingers of his hand up to the knuckles into his throat, but nevertheless could not vomit. His face was flushed.

The other two experimental subjects had already early shown a pale face. The other symptoms were the same. The motor unrest increased so much that the persons flung themselves up and then down, rolled their eyes and made meaningless motions with their hands and arms. Finally the agitation subsided, the pupils dilated to the maximum, and the condemned lay motionless. . . . Death occurred 121, 123, and 129 minutes after entry of the projectile.

INCENDIARY BOMB EXPERIMENTS

These experiments were likewise carried out at Buchenwald, and the Ding diary gives us the facts. In November 1943 five persons were deliberately burned with phosphorus material taken from an English incendiary bomb. The victims were permanently and seriously injured.

JEWISH SKELETON COLLECTION

I come now to charges stated in paragraphs 7 and 11 of the indictment. These are perhaps the most utterly repulsive charges in the entire indictment. They concern the defendants Rudolf Brandt and Sievers. Sievers and his associates in the Ahnenerbe Society were completely obsessed by all the vicious and malignant Nazi racial theories. They conceived the notion of applying these nauseous theories in the field of anthropology. What ensued was murderous folly.

In February 1942, Sievers submitted to Himmler, through Rudolf Brandt, a report, from which the following is an extract:

> We have a nearly complete collection of skulls of all races and peoples at our disposal. Only very few specimens of skulls of the Jewish race, however, are available, with the result that it is impossible to arrive at precise conclusions from examining them. The war in the East now presents us with the opportunity to overcome this deficiency. By procuring the skulls of the Jewish-Bolshevik Commissars, who represent the prototype of the repulsive but characteristic subhuman, we have the chance now to obtain a palpable, scientific document.
>
> The best practical method for obtaining and collecting this skull material could be handled by directing the Wehrmacht to turn over alive all captured Jewish-Bolshevik Commissars to the Field Police. They, in turn, are to be given special directives to inform a certain office at regular intervals of the number and place of detention of these captured Jews and to give them special close attention and care until a special delegate arrives. This special delegate, who will be in charge of securing the "material," has the job of taking a series of previously established

photographs, anthropological measurements, and in addition has to determine, as far as possible, the background, date of birth, and other personal data of the prisoner. Following the subsequently induced death of the Jew, whose head should not be damaged, the delegate will separate the head from the body and will forward it to its proper point of destination in a hermetically sealed tin can, especially produced for this purpose and filled with a conserving fluid.

Having arrived at the laboratory, the comparison tests and anatomical research on the skull, as well as determination of the race membership of pathological features of the skull form, the form and size of the brain, etc., can proceed. The basis of these studies will be the photos, measurements, and other data supplied on the head, and finally the tests of the skull itself.

After extensive correspondence between Himmler and the defendants Sievers and Rudolf Brandt, it was decided to procure the skulls from inmates of the Auschwitz concentration camp instead of at the front. The hideous program was actually carried out, as is shown by a letter from Sievers written in June 1943, which states in part:

> I wish to inform you that our associate, Dr. Beger, who was in charge of the above special project, has interrupted his experiments in the concentration camp Auschwitz because of the existing danger of epidemics. Altogether 115 persons were worked on, 79 were Jews, 30 were Jewesses, 2 were Poles, and 4 were Asiatics. At the present time these prisoners are segregated by sex and are under quarantine in the two hospital buildings of Auschwitz.

After the death of these wretched Jews had been "induced" their corpses were sent to Strasbourg. A year elapsed, and the Allied armies were racing across France and were nearing Strasbourg where this monstrous exhibit of the culture of the master race reposed. Alarmed, Sievers sent a telegram to Rudolf Brandt in September 1944, from which I quote:

> According to the proposal of 9 February 1942, and your approval of 23 February 1942, Professor Dr. Hirt has assembled a skeleton collection which has never been in existence before. Because of the vast amount of scientific research that is connected with this project, the job of reducing the corpses to skeletons has not yet been completed. Since it might require some time to process 80 corpses, Hirt requested a decision pertaining to the treatment of the collection stored in the morgue of the Anatomy, in case Strasbourg should be endangered. The collection can be defleshed and rendered unrecognizable. This, however, would mean that the whole work had been done for nothing — at least in part — and that this singular collection would be lost to science, since it would be impossible to make plaster casts afterwards. The skeleton collection, as such, is inconspicuous. The flesh parts could be declared as having been left by the French at the time we took over the Anatomy and would be turned over for cremating. Please advise me which of the following three proposals is to be carried out:
>
> (1) The collection as a whole is to be preserved.
> (2) The collection is to be dissolved in part.
> (3) The collection is to be completely dissolved.

The final chapter of this barbaric enterprise is found in a note in Himmler's files addressed to Rudolf Brandt stating that:

> During his visit at the Operational Headquarters on 21 November 1944, Sievers told me that the collection in Strasbourg had been completely dissolved in conformance with the directive given him at the time. He is of the opinion that this arrangement is for the best in view of the whole situation.

These men, however, reckoned without the hand of fate. The bodies of these unfortunate people were not completely disposed of, and this Tribunal will hear the testimony of witnesses and see pictorial exhibits depicting the charnel house that was the Anatomy Institute of the Reich University of Strasbourg.

I have now completed the sketch of some of the foul crimes that these defendants committed in the name of research. The horrible record of their degradation needs no underlining. But German medical science was in past years honored throughout the world, and many of the most illustrious names in medical research are German. How did these things come to pass? I will outline briefly the historical evidence which we will offer and which, I believe, will show that these crimes were the logical and inevitable outcome of the prostitution of German medicine under the Nazis. . . .

SUMMARY

I have outlined the particular charges against the defendants under counts two, three, and four of the indictment; and I have sketched the general nature of the evidence that we will present. But we must not overlook that the medical experiments were not an assortment of unrelated crimes. On the contrary, they constituted a well-integrated criminal program in which the defendants planned and collaborated among themselves and with others.

We have here, in other words, a conspiracy and a common design, as is charged in count one of the indictment, to commit the criminal experiments set forth in paragraphs 6 and 11 thereof. There was a common design to discover, or improve, various medical techniques. There was a common design to utilize for this purpose the unusual resources which the defendants had at their disposal, consisting of numberless unfortunate victims of Nazi conquest and Nazi ideology. The defendants conspired and agreed together to utilize these human resources for nefarious and murderous purposes, and proceeded to put their criminal design into execution. Numbered among the countless victims of the conspiracy and the crimes are Germans, and nationals of countries overrun by Germany, and Gypsies, and prisoners of war, and Jews of many nationalities. All the elements of a conspiracy to commit the crimes charged in paragraphs 6 and 11 are present, and all will be clearly established by the proof.

There were many co-conspirators who are not in the dock. Among the planners and leaders of this plot were Conti and Grawitz, and Hippke whose whereabouts is unknown. Among the actual executioners, Dr. Ding is dead and Rascher is thought to be dead. There were many others.

Final judgment as to the relative degrees of guilt among those in the dock must await the presentation of the proof in detail. Nevertheless, before the introduction of evidence, it will be helpful to look again at the defendants and their part in the conspiracy. What manner of men are they, and what was their major role?

The 20 physicians in the dock range from leaders of German scientific medicine, with excellent international reputations, down to the dregs of the German medical profession. All of them have in common a callous lack of consideration and human regard for, and an unprincipled willingness to abuse their power over, the poor, unfortunate, defenseless creatures who have been deprived of their rights by the ruthless and criminal government. All of them violated the Hippocratic commandments which they had solemnly sworn to uphold and abide by, including the fundamental principle never to do harm — *"primum non nocere."*

Outstanding men of science, distinguished for their scientific ability in Germany and abroad, are the defendants Rostock and Rose. Both exemplify, in their training and practice alike, the highest traditions of German medicine. Rostock headed the Department of Surgery at the University of Berlin and served as dean of its medical school. Rose studied under the famous surgeon, Enderlen, at Heidelberg and then became a distinguished specialist in the fields of public health and tropical diseases. Handloser and Schroeder are outstanding medical administrators. Both of them made their careers in military medicine and reached the peak of their profession. Five more defendants are much younger men who are nevertheless already known as the possessors of considerable scientific ability, or capacity in medical administration. These include the defendants Karl Brandt, Ruff, Beiglboeck, Schaefer, and Becker-Freyseng.

A number of the others such as Romberg and Fischer are well trained, and several of them attained high professional positions. But among the remainder few were known as outstanding scientific men. Among them at the foot of the list is Blome who has published his autobiography, entitled *Embattled Doctor*, in which he sets forth that he eventually decided to become a doctor because a medical career would enable him to become "master over life and death."

The part that each of these 20 physicians and their 3 lay accomplices played in the conspiracy and its execution corresponds closely to his professional interests in his place in the hierarchy of the Third Reich, as shown in the chart. The motivating force for this conspiracy came from two principal sources. Himmler, as head of the SS, a most terrible machine of oppression with vast resources, could provide numberless victims for the experiments. By doing so, he enhanced the prestige of his organization and was able to give free rein to the Nazi racial theories of which he was a leading protagonist and to develop new techniques for mass exterminations which were dear to his heart. The German military leaders, as the other main driving force, caught up the opportunity which Himmler presented them with and ruthlessly capitalized on Himmler's hideous overtures in an endeavor to strengthen their military machine.

And so the infernal drama was played just as it had been conceived in the minds of the authors. Special problems which confronted the German military or civilian authorities were, on the orders of the medical leaders, submitted for solution in the concentration camps. Thus we find Karl Brandt stimulating the epidemic jaundice experiments, Schroeder demanding "40 healthy experimental subjects" for the sea-water experiments, Handloser providing the impetus for Ding's fearful typhus researches, and Milch and Hippke at the root of the freezing experiments. Under Himmler's authority, the medical leaders of the SS — Grawitz, Genzken, Gebhardt, and others — set the wheels in motion. They arranged for the procurement of victims through other branches of the SS and gave directions to their underlings in the SS medical service such as Hoven and Fischer. Himmler's administrative assistants, Sievers and Rudolf Brandt passed on the Himmler orders, gave a push here and a shove there and kept the machinery oiled. Blome and Brack assisted from the side of the civilian and party authorities.

The Wehrmacht provided supervision and technical assistance for those experiments in which it was most interested. A low-pressure chamber was furnished for the high-altitude tests, the services of Weltz, Ruff, Romberg, and Rascher for the high-altitude and freezing experiments, and those of Becker-Freyseng, Schaefer, and Beiglboeck for sea water. In the important but sinister typhus researches, the eminent Dr. Rose appeared for the Luftwaffe to give expert guidance to Ding.

The proper steps were taken to ensure that the results were made available to those who needed to know. Annual meetings of the consulting physicians of the Wehrmacht held under Handloser's direction were favored, with lectures on some of the experiments. The report on the high-altitude experiment was sent to Field Marshal Milch, and a moving picture about them was shown at the Air Ministry in Berlin. Weltz spoke on the effects of freezing at a medical conference in Nuernberg, the same symposium at which Rascher and others passed on their devilish knowledge.

There could, we submit, be no clearer proof of conspiracy. This was the medical service of the Third Reich at work. Among the defendants in the box sit the surviving leaders of that service. We will ask the Tribunal to determine that neither scientific eminence nor superficial respectability shall shield them against the fearful consequences of the orders they gave.

I intend to pass very briefly over matters of medical ethics, such as the conditions under which a physician may lawfully perform a medical experiment upon a person who has voluntarily subjected himself to it, or whether experiments may lawfully be performed upon criminals who have been condemned to death. This case does not present such problems. No refined questions confront us here.

None of the victims of the atrocities perpetrated by these defendants were volunteers, and this is true regardless of what these unfortunate people may have said or signed before their tortures began. Most of the victims had not been condemned to death, and those who had been were not criminals, unless it be a crime to be a Jew, or a Pole, or a Gypsy, or a Russian prisoner of war.

Whatever book or treatise on medical ethics we may examine, and whatever expert on forensic medicine we may question, will say that it is a fundamental and inescapable obligation of every physician under any known system of law not to perform a dangerous experiment without the subject's consent. In the tyranny that was Nazi Germany, no one could give such a consent to the medical agents of the State; everyone lived in fear and acted under duress. I fervently hope that none of us here in the courtroom will have to suffer in silence while it is said on the part of these defendants that the wretched and helpless people whom they froze and drowned and burned and poisoned were volunteers. If such a shameless lie is spoken here, we need only remember the four girls who were taken from the Ravensbrueck concentration camp and made to lie naked with the frozen and all but dead Jews who survived Dr. Rascher's tank of ice water. One of these women, whose hair and eyes and figure were pleasing to Dr. Rascher, when asked by him why she had volunteered for such a task, replied, "rather half a year in a brothel than half a year in a concentration camp."

Were it necessary, one could make a long list of the respects in which the experiments that these defendants performed departed from every known standard of medical ethics. But the gulf between these atrocities and serious research in the healing art is so patent that such a tabulation would be cynical.

We need look no further than the law which the Nazis themselves passed on the 24th of November 1933 for the protection of animals. This law states explicitly that it is designed to prevent cruelty and indifference of man towards animals and to awaken and develop sympathy and understanding for animals as one of the highest moral values of a people. The soul of the German people should abhor the principle of mere utility without consideration of the moral aspects. The law states further that all operations or treatments which are associated with pain or injury, especially experiments involving the use of cold, heat, or infection, are prohibited, and can be permitted only under special exceptional circumstances. Special written authorization by the head of the department is necessary in every case, and experimenters are prohibited from performing experiments according to their own free judgment. Experiments for the purpose of teaching must be reduced to a minimum. Medico-legal tests, vaccinations, withdrawal of blood for diagnostic purposes, and trial of vaccines prepared according to well-established scientific principles are permitted, but the animals have to be killed immediately and painlessly after such experiments. Individual physicians are not permitted to use dogs to increase their surgical skill by such practices. National Socialism regards it as a sacred duty of German science to keep down the number of painful animal experiments to a minimum.

If the principles announced in this law had been followed for human beings as well, this indictment would never have been filed. It is perhaps the deepest shame of the defendants that it probably never even occurred to them that human beings should be treated with at least equal humanity.

This case is one of the simplest and clearest of those that will be tried in this building. It is also one of the most important. It is true that the defendants in the box were not among the highest leaders of the Third Reich. They are not the war lords who assembled and drove the German military machine, nor the industrial barons who made the parts, nor the Nazi politicians who debased and brutalized the minds of the German people. But this case, perhaps more than any other we will try, epitomizes Nazi thought and the Nazi way of life, because these defendants pursued the savage premises of Nazi thought so far. The things that these defendants did, like so many other things that happened under the Third Reich, were the result of the noxious merger of German militarism and Nazi racial objectives. We will see the results of this merger in many other fields of German life; we see it here in the field of medicine.

Germany surrendered herself to this foul conjunction of evil forces. The nation fell victim to the Nazi scourge because its leaders lacked the wisdom to foresee the consequences and the courage to stand firm in the face of threats. Their failure was the inevitable outcome of that sinister undercurrent of German philosophy that preaches the supreme importance of the state and the complete subordination of the individual. A nation in which the individual means nothing will find few leaders courageous and able enough to serve its best interests.

Individual Germans did indeed give warning of what was in store, and German doctors and scientists were numbered among the courageous few. At a meeting of Bavarian psychiatrists held in Munich in 1931, when the poisonous doctrines of the Nazis were already sweeping Germany, there was a discussion of mercy killings and sterilization, and the Nazi views on these matters, with which we are now familiar, were advanced. A German professor named Oswald Bumke rose and made a reply more eloquent and prophetic than anyone could have possibly realized at the time. He said:

> I should like to make two additional remarks. One of them is please for God's sake leave our present financial needs out of all these considerations. This is a problem which concerns the entire future of our people, indeed, one may say without being overemotional about it, the entire future of humanity. One should approach this problem neither from the point of view of our present scientific opinion nor from the point of view of the still more ephemeral economic crises. If by sterilization we can prevent the occurrence of mental disease then we should certainly do it, not in order to save money for the government but because every

case of mental disease means infinite suffering to the patient and to his relatives. But to introduce economic points of view is not only inappropriate but outright dangerous because the logical consequence of the thought that for financial reasons all these human beings, who could be dispensed with for the moment, should be exterminated, is a quite monstrous logical conclusion; we would then have to put to death not only the mentally sick and the psychopathic personalities but all the crippled, including the disabled veterans, all old maids who do not work, all widows whose children have completed their education, and all those who live on their income or draw pensions. That would certainly save a lot of money but the probability is that we will not do it.

The second point of advice is to use utmost restraint, at least until the political atmosphere here in this country shall have improved, and scientific theories concerning heredity and race can no longer be abused for political purposes. Because, if the discussion about sterilization today is carried into the arena of political contest, then pretty soon we will no longer hear about the mentally sick but, instead, about Aryans and non-Aryans, about the blonde Germanic race and about inferior people with round skulls. That anything useful could come from that is certainly improbable; but science in general and genealogy and eugenics in particular would suffer an injury which could not easily be repaired again.

I said at the outset of this statement that the Third Reich died of its own poison. This case is a striking demonstration not only of the tremendous degradation of German medical ethics which Nazi doctrine brought about, but of the undermining of the medical art and thwarting of the techniques which the defendants sought to employ. The Nazis have, to a certain extent, succeeded in convincing the peoples of the world that the Nazi system, although ruthless, was absolutely efficient; that although savage, it was completely scientific; that although entirely devoid of humanity, it was highly systematic — that "it got things done." The evidence which this Tribunal will hear will explode this myth. The Nazi methods of investigation were inefficient and unscientific, and their techniques of research were unsystematic.

These experiments revealed nothing which civilized medicine can use. It was, indeed, ascertained that phenol or gasoline injected intravenously will kill a man inexpensively and within 60 seconds. This and a few other "advances" are all in the field of thanatology. There is no doubt that a number of these new methods may be useful to criminals everywhere and there is no doubt that they may be useful to a criminal state. Certain advances in destructive methodology we cannot deny, and indeed from Himmler's standpoint this may well have been the principal objective.

Apart from these deadly fruits, the experiments were not only criminal but a scientific failure. It is indeed as if a just deity had shrouded the solutions which they attempted to reach with murderous means. The moral shortcomings of the defendants and the precipitous ease with which they decided to commit murder in quest of "scientific results" dulled also that scientific hesitancy, that thorough thinking-through, that responsible weighing of every single step which alone can ensure scientifically valid results. Even if they had merely been forced to pay as little as two dollars for human experimental subjects, such as American investigators may have to pay for a cat, they might have thought twice before wasting unnecessary numbers, and thought of simpler and better ways to solve their problems. The fact that these investigators had free and unrestricted access to human beings to be experimented upon misled them to the dangerous and fallacious conclusion that the results would thus be better and more quickly obtainable than if they had gone through the labor of preparation, thinking, and meticulous preinvestigation.

A particularly striking example is the sea-water experiment. I believe that three of the accused — Schaefer, Becker-Freyseng, and Beiglboech — will today admit that this problem could have been solved simply and definitively within the space of one afternoon. On 20 May 1944 when these accused convened to discuss the problem, a thinking chemist could have solved it right in the presence of the assembly within the space of a few hours by the use of nothing more gruesome than a piece of jelly, a semipermeable membrane and a salt solution, and the German Armed Forces would have had the answer on 21 May 1944. But what happened instead? The vast armies of the disenfranchised slaves were at the beck and call of this sinister assembly; and instead of thinking, they simply relied on their power over human beings rendered rightless by a criminal state and government. What time, effort and staff did it take to get that machinery in motion! Letters had to be written, physicians, of whom dire shortage existed in the German Armed Forces whose soldiers went poorly attended, had to be taken out of hospital positions and dispatched hundreds of miles away to obtain the answer which should have been known in a few hours, but which thus did not become available to the German Armed Forces until after the completion of the gruesome show, and until 42 people had been subjected to the tortures of the damned, the very tortures which Greek mythology had reserved for Tantalus.

In short, this conspiracy was a ghastly failure as well as a hideous crime. The creeping paralysis of Nazi superstition spread through the German medical profession and, just as it destroyed character and morals, it dulled the mind.

Guilt for the oppression and crimes of the Third Reich is widespread, but it is the guilt of the leaders that is deepest and most culpable. Who could German medicine look to to keep the profession true to its traditions and protect it from the ravaging inroads of Nazi pseudo-science? This was the supreme responsibility of the leaders of German medicine — men like Rostock and Rose and Schroeder and Handloser. That is why their guilt is greater than that of any of the other defendants in the dock. They are the men who utterly failed their country and their profession, who showed neither courage nor wisdom nor the vestiges of moral character. It is their failure, together with the failure of the leaders of Germany in other walks of life, that debauched Germany and led to her defeat. It is because of them and others like them that we all live in a stricken world.[1]

NOTES

1. *Trials of War Criminals Before the Nuremberg Military Tribunals Under Control Council Law 10*, Vol. 1 (Washington, D.C.: Superintendent of Documents, U.S. Government Printing Office, 1950); Military Tribunal, Case 1, *United States v. Karl Brandt et al.*, October 1946–April 1949, pp. 27–74.

6

Judgment and Aftermath

[Editors' Note: These historical documents are reproduced as written. Spelling errors are silently corrected.]

Military Tribunal I was established on 25 October 1946 under General Orders No. 68 issued by command of the United States Military Government for Germany. It was the first of several military tribunals constituted in the United States Zone of Occupation pursuant to Military Government Ordinance No. 7, for the trial of offenses recognized as crimes by Law No. 10 of the Control Council for Germany.

By the terms of the order which established the Tribunal and designated the undersigned as members thereof, Military Tribunal I was ordered to convene at Nuernberg, Germany, to hear such cases as might be filed by the Chief of Counsel for War Crimes or his duly designated representative.

On 25 October 1946 the Chief of Counsel for War Crimes lodged an indictment against the defendants named in the caption above [see pp. 63–65] in the Office of the Secretary General of Military Tribunal at the Palace of Justice, Nuernberg, Germany. A copy of the indictment in the German language was served on each defendant on 5 November 1946. Military Tribunal I arraigned the defendants on 21 November 1946, each defendant entering a plea of "not guilty" to all the charges preferred against him.

The presentation of evidence to sustain the charges contained in the indictment was begun by the prosecution on 9 December 1946. At the conclusion of the prosecution's case in chief the defendants began the presentation of their evidence. All evidence in the case was concluded on 3 July 1947. During the week beginning 14 July 1947 the Tribunal heard arguments by counsel for the prosecution and defense. The personal statements of the defendants were heard on 19 July 1947 on which date the case was finally concluded.

The trial was conducted in two languages—English and German. It consumed 139 trial days, including 6 days allocated for final arguments and the personal statements of the defendants. During the 133 trial days used for the presentation of evidence 32 witnesses gave oral evidence for the prosecution and 53 witnesses, including the 23 defendants, gave oral evidence for the defense. In addition, the prosecution put in evidence as exhibits a total of 570 affidavits, reports, and documents; the defense put in a total number of 901 — making a grand total of 1,471 documents received in evidence.

Copies of all exhibits tendered by the prosecution in their case in chief were furnished in the German language to the defendants prior to the time of the reception of the exhibits in evidence.

Each defendant was represented at the arraignment and trial by counsel of his own selection.

Whenever possible, all applications by defense counsel for the procuring of the personal attendance of persons who made affidavits in behalf of the prosecution were granted and the persons brought to Nuernberg for interrogation or cross-examination by defense counsel. Throughout the trial great latitude in presenting evidence was allowed defense counsel, even to the point at times of receiving in evidence certain matters of but scant probative value.

All of these steps were taken by the Tribunal in order to allow each defendant to present his defense completely, in accordance with the spirit and intent of Military Government Ordinance No. 7, which provides that a defendant shall have the right to be represented by counsel, to cross-examine prosecution witnesses, and to offer in the case all evidence deemed to have probative value.

The evidence has now been submitted, final arguments of counsel have been concluded, and the Tribunal has heard personal statements from each of the defendants. All that remains to be accomplished in the case is the rendition of judgment and the imposition of sentence.

THE JURISDICTION OF THE TRIBUNAL

The jurisdiction and powers of this Tribunal are fixed and determined by Law No. 10 of the Control Council for Germany. The pertinent portions of the Law with which we are concerned provide as follows:

Article II

1. Each of the following acts is recognized as a crime:

. . . .

(b) *War Crimes*. Atrocities or offenses against persons or property constituting violations of the laws or customs of war, including but not limited to, murder, ill-treatment or deportation to slave labor or for any other purpose, of civilian population from occupied territory, murder or ill-treatment of prisoners of war or persons on the seas, killing of hostages, plunder of public or private property, wanton destruction of cities, towns, or villages, or devastation not justified by military necessity.

(c) *Crimes against Humanity*. Atrocities and offenses, including but not limited to murder, extermination, enslavement, deportation, imprisonment, torture,
rape, or other inhumane acts committed against any civilian population, or persecutions on political, racial or religious grounds, whether or not in violation of the
domestic laws of the country where perpetrated.

(d) Membership in categories of a criminal group or organization declared
criminal by the International Military Tribunal.

2. Any person without regard to nationality or the capacity in which he acted is
deemed to have committed a crime as defined in . . . this Article, if he (a) was a
principal or (b) was an accessory to the commission of any such crime or ordered
or abetted the same or (c) took a consenting part therein or (d) was connected
with plans or enterprises involving its commission or (e) was a member of any
organization or group connected with the commission of any such crime. . . .

. . . .

(4). (a) The official position of any person, whether as Head of State or as a
responsible official in a Government Department, does not free him from responsibility for a crime or entitle him to mitigation of punishment.

(b) The fact that any person acted pursuant to the order of his Government or
of a superior does not free him from responsibility for a crime, but may be
considered in mitigation.

The indictment in the case at bar is filed pursuant to these provisions.

THE CHARGE

The indictment is framed in four counts.

COUNT ONE — *The Common Design or Conspiracy*. The first count of
the indictment charges that the defendants, acting pursuant to a common
design, unlawfully, willfully, and knowingly did conspire and agree together
to commit war crimes and crimes against humanity, as defined in Control
Council Law No. 10.

During the course of the trial the defendants challenged the first count of
the indictment, alleging as grounds for their motion the fact that under the
basic law the Tribunal did not have jurisdiction to try the crime of conspiracy considered as a separate substantive offense. The motion was set down
for argument and duly argued by counsel for the prosecution and the defense. Thereafter, in one of its trial sessions the Tribunal granted the motion.
That this judgment may be complete, the ruling made at that time is incorporated in this judgment. The order which was entered on the motion is as
follows:

It is the ruling of this Tribunal that neither the Charter of the International
Military Tribunal nor Control Council Law No. 10 has defined conspiracy to
commit a war crime or crime against humanity as a separate substantive crime;
therefore, this Tribunal has no jurisdiction to try any defendant upon a charge of
conspiracy considered as a separate substantive offense.

Count I of the indictment, in addition to the separate charge of conspiracy, also alleges unlawful participation in the formulation and execution of plans to commit war crimes and crimes against humanity which actually involved the commission of such crimes. We, therefore, cannot properly strike the whole of count I from the indictment, but, insofar as count I charges the commission of the alleged crime of conspiracy as a separate substantive offense, distinct from any war crime or crime against humanity, the Tribunal will disregard that charge.

This ruling must not be construed as limiting the force or effect of Article 2, paragraph 2 of Control Council Law No. 10, or as denying to either prosecution or defense the right to offer in evidence any facts or circumstances occurring either before or after September 1939, if such facts or circumstances tend to prove or to disprove the commission by any defendant of war crimes or crimes against humanity as defined in Control Council Law No. 10.

COUNTS TWO AND THREE — *War Crimes and Crimes Against Humanity*. The second and third counts of the indictment charge the commission of war crimes and crimes against humanity. The counts are identical in content, except for the fact that in count two the acts which are made the basis for the charges are alleged to have been committed on "civilians and members of the armed forces [of nations] then at war with the German Reich . . . in the exercise of belligerent control," whereas in count three the criminal acts are alleged to have been committed against "German civilians and nationals of other countries." With this distinction observed, both counts will be treated as one and discussed together.

Counts two and three allege, in substance, that between September 1939 and April 1945 all of the defendants "were principals in, accessories to, ordered, abetted, took a consenting part in, and were connected with plans and enterprises involving medical experiments without the subjects' consent . . . in the course of which experiments the defendants committed murders, brutalities, cruelties, tortures, atrocities, and other inhuman acts." It is averred that "such experiments included, but were not limited to" the following:

(A) *High-Altitude Experiments*. From about March 1942 to about August 1942 experiments were conducted at the Dachau concentration camp, for the benefit of the German Air Force, to investigate the limits of human endurance and existence at extremely high altitudes. The experiments were carried out in a low-pressure chamber in which the atmospheric conditions and pressures prevailing at high altitude (up to 68,000 feet) could be duplicated. The experimental subjects were placed in the low-pressure chamber and thereafter the simulated altitude therein was raised. Many victims died as a result of these experiments and others suffered grave injury, torture, and ill-treatment. The defendants Karl Brandt, Handloser, Schroeder, Gebhardt, Rudolf Brandt, Mrugowsky, Poppendick, Sievers, Ruff, Romberg, Becker-Freyseng, and Weltz are charged with special responsibility for and participation in these crimes.

(B) *Freezing Experiments*. From about August 1942 to about May 1943 experiments were conducted at the Dachau concentration camp, primarily for the benefit of the German Air Force, to investigate the most effective means of treating persons who had been severely chilled or frozen. In one series of experiments the subjects were forced to remain in a tank of ice water for periods up to 3 hours. Extreme rigor developed in a short time. Numerous victims died in the course of these experiments. After the survivors were severely chilled, rewarming was attempted by various means. In other series of experiments, the subjects were kept naked outdoors for many hours at temperatures below freezing. . . . The defendants Karl Brandt, Handloser, Schroeder, Gebhardt, Rudolf Brandt, Mrugowsky, Poppendick, Sievers, Becker-Freyseng, and Weltz are charged with special responsibility for and participation in these crimes.

(C) *Malaria Experiments.* From about February 1942 to about April 1945 experiments were conducted at the Dachau concentration camp in order to investigate immunization for treatment of malaria. Healthy concentration camp inmates were infected by mosquitoes or by injections of extracts of the mucous glands of mosquitoes. After having contracted malaria, the subjects were treated with various drugs to test their relative efficacy. Over 1,000 involuntary subjects were used in these experiments. Many of the victims died and others suffered severe pain and permanent disability. The defendants Karl Brandt, Handloser, Rostock, Gebhardt, Blome, Rudolf Brandt, Mrugowsky, Poppendick, and Sievers are charged with special responsibility for and participation in these crimes.

(D) *Lost (Mustard) Gas Experiments.* At various times between September 1939 and April 1945 experiments were conducted at Sachsenhausen, Natzweiler, and other concentration camps for the benefit of the German Armed Forces to investigate the most effective treatment of wounds caused by Lost gas. Lost is a poison gas which is commonly known as mustard gas. Wounds deliberately inflicted on the subjects were infected with Lost. Some of the subjects died as a result of these experiments and others suffered intense pain and injury. The defendants Karl Brandt, Handloser, Blome, Rostock, Gebhardt, Rudolf Brandt, and Sievers are charged with special responsibility for and participation in these crimes.

(E) *Sulfanilamide Experiments.* From about July 1942 to about September 1943 experiments to investigate the effectiveness of sulfanilamide were conducted at the Ravensbrueck concentration camp for the benefit of the German Armed Forces. Wounds deliberately inflicted on the experimental subjects were infected with bacteria such as streptococcus, gas gangrene, and tetanus. Circulation of blood was interrupted by tying off blood vessels at both ends of the wound to create a condition similar to that of a battlefield wound. Infection was aggravated by forcing wood shavings and ground glass into the wounds. The infection was treated with sulfanilamide and other drugs to determine their effectiveness. Some subjects died as a result of these experiments and others suffered serious injury and intense agony. The defendants Karl Brandt, Handloser, Rostock, Schroeder, Genzken, Gebhardt, Blome, Rudolf Brandt, Mrugowsky, Poppendick, Becker-Freyseng, Oberheuser, and Fischer are charged with special responsibility for and participation in these crimes.

(F) *Bone, Muscle, and Nerve Regeneration and Bone Transplantation Experiments.* From about September 1942 to about December 1943 experiments were conducted at the Ravensbrueck concentration camp, for the benefit of the German Armed Forces, to study bone, muscle, and nerve regeneration, and bone transplantation from one person to another. Sections of bones, muscles, and nerves were removed from the subjects. As a result of these operations, many victims suffered intense agony, mutilation, and permanent disability. The defendants Karl Brandt, Handloser, Rostock, Gebhardt, Rudolf Brandt, Oberheuser, and Fischer are charged with special responsibility for and participation in these crimes.

(G) *Sea-Water Experiments.* From about July 1944 to about September 1944 experiments were conducted at the Dachau concentration camp, for the benefit of the German Air Force and Navy, to study various methods of making sea water drinkable. The subjects were deprived of all food and given only chemically processed sea water. Such experiments caused great pain and suffering and resulted in serious bodily injury to the victims. The defendants Karl Brandt, Handloser, Rostock, Schroeder, Gebhardt, Rudolf Brandt, Mrugowsky, Poppendick, Sievers, Becker-Freyseng, Schaefer, and Beiglboeck are charged with special responsibility for and participation in these crimes.

(H) *Epidemic Jaundice Experiments.* From about June 1943 to about January 1945 experiments were conducted at the Sachsenhausen and Natzweiler concentration camps, for the benefit of the German Armed Forces, to investigate the causes of, and inoculations against, epidemic jaundice. Experimental subjects were deliberately infected with epidemic jaundice, some of whom died as a result, and others were caused great pain and suffering. The defendants Karl Brandt, Handloser, Rostock, Schroeder, Gebhardt, Rudolf Brandt, Mrugowsky, Poppendick, Sievers, Rose, and Becker-Freyseng are charged with special responsibility for and participation in these crimes.

(I) *Sterilization Experiments.* From about March 1941 to about January 1945 sterilization experiments were conducted at the Auschwitz and Ravensbrueck concentration camps, and other places. The purpose of these experiments was to develop a method of sterilization which would be suitable for sterilizing millions of people with a minimum of time and effort. These experiments were conducted by means of X-ray, surgery, and various drugs. Thousands of victims were sterilized and thereby suffered great mental and physical anguish. The defendants Karl Brandt, Gebhardt, Rudolf Brandt, Mrugowsky, Poppendick, Brack, Pokorny, and Oberheuser are charged with special responsibility for and participation in these crimes.

(J) *Spotted Fever (Fleckfieber)* * Experiments.* From about December 1941 to about February 1945 experiments were conducted at the Buchenwald and Natzweiler concentration camps for the benefit of the German Armed Forces, to investigate the effectiveness of spotted fever and other vaccines. At Buchenwald, numerous healthy inmates were deliberately infected with spotted fever virus in order to keep the virus alive; over 90 percent of the victims died as a result. Other healthy inmates were used to determine the effectiveness of different spotted fever vaccines and of various chemical substances. In the course of these experiments 75 percent of the selected number of inmates were vaccinated with one of the vaccines or nourished with one of the chemical substances and, after a period of 3 to 4 weeks, were infected with spotted fever germs. The remaining 25 percent were infected without any previous protection in order to compare the effectiveness of the vaccines and the chemical substances. As a result, hundreds of the persons experimented upon died. Experiments with yellow fever, smallpox, typhus, paratyphus A and B, cholera, and diphtheria were also conducted. Similar experiments with like results were conducted at Natzweiler concentration camp. The defendants Karl Brandt, Handloser, Rostock, Schroeder, Genzken, Gebhardt,

*A more correct translation is typhus.

Rudolf Brandt, Mrugowsky, Poppendick, Sievers, Rose, Becker-Freyseng, and Hoven are charged with special responsibility for and participation in these crimes.

(K) *Experiments with Poison.* In or about December 1943 and in or about October 1944 experiments were conducted at the Buchenwald concentration camp to investigate the effect of various poisons upon human beings. The poisons were secretly administered to experimental subjects in their food. The victims died as a result of the poison or were killed immediately in order to permit autopsies. In or about September 1944 experimental subjects were shot with poison bullets and suffered torture and death. The defendants Genzken, Gebhardt, Mrugowsky, and Poppendick are charged with special responsibility for and participation in these crimes.

(L) *Incendiary Bomb Experiments.* From about November 1943 to about January 1944 experiments were conducted at the Buchenwald concentration camp to test the effect of various pharmaceutical preparations on phosphorus burns. These burns were inflicted on experimental subjects with phosphorus matter taken from incendiary bombs, and caused severe pain, suffering, and serious bodily injury. The defendants Genzken, Gebhardt, Mrugowsky, and Poppendick are charged with special responsibility for and participation in these crimes.

In addition to the medical experiments, the nature and purpose of which have been outlined as alleged, certain of the defendants are charged with criminal activities involving murder, torture, and ill-treatment of non-German nationals as follows:

7. Between June 1943 and September 1944 the defendants Rudolf Brandt and Sievers . . . were principals in, accessories to, ordered, abetted, took a consenting part in, and were connected with plans and enterprises involving the murder of civilians and members of the armed forces of nations then at war with the German Reich and who were in the custody of the German Reich in exercise of belligerent control. One hundred twelve Jews were selected for the purpose of completing a skeleton collection for the Reich University of Strasbourg. Their photographs and anthropological measurements were taken. Then they were killed. Thereafter, comparison tests, anatomical research, studies regarding race, pathological features of the body, form and size of the brain, and other tests were made. The bodies were sent to Strasbourg and defleshed.

8. Between May 1942 and January 1944 the defendants Blome and Rudolf Brandt . . . were principals in, accessories to, ordered, abetted, took a consenting part in, and were connected with plans and enterprises involving the murder and mistreatment of tens of thousands of Polish nationals who were civilians and members of the armed forces of a nation then at war with the German Reich in exercise of belligerent control. These people were alleged to be infected with incurable tuberculosis. On the ground of ensuring the health and welfare of Germans in Poland, many tubercular Poles were ruthlessly exterminated while others were isolated in death camps with inadequate medical facilities.

9. Between September 1939 and April 1945 the defendants Karl Brandt, Blome, Brack, and Hoven . . . were principals in, accessories to, ordered, abetted, took a consenting part in, and were connected with plans and enterprises involving the execution of the so-called 'euthanasia' program of the German

Reich in the course of which the defendants herein murdered hundreds of thousands of human beings, including nationals of German-occupied countries. This program involved the systematic and secret execution of the aged, insane, incurably ill, of deformed children, and other persons, by gas, lethal injections, and diverse other means in nursing homes, hospitals, and asylums. Such persons were regarded as 'useless eaters' and a burden to the German war machine. The relatives of these victims were informed that they died from natural causes, such as heart failure. Germans doctors involved in the 'euthanasia' program were also sent to the eastern occupied countries to assist in the mass extermination of Jews.

Counts two and three of the indictment conclude with the averment that the crimes and atrocities which have been delineated "constitute violations of international conventions . . . , the laws and customs of war, the general principles of criminal law as derived from the criminal laws of all civilized nations, the internal penal laws of the countries in which such crimes were committed, and of Article II of Control Council Law No. 10."

COUNT FOUR—*Membership in a Criminal Organization:* The fourth count of the indictment alleges that the defendants Karl Brandt, Genzken, Gebhardt, Rudolf Brandt, Mrugowsky, Poppendick, Sievers, Brack, Hoven, and Fischer are guilty of membership in an organization declared to be criminal by the International Military Tribunal, in that each of these named defendants was a member of the SCHUTZSTAFFELN DER NATIONAL SOZIALISTISCHEN DEUTSCHEN ARBEITERPARTEI (commonly known as the SS) after 1 September 1939, in violation of paragraph 1 (d) Article II of Control Council Law No. 10.

Before turning our attention to the evidence in the case, we shall state the law announced by the International Military Tribunal with reference to membership in an organization declared criminal by the Tribunal:

> In dealing with the SS the Tribunal includes all persons who had been officially accepted as members of the SS including the members of the Allgemeine SS, members of the Waffen SS, members of the SS Totenkopf Verbaende, and the members of any of the different police forces who were members of the SS. The Tribunal does not include the so-called riding units. . . .
>
> The Tribunal declares to be criminal within the meaning of the Charter the group composed of those persons who had been officially accepted as members of the SS as enumerated in the preceding paragraph who became or remained members of the organization with knowledge that it was being used for the commission of acts declared criminal by Article 6 of the Charter, or who were personally implicated as members of the organization in the commission of such crimes excluding, however, those who were drafted into membership by the State in such a way as to give them no choice in the matter, and who had committed no such crimes. The basis of this finding is the participation of the organization in war crimes and crimes against humanity connected with the war; this group declared criminal cannot include, therefore, persons who had ceased to belong to the organization enumerated in the preceding paragraph prior to 1 September 1939.

THE PROOF AS TO WAR CRIMES AND CRIMES AGAINST HUMANITY

Judged by any standard of proof the record clearly shows the commission of war crimes and crimes against humanity substantially as alleged in counts two and three of the indictment. Beginning with the outbreak of World War II criminal medical experiments on non-German nationals, both prisoners of war and civilians, including Jews and "asocial" persons, were carried out on a large scale in Germany and the occupied countries. These experiments were not the isolated and causal acts of individual doctors and scientists working solely on their own responsibility, but were the product of coordinated policy-making and planning at high governmental, military, and Nazi Party levels, conducted as an integral part of the total war effort. They were ordered, sanctioned, permitted, or approved by persons in positions of authority who under all principles of law were under the duty to know about these things and to take steps to terminate or prevent them.

PERMISSIBLE MEDICAL EXPERIMENTS

The great weight of the evidence before us is to the effect that certain types of medical experiments on human beings, when kept within reasonably well-defined bounds, conform to the ethics of the medical profession generally. The protagonists of the practice of human experimentation justify their views on the basis that such experiments yield results for the good of society that are unprocurable by other methods or means of study. All agree, however, that certain basic principles must be observed in order to satisfy moral, ethical and legal concepts:

1. The voluntary consent of the human subject is absolutely essential.

    This means that the person involved should have legal capacity to give consent; should be so situated as to be able to exercise free power of choice, without the intervention of any element of force, fraud, deceit, duress, over-reaching, or other ulterior form of constraint or coercion; and should have sufficient knowledge and comprehension of the elements of the subject matter involved as to enable him to make an understanding and enlightened decision. This latter element requires that before the acceptance of an affirmative decision by the experimental subject there should be made known to him the nature, duration, and purpose of the experiment; the method and means by which it is to be conducted; all inconveniences and hazards reasonably to be expected; and the effects upon his health or person which may possibly come from his participation in the experiment.

    The duty and responsibility for ascertaining the quality of the consent rests upon each individual who initiates, directs, or engages in the experiment. It is a personal duty and responsibility which may not be delegated to another with impunity.

2. The experiment should be such as to yield fruitful results for the good of society, unprocurable by other methods or means of study, and not random and unnecessary in nature.

3. The experiment should be so designed and based on the results of animal experimentation and a knowledge of the natural history of the disease or other problem under study that the anticipated results will justify the performance of the experiment.

4. The experiment should be so conducted as to avoid all unnecessary physical and mental suffering and injury.

5. No experiment should be conducted where there is an *a priori* reason to believe that death or disabling injury will occur; except, perhaps, in those experiments where the experimental physicians also serve as subjects.

6. The degree of risk to be taken should never exceed that determined by the humanitarian importance of the problem to be solved by the experiment.

7. Proper preparations should be made and adequate facilities provided to protect the experimental subject against even remote possibilities of injury, disability, or death.

8. The experiment should be conducted only by scientifically qualified persons. The highest degree of skill and care should be required through all stages of the experiment of those who conduct or engage in the experiment.

9. During the course of the experiment the human subject should be at liberty to bring the experiment to an end if he has reached the physical or mental state where continuation of the experiment seems to him to be impossible.

10. During the course of the experiment the scientist in charge must be prepared to terminate the experiment at any stage, if he has probable cause to believe, in the exercise of the good faith, superior skill and careful judgment required of him that a continuation of the experiment is likely to result in injury, disability, or death to the experimental subject.

Of the ten principles which have been enumerated, our judicial concern, of course, is with those requirements which are purely legal in nature — or which at least are so clearly related to matters legal that they assist us in determining criminal culpability and punishment. To go beyond that point would lead us into a field that would be beyond our sphere of competence. However, the point need not be labored. We find from the evidence that in the medical experiments which have been proved, these ten principles were much more frequently honored in their breach than in their observance. Many of the concentration camp inmates who were the victims of these atrocities were citizens of countries other than the German Reich. They were non-German nationals, including Jews and "asocial persons," both prisoners of war and civilians, who had been imprisoned and forced to submit to these tortures and barbarities without so much as a semblance of trial. In every single instance appearing in the record, subjects were used who did not consent to the experiments; indeed, as to some of the experiments, it is not even contended by the defendants that the subjects occupied the status of volunteers. In no case was the experimental subject at liberty of his own free choice to withdraw from any experiment. In many cases, experiments were performed by unqualified persons; were conducted at random for no adequate scientific reason, and under revolting physical conditions. All of the experiments were conducted with unnecessary suffering and injury and but very little, if any, precautions were taken to protect or safeguard the human subjects from the possibilities of injury, disability, or death. In every one of the experiments the subjects experienced extreme pain or torture, and in most of them they suffered permanent injury, mutilation, or death, either as a direct result of the experiments or because of lack of adequate follow-up care.

Obviously all of these experiments involving brutalities, tortures, disabling injury, and death were performed in complete disregard of international conventions, the laws and customs of war, the general principles of criminal law as derived from the criminal laws of all civilized nations, and Control Council Law No. 10. Manifestly human experiments under such conditions are contrary to "the principles of the law of nations as they result from the usages established among civilized peoples, from the laws of humanity, and from the dictates of public conscience."

Whether any of the defendants in the dock are guilty of these atrocities is, of course, another question.

Under the Anglo-Saxon system of jurisprudence every defendant in a criminal case is presumed to be innocent of an offense charged until the prosecution, by competent, credible proof, has shown his guilt to the exclusion of every reasonable doubt. And this presumption abides with a defendant through each stage of his trial until such degree of proof has been adduced. A "reasonable doubt" as the name implies is one conformable to reason—a doubt which a reasonable man would entertain. Stated differently, it is that state of a case which, after a full and complete comparison and consideration of all the evidence, would leave an unbiased, unprejudiced, reflective person, charged with the responsibility for decision, in the state of mind that he could not say that he felt an abiding conviction amounting to a moral certainty of the truth of the charge.

If any of the defendants are to be found guilty under counts two or three of the indictment it must be because the evidence has shown beyond a reasonable doubt that such defendant, without regard to nationality or the capacity in which he acted, participated as a principal in, accessory to, ordered, abetted, took a consenting part in, or was connected with plans or enterprises involving the commission of at least some of the medical experiments and other atrocities that are the subject matter of these counts. Under no circumstances may he be convicted. . . . [1]

Epilogue:
Seven Were Hanged

ALEXANDER MITSCHERLICH
FRED MIELKE

The trial known as "The Case Against the Nazi Physicians" was completed on August 20, 1947. Fifteen of the 23 defendants were found guilty. Seven were found not guilty. One (Poppendick) was acquitted of the charges of having performed medical experiments but was found guilty of SS membership.

Sentence was pronounced the following day. Karl Brandt, Gebhardt, Mrugowsky, Rudolf Brandt, Sievers, Brack and Hoven (the last three being nonphysicians) were sentenced to death by hanging. Life imprisonment sentences were imposed on Handloser, Schoeder, Genzken, Rose, and Fischer.

Herta Oberheuser, the only woman among the defendants, was sentenced to 20 years, as was Becker-Freysing. Bieglböck was sentenced to 15 years, Poppendick to 10 years for SS membership. Rostock, Blome, Ruff, Romberg, Weltz, Schäfer, and Pokorny were acquitted and freed.

A few days previously, 31 lesser fry of the staff of the Buchenwald concentration camp had been found guilty on all counts, and 22 of them had been sentenced to hang. Among them was Ilse Koch, the notorious "Bitch of Buchenwald," whose life sentence has since been commuted to four years.

One of the condemned among the medical underlings was Edwin Katzenellenbogen, erstwhile member of the faculty of Harvard Medical School. He asked the court for the death sentence in the following words: "You have placed the mark of Cain on my forehead. Any physician who committed the crimes I am charged with deserves to be killed. Therefore I ask for only one grace. Apply to me the highest therapy that is in your hands." He was given life imprisonment. Another of these lesser torturers of humans, Dr. Ilans Elsor, is reported to have said that if he was found guilty the court "should not confine me to prison, but rather to an insane asylum."

Neither this horror at the character of their crimes, nor this disbelief in their own ability to take part in such monstrosities, was shared by the major

Nazi medical criminals convicted at Nuremberg. To the end, they did not acknowledge that they had done any wrong.

The hangings took place on June 2, 1948. The scene was the prison at Landsberg, in the American zone. Here Hitler had been imprisoned while he wrote *Mein Kampf.*

History records that the hangings took 62 minutes. Two black gallows were created in the prison courtyard. Karl Brandt was the only one of the seven who refused religious solace.

Karl Brandt had boasted he was "one German the Americans will never hang." He tried to cheat the gallows by offering his living body for medical experiments like those he had conducted. To his surprise, the American authorities rejected his offer. Beside the gallows, he made a final speech, declaring his conviction was "nothing but political revenge." Cried Brandt: "It is no shame to stand on this scaffold. I served my fatherland as others before me." He refused to end his speech, and finally the black hood was dropped over in mid-sentence. He was 43.

Mrugowsky shouted: "I die as a German officer sentenced by a brutal enemy and conscious I never committed the crimes charged against me." He was 43.

Gebhardt, 50-year-old former head of the German Red Cross, said: "I die without bitterness but regret there is still injustice in the world."

The last words of the other murderers were not reported. In any event, 7 were hanged, only 4 of them physicians — 7 out of the 23, and out of the many more who, as Dr. Mitscherlich's narrative makes clear, were involved in the Nazi medical crimes. It can never be said that the quality of American mercy had been strained.[2]

UPDATE

Between 1945 and 1955 the United States operated a special project entitled "Paperclip."[3] This project employed 765 German and Austrian scientists, engineers, and technicians in an attempt to exploit their expertise and to prevent the remilitarization of post-war Germany. Four of the Nazi defendants at the Nuremberg Medical Trials were at some point employed by the U.S. Military. Defendants Becker-Freysing, Ruff, and Shaefer were employed by Army Air Force up until they were arrested and taken to the Nuremberg prison to stand trial for war crimes and crimes against humanity.[4] Hermann Becker-Freysing was subsequently found guilty and sentenced to 20 years' imprisonment for his participation in the high altitude, freezing, sulfanilamide, seawater, epidemic jaundice and typhus experiments.[5] After the trial, in 1949, the U.S. Air Force brought acquitted defendant Konrad Shaefer to Randolph Field, Texas under Paperclip. He was subsequently repatriated to Germany in 1951.[6] Nuremberg defendant Kurt Blome, who in 1943 had been ordered by SS Chief Himmler to conduct plague vaccine experiments on concentration camps inmates, was contracted to work for the U.S. Army Chemical Corps under "Project 63" on August 21, 1951. The U.S. consul in Frankfurt denied Blome immigration clearance and he was subsequently given a camp doctor position at the European Command Intelligence Center in Oberusal.[7] Several of the Nuremberg physician defendants continued to practice medicine after the war and some went to work for the German pharmaceutical industry.[8] A small number of survivors were eventually compensated.[9]

NOTES

1. *Trials of War Criminals Before the Nuremberg Military Tribunals Under Control Council Law 10* (Washington, D.C.: Superintendent of Documents, U.S. Government Printing Office, 1950); Military Tribunal Case 1, *United States v. Karl Brandt et al.*, October 1946–April 1949, pp. 171–184.

2. A. Mitscherlich and F. Mielke, *Doctors of Infamy* (New York: Henry Schuman, 1949), pp. 146–148. Alexander Mitscherlich, MD was the former head of the German Medical Commission and Fred Mielke was observer to Military Tribunal No. 1, Nuremberg.

3. See T. Bower, *The Paperclip Conspiracy: The Hunt for Nazi Scientists* (Boston: Little, Brown, 1987).

4. See L. Hunt, *Secret Agenda: The United States Government, and the Project Paperclip, 1945–1990* (New York: St Martin's Press, 1991), pp. 78–93, and L. Hunt, "U.S. Coverup of Nazi Scientists," *Bulletin of the Atomic Scientists* (April 1985):16–24.

5. Ibid.

6. Ibid.

7. Ibid.

8. Personal communication, Dr. Christian Pross, West German Medical Society, West Berlin, Germany, October 11, 1991.

9. B. B. Ferencz, *Less Than Slaves: Jewish Forced Labor and the Quest for Compensation* (Cambridge, Mass.: Harvard University Press, 1979), pp. 58–59, and N. Cousins, "Report on the Ladies," *Saturday Review*, Feb. 16, 1963, p. 22.

PHOTOS AND EXHIBITS

PROSECUTION COUNSEL

Chief of Counsel:
    BRIGADIER GENERAL TELFORD TAYLOR
Chief Prosecutor:
    MR. JAMES M. McHANEY
Associate Counsel:
    MR. ALEXANDER G. HARDY
    MR. ARNOST HORLIK-HOCHWALD
Assistant Counsel:
    MR. GLEN J. BROWN
    MISS ESTHER J. JOHNSON
    MR. JACK W. ROBBINS
    MR. DANIEL J. SHILLER

DEFENSE COUNSEL

Defendants	Defense Counsel	Associate Defense Counsel
BRANDT, KARL	DR. ROBERT SERVATIUS	DR. RUDOLF SCHMIDT
HANDLOSER, SIEGFRIED	DR. OTTO NELTE	
ROSTOCK, PAUL	DR. HANS PRIBILLA	
SCHROEDER, OSKAR	DR. HANNS MARX	DR. WALTER DEHNER
GENZKEN, KARL	DR. RUDOLF MERKEL	DR. ALFRED BRENNER
GEBHARDT, KARL	DR. ALFRED SEIDL	DR. GEORG GIERL
BLOME, KURT	DR. FRITZ SAUTER	
BRANDT, RUDOLF	DR. KURT KAUFFMANN	
MRUGOWSKY, JOACHIM	DR. FRITZ FLEMMING	
POPPENDICK, HELMUT	DR. GEORG BOEHM	DR. HELMUT DUERR
SIEVERS, WOLFRAM	DR. JOSEF WEISGERBER	DR. ERICH BERGLER
ROSE, GERHARD	DR. HANS FRITZ	
RUFF, SIEGFRIED	DR. FRITZ SAUTER	
ROMBERG, HANS WOLFGANG	DR. BERND VORWERK	
BRACK, VIKTOR	DR. GEORG FROESCHMANN	
BECKER-FREYSENG, HERMANN	DR. HANNS MARX	DR. WALTER DEHNER
WELTZ, GEORG AUGUST	DR. SIEGFRIED WILLE	
SCHAEFER, KONRAD	DR. HORST PELCKMANN	
HOVEN, WALDEMAR	DR. HANS GAWLIK	DR. GERHARD KLINNERT
BEIGLBOECK, WILHELM	DR. GUSTAV STEINBAUER	
POKORNY, ADOLF	DR. KARL HOFFMANN	DR. HANS-GUNTHER SERAPHIM
OBERHEUSER, HERTA	DR. ALFRED SEIDL	DR. GEORG GIERL
FISCHER, FRITZ	DR. ALFRED SEIDL	DR. GEORG GIERL

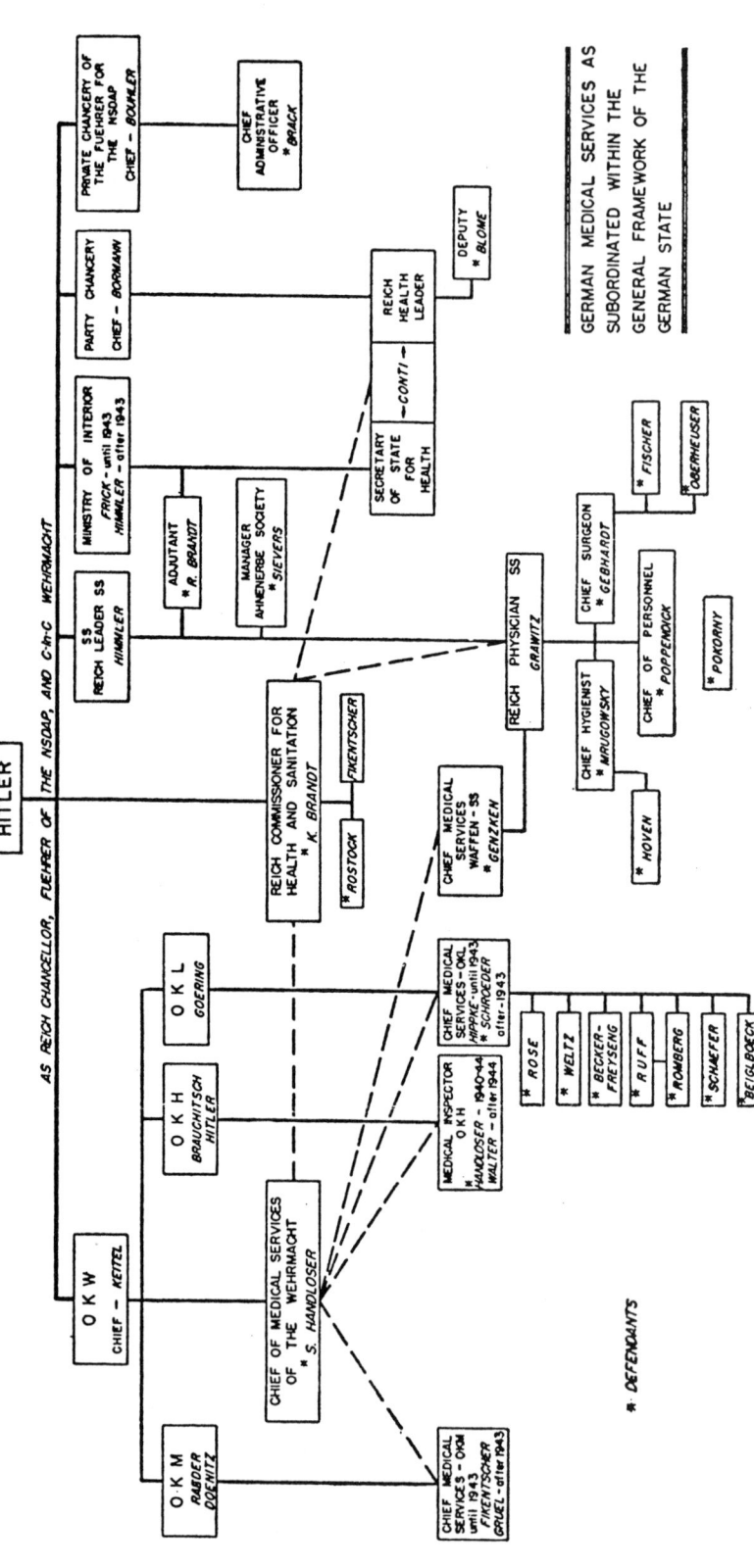

The organization of the German medical system. This chart was used by the prosecution in the course of its opening statement in order to show graphically the way the individual defendants fitted into the system. OKW = the High Command of the German Armed Forces, OKM = the High Command of the Navy, OKH = the High Command of the Army, and OKL = the High Command of the Air Force. (Public Information Photo Section, Office Chief of Counsel for War Crimes, Nuremberg)

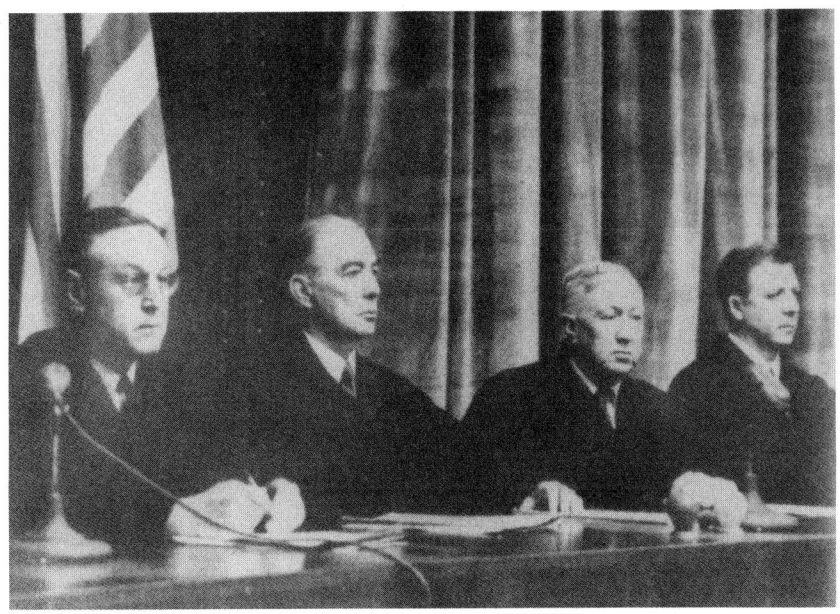

Judges of U.S. Military Tribunal No. 1. These four prominent American judges, appointed by President Truman, are shown listening to testimony during the trial of the 23. Left to right: Harold L. Sebring, justice of the Supreme Court of Florida; Walter B. Beals (presiding judge), justice of the Supreme Court of the state of Washington; Johnson T. Crawford, former justice of the Oklahoma District Court in Ada, Oklahoma; and Victor C. Swearingen, alternate member, former assistant attorney general of Michigan, from Detroit. (Wide World Photo)

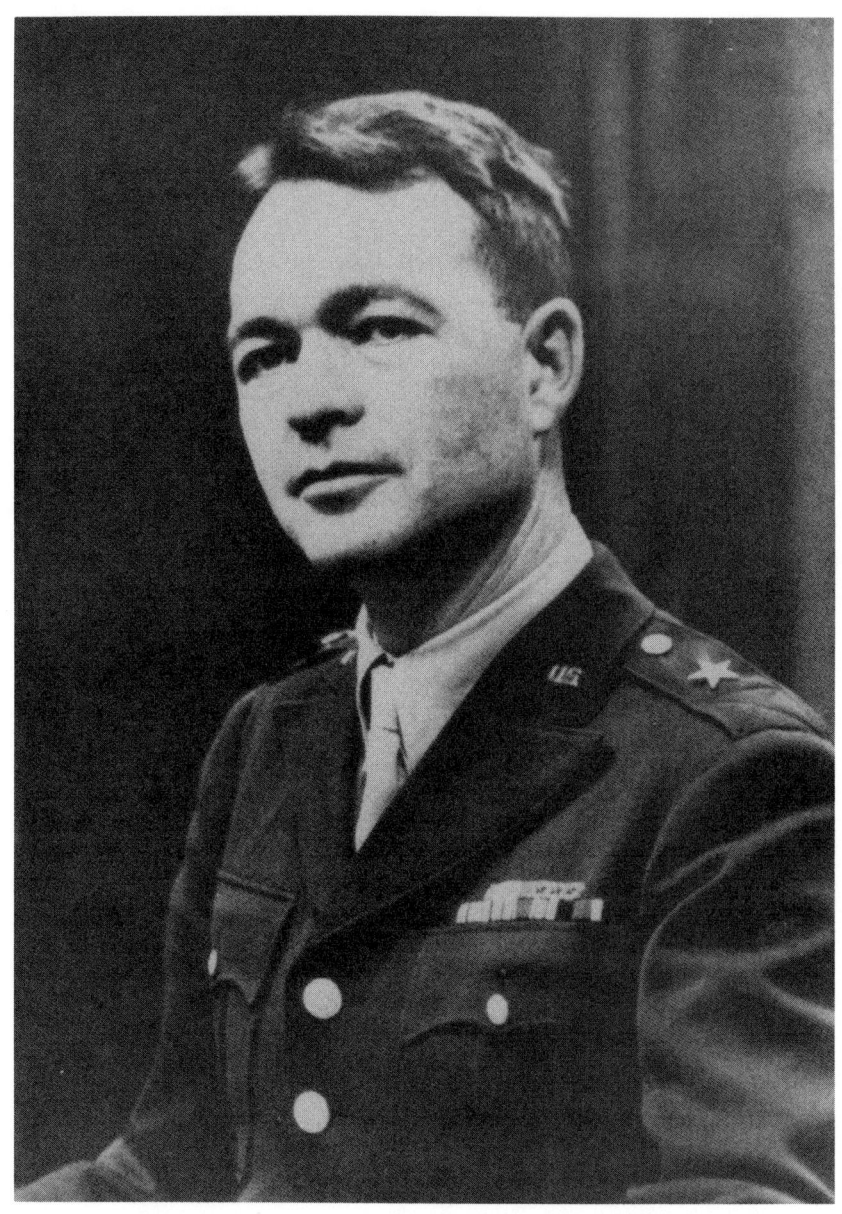

*Brig. Gen. Telford Taylor, Chief of Counsel for War Crimes, is here pictured at the trial. (*Acme Photo*)*

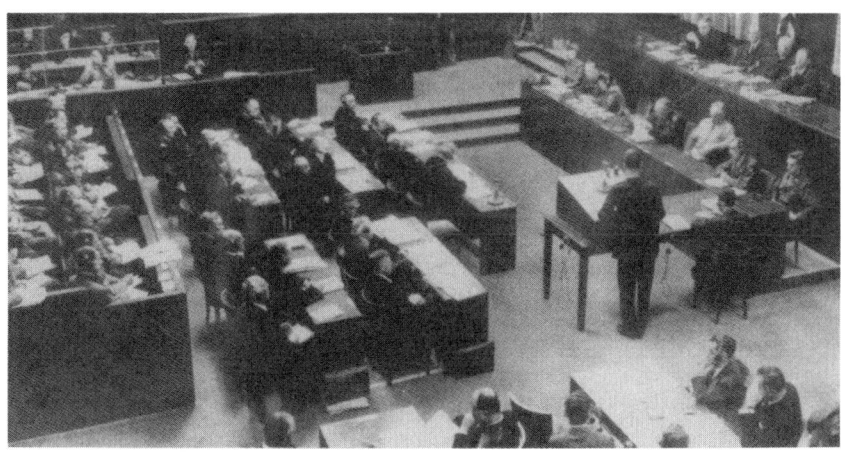

General view of courtroom on opening day of trial. Upper left: Court reporter and translators. Left: *Defendants and defense counsel.* At rostrum: *Brigadier General Telford Talyor, Chief of Counsel for War Crimes.* Right: *Judges and court clerks of Tribunal I.* Foreground: *Members of the prosecution staff with Mr. James McHaney, Chief Prosecutor, and Mr. Alexander Hardy, Associate Prosecutor, seated at table directly behind Brigadier General Taylor. (*Public Information Photo Section, *Office Chief of Counsel for War Crimes, Nuremberg)*

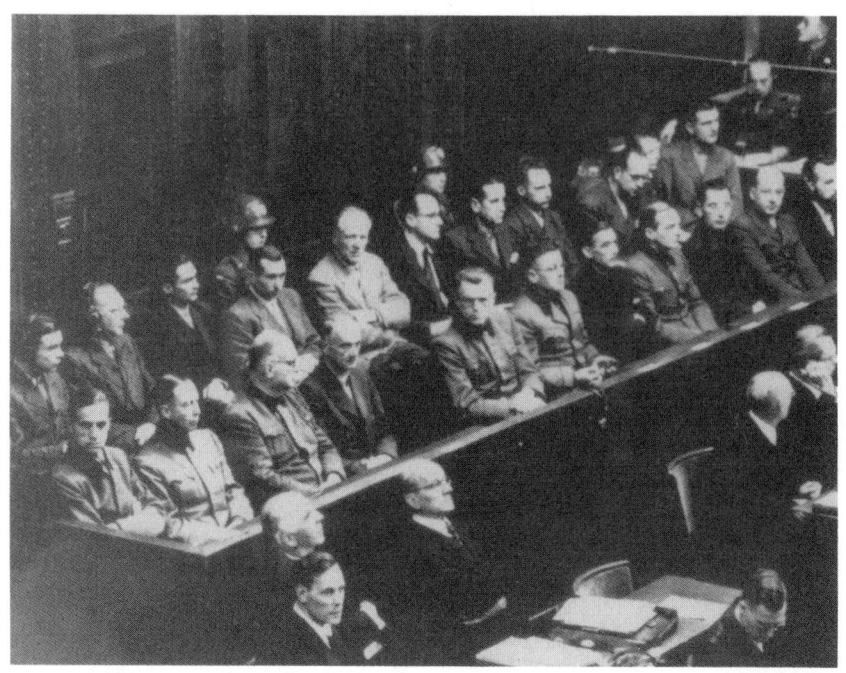

The "Dock" of defendant physicians at the "Doctor's Trial," November 1946
(UPI/Bettmann Newsphotos)

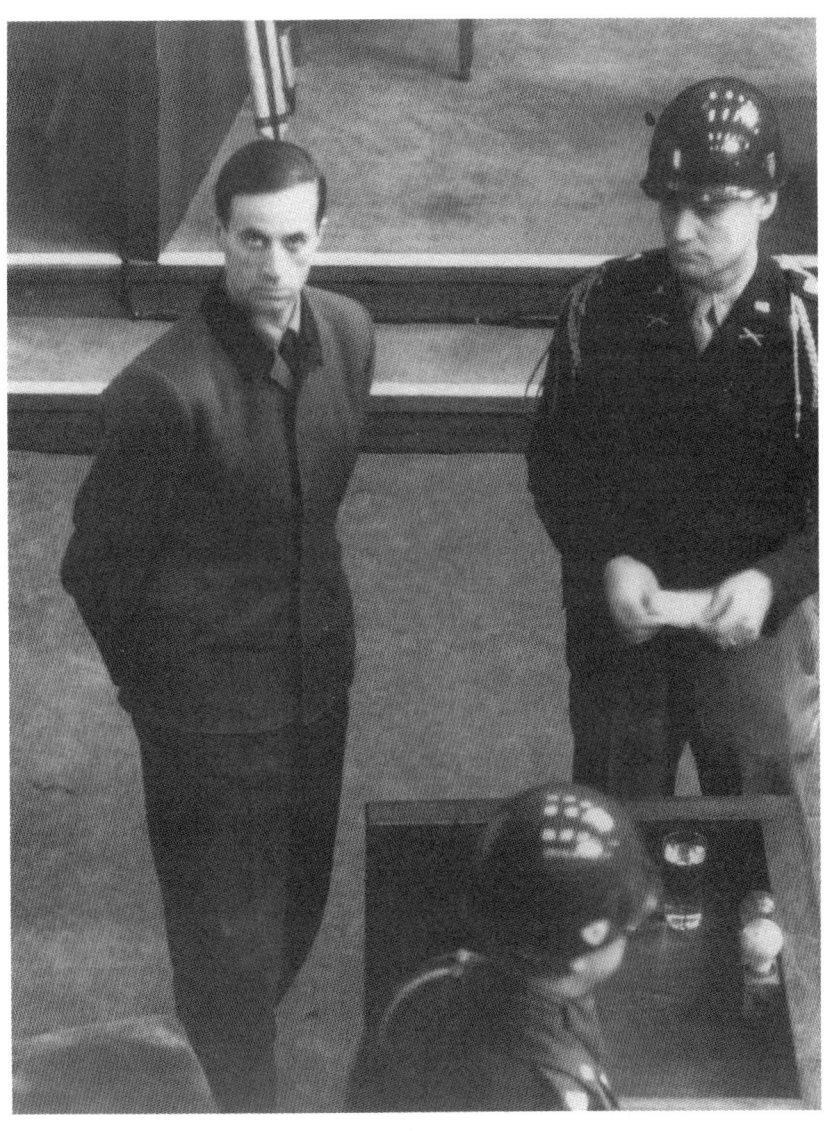

*Karl Brandt, personal physician to Adolph Hitler and Reich Commissioner for Health and Sanitation, sentenced to death by hanging. (*U.S. Army Photo, Ray D'Addario*)*

Tippe + Kurragan during the trial. D urged that he Became involved in genocide from a sense of duty to protect the state against the threat posed by groups such as Jews

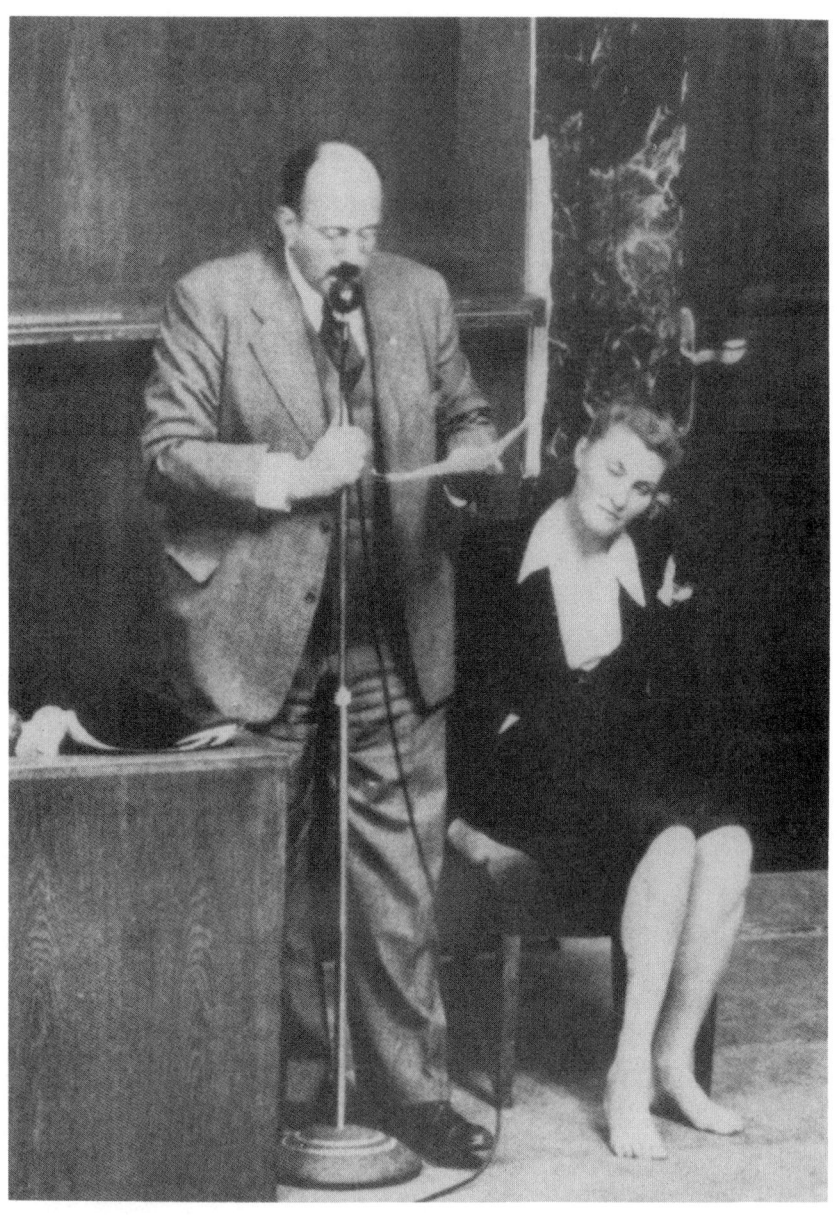

Dr. Leo Alexander, Boston neurologist and psychiatrist who served as consultant to the Secretary of War and to the Chief of Counsel for War Crimes at the trial, examines a Polish girl who was permanently crippled by physician experiments. (World Wide Photo)

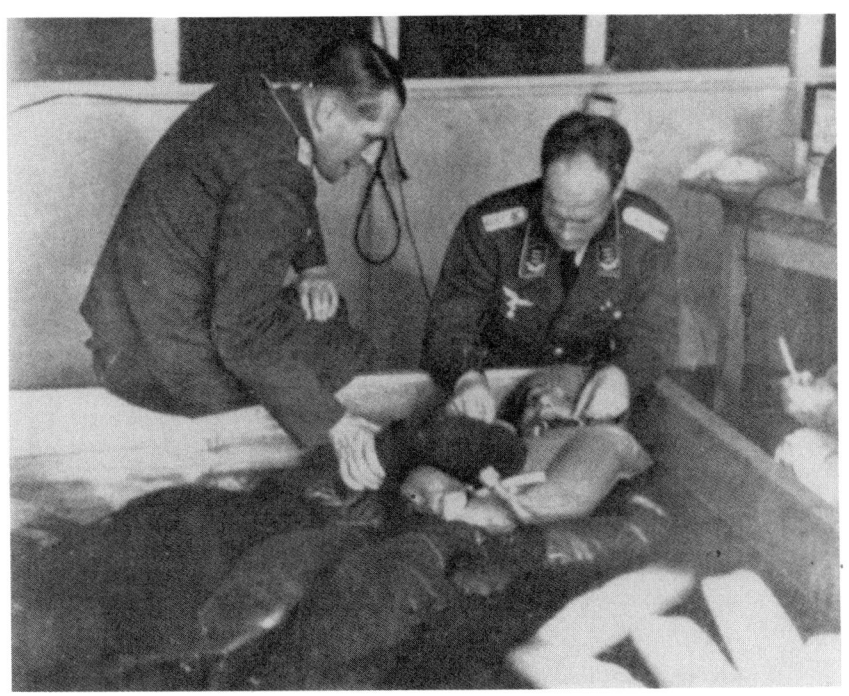

*A freezing experiment at Dachau concentration camp. Dr. E. Holzlöhner, left, professor of physiology at the Medical School of the University of Kiel, and Dr. Sigmund Rascher, right, observe a victim immersed in ice water. This particular man was a political prisoner. (*Trial Exhibit—Office Chief of Counsel for War Crimes, Nuremberg*)

SENTENCES AND COMMUTATIONS

This case charged 24 defendants with performing medical experiments on concentration camp inmates and other living human subjects. Eight defendants were acquitted.

Defendants	Sentences	Commutations
Karl Brandt	Death	—
Siegfried Handloser	Life	20 years
Oskar Schröder	Life	15 years
Karl Genzken	Life	20 years
Karl Gebhardt	Death	—
Rudolf Brandt	Death	—
Joachim Mrugowsky	Death	—
Helmut Poppendick	10 years	Time served
Wolfram Sievers	Death	—
Gerhard Rose	Life	15 years
Viktor Brack	Death	—
Hermann Becker-Freyseng	20 years	10 years
Waldemar Hoven	Death	—
Wilhelm Beiglböck	15 years	10 years
Herta Oberheuser	20 years	10 years
Fritz Fischer	Life	15 years

From: *War Crimes, War Criminals and War Crimes Trials*, An Annotated Bibliography and Source Book Compiled and Edited by Norman Tutoren, Greenwood Press, Westport, Conn. 1986, pg. 469.

7

Historical Origins of
the Nuremberg Code

MICHAEL A. GRODIN

The Nuremberg Code consists of 10 principles enumerated in the final judgment of the Doctors' Trial or Medical Case.[1] These principles were formulated in an attempt to establish the substantive standards and procedural guidelines for permissible medical experimentation with humans. They were not identified as a code of medical ethics but rather appear as part of the final legal judgment, where it is claimed that they are derived from the "natural law" of all people. (George Annas discusses the legal standing of the Nuremberg Code in U.S. law in Chapter 11.)

The 10 principles articulating the acceptable limits of human experimentation must be understood in the context of the criminal trials. Nazi physicians and scientists had carried out extensive human experimentation and murders during the war. (Chapter 5 describes the extent of Nazi experimentation as part of the indictments for crimes against humanity. Eva Mozes-Kor presents a personal account of the Mengele twin experiments carried out at the Birkenau concentration camp in Chapter 4.) The appropriate standards for the conduct of human experimentation were a major theme recurring throughout the trial. While the tribunal's focus was on the criminal nature of the Nazi experiments, the judges were also grappling with much broader ethical concerns regarding medical research. The trial court sought a historical framework of medical standards from which to judge the Nazi physicians and attempted to elucidate the scope of medical experimentation undertaken by the Nazis, and other physicians and scientists, during World War II. Finally, the trial court attempted to establish a set of principles of human experimentation that could serve as a code of research ethics.

This chapter focuses on the historical origins of the 10 principles later known as the Nuremberg Code. An attempt is made to place the code in context by analyzing earlier German and non-German medical codes. Significant questions are raised concerning the standing, scope, impact, and enforceability of all of the codes, which may address diverse populations and circumstances. The codes of human experimentation all appear to have been developed in response to specific abuses and perceived needs. In all cases, violations continued to surface after their promulgation. Most of the codes do not distinguish therapeutic from nontherapeutic human experimentation because experimentation carried out in the context of patient care was rarely considered research. All of the codes appear to accept a universal necessity to continue scientific inquiry through experimentation.

The Nuremberg Code was not the first code of human experimentation, nor was it the most comprehensive. Even pre-German codes are more extensive in their concern for the ethics of human experimentation. Perhaps it was the unprecedented nature of the atrocities committed by Nazi physicians that has made the Nuremberg Code the hallmark for all subsequent discourse on the ethics of human experimentation. Because the code was written in response to the acts of a scientific and medical community out of control, it is not surprising that voluntary informed consent was its critical centerpiece and the protection of human subjects its paramount concern.

EARLY MEDICAL CODES AND ETHICAL STATEMENTS AS THE BASIS FOR THE NUREMBERG CODE

The Nuremberg Code was based on a convergence of historical documents and circumstances. During the trial, both the prosecution and the defense repeatedly cited and analyzed past experiences and standards of ethical human experimentation. The defense counsel cited examples of widespread misuse of human subjects for research, as well as the existing medical ethics literature.[2]

The prosecution used its two primary medical expert witnesses, Leo Alexander and Andrew Ivy, as the sources for the history and ethical standards of human experimentation.[3] It is particularly important to understand the testimony of these witnesses, for we will see later that they were the primary sources of the principles upon which the Nuremberg Code is based. All of the physician witnesses and defendants at the trial based their views of medical ethics on the history of human experimentation and on historical documents. This section analyzes four historical documents that were well known and undoubtedly influenced the thinking of Ivy and Alexander. These documents are the oaths, codes, and writings of Hippocrates, Percival, Beaumont, and Bernard.

Ivy and Alexander specifically cited Hippocrates as the major foundation for their views on medical ethics.[4] At the trial, Ivy was asked the sources of his belief in the acceptability of human experimentation. He responded:

I base that opinion on the principles of ethics and morals contained in the oath of Hippocrates. I think it should be obvious that a state cannot follow a physician around in his daily administration to see that the moral responsibility inherent therein is properly carried out. This moral responsibility that controls or should control the conduct of a physician should be inculcated into the minds of physicians just as moral responsibility of other sorts, and those principles are clearly depicted or enunciated in the oath of Hippocrates, with which every physician should be acquainted. According to my knowledge, it represents the Golden Rule of the medical profession. It states how one doctor would like to be treated by another doctor in case he is ill. And in that way how a doctor should treat his patient or experimental subjects. He should treat them as though he were serving as a subject.[5]

Alexander further noted:

Every professional relationship between the physician and another human being, irrespective of whether the physician treats the patient, examines him or performs an experiment upon him with his permission, is bound by the principles laid down in the Hippocrates oath.[6]

It is interesting, but not surprising, that both Leo Alexander and Andrew Ivy cite the Hippocratic oath as the basis of their views on medical ethics. The Hippocratic oath was written (probably not by Hippocrates) some time between 470 and 360 B.C.E. It has had profound significance for the general ethos of medical practice and medical ethics.[7] It explicitly states that the physician should work to the best of his ability for the good of his patients:

I will follow that system of regimes which, according to my ability and judgment, I consider for the benefit of my patients, and abstain from whatever is deleterious and mischievous.[8]

The primary thrust of the Hippocratic oath, and its most critical point, is the obligation to benefit the patient. During the Hippocratic period, however, benefit to the patient was determined by the physician; today's medical ethicists are concerned with benefit as determined by the patient or the patient's proxy.[9]

The most striking problem, however, with using the Hippocratic oath as the foundation for the Nuremberg Code on human experimentation is that it does not deal with research. The oath deals with patients, not with experimental human subjects. Benefit to the patient is most problematic in the area of human experimentation, particularly in nontherapeutic research, where there is no claim of benefit for the subject at all. The risks to the subject are balanced against the benefits to society at large. In addition, no discussion of the principle of informed consent is found within the oath. This is particularly relevant in that consent is believed by many to be the key principle of the Nuremberg Code (see Chapter 12 for a discussion of the importance of informed consent to the Nuremberg Code and the ethics of human experimentation). It is also of interest that during the Hippocratic period, animals were considered sacred and human autopsies were outlawed. This is important because the Nuremberg Code explicitly states that animal experimentation should be done before humans become subjects. Alexander and Ivy confused therapeutic treatment of patients with nontherapeutic experimentation on prisoners and thus incorrectly cited Hippocrates as the source for the ethics of human experimentation.

Medicine had hardly advanced, with regard to effective therapies, from the time of Hippocrates until the end of the eighteenth century.[10] During the intervening centuries, human experimentation was performed in an uncontrolled, unscientific manner. Reports of medical experiments on condemned criminals in ancient times and of human vivisection are now well documented.[11] Some of these early examples of human experimentation focused on the use of variolation vaccinations. In England in 1721, condemned prisoners at Newgate Prison were offered a pardon if they participated in inoculations.[12] Perhaps the earliest evidence of experimentation on children dates from 1776, when Edward Jenner inoculated an 8-year-old boy with cowpox material.[13] It should be noted that up to the nineteenth century, almost all medical practice may be considered uncontrolled, unstandardized, and innovative therapeutics or, quite simply, human experimentation of a purely empirical nature.

One of the earliest codes to include specific directives with respect to research ethics was written by Thomas Percival, an English physician, in 1803. Percival's code of medical ethics was the source for the first American Medical Association Code of Ethics in the United States in 1847. Andrew Ivy, as the representative of the American Medical Association at the Nuremberg Tribunals, was well aware of the Association's Code and its roots in the English Code of Percival. It is of interest that the first American Medical Association Code of Ethics does not identify human experimentation as a distinct area of concern.[14]

While Percival's code deals primarily with the clinical practice of medicine, it does include specific directives to the physician who is planning to perform human experiments. Percival notes:

> Whenever cases occur, attended with circumstances not heretofore observed, or in which the ordinary modes of practice have been attempted without success, it is for the public good, and in especial degree advantageous to the poor (who, being the most numerous class of this society, are the greatest beneficiaries of the healing art) that new remedies *and new methods of chirurgical treatment* should be devised but, in the accomplishment of the salutary purpose, the gentlemen of the faculty should be *scrupulously and conscientiously governed by sound reason, just analogy, or well-authenticated facts*. And no such trials should be instituted without a previous consultation of the physicians or surgeons according to the nature of the case.[15]

Percival's code clearly states the need to devise new remedies and new, innovative therapies. In his view, this research must be based on conscientious and scrupulous reasoning and careful investigation of facts, and action should be taken only after consultation with one's fellow physicians. The focus, then, of this early guide to research ethics is on good methodology and competent investigators. While both are crucial, there is no mention in Percival's code of the need for the protection of human subjects, nor is there any discussion of consent at all.

Some have cited the code of William Beaumont in 1833 as the oldest American document dealing with the ethics of human experimentation.[16] Beaumont was a physician who carried out extensive nontherapeutic experiments with his patient, Alexis St. Martin. St. Martin had suffered an accidental gunshot wound to his abdomen that, in healing, had left an open fistula tract. Beaumont utilized this tract to study the physiology of the stomach. In an attempt to justify his human experiments, Beaumont set forth a set of principles to guide the researcher.

William Beaumont's code includes the following points:

1. There must be recognition of an area where experimentation in man is needed. . . .
2. Some experimental studies in man are justifiable when the information cannot otherwise be obtained.
3. The investigator must be conscientious and responsible . . . for a well-considered, methodological approach is required so that as much information as possible will be obtained whenever a human subject is used. No random studies are to be made.
4. The voluntary consent of the subject is necessary. . . .
5. The experiment is to be discontinued when it causes distress to the subject. . . .
6. The project must be abandoned when the subject becomes dissatisfied.[17]

Beaumont's code resembles Percival's in claiming that human experimentation is needed, and that the investigator must be conscientious and responsible and must use a sound methodological approach. Of particular importance, however, is its further statement that the voluntary consent of the subject is necessary and that the project should be abandoned if the subject is distressed by it. These requirements reflect the fact that Beaumont's subject was not a prisoner but an alert, competent adult, so that consent would seem to be a prerequisite to enlisting his cooperation.

The influential French physiologist Claude Bernard wrote extensively on experimental medicine, including the guidelines governing human experimentation. His work was known to both Ivy and Alexander.[18]

In his famous text, *An Introduction to the Study of Experimental Medicine*, published in 1865, Bernard lays down his principles for the ethical pursuit of human experimentation:

> It is our duty and our right to perform an experiment on man whenever it can save his life, cure him or gain him some personal *benefit*. The principle of medical and surgical morality, therefore, consists in never performing on man an experi-

ment which might be harmful to him to any extent, even though the result might be highly advantageous to science, i.e., to the health of others. . . . Christian morals forbid only one thing, doing ill to one's neighbor. So, among the experiments that might be tried on man, those that can only *harm* are forbidden. Those that are innocent are permissible, and those that may do good are obligatory.[19]

Bernard's writings suggest a merging of patient care, innovative therapy, and therapeutic experimentation. He appears to exclude any nontherapeutic research by demanding the personal benefit of the subject. In the context of medical care, he believes that it is imperative to perform scientifically vigorous experimentation in order to gain that benefit. The benefit, however, is to be determined by the physician.

The limits of acceptable research condoned by Bernard can be surmised from the following two cases. He supported the use of dying patients in human experimentation that caused no suffering. He also endorsed the administration of the larvae of intestinal worms to a condemned women with the goal of postmortem examination. These cases seem to call into question Bernard's prohibition of nonbeneficial experimentation.[20]

The codes of Hippocrates, Percival, Beaumont, and Bernard are all concerned with a physician's responsibility to benefit the patient/subject. While Hippocrates deals only with the physician–patient relationship, Percival addresses innovative therapies, Beaumont covers nontherapeutic experimentation, and Bernard focuses on the scientific method and therapeutic research. Beaumont and Bernard are also concerned with acceptable experimental risk. Only Beaumont provides any discussion of voluntary consent as a necessity for human experimentation.

Alexander and Ivy had read the works of Hippocrates, Percival, Beaumont, and Bernard. Beyond these documents, Alexander was most interested in American statements and court decisions on cases involving the use of new medical or surgical techniques and the administration of new and unproven drugs. Alexander cites several reviews and cases as important foundations for his ethical formulations.[21] These law review articles and cases identify the liability of the physician who subjects a patient to experimental methods of treatment without making a full disclosure of the material facts so that the patient may assume or reject the risk. The law review articles also specify the legal responsibility for human experimentation involving risk to life without compensating social or scientific interests.[22]

Ivy and Alexander, as medical experts at the Nuremberg trial, were also cognizant of some of the prewar German literature on the ethics of human experimentation. Alexander specifically cites a German book by Ebermayer, written in 1930, as an influence on his views of the ethics of human experimentation.[23] Insofar as the German physicians on trial at Nuremberg claimed that the ethics of their human experimentation must first be judged on the basis of German standards and codes, it is relevant to examine the nature of medical ethics and the ethics of human experimentation in prewar Germany.

THE ETHICS OF HUMAN EXPERIMENTATION IN
PRE-NUREMBERG GERMANY

The earliest piece of legislation in Germany concerning the ethics of human experimentation was a directive issued on December 29, 1900, by the Prussian Minister of Religious, Educational and Medical Affairs. This document may, in fact, be the first reported regulatory action relating specifically to the field of human experimentation (see the discussion in Chapter 8 of this volume). The directive reads:

I. I wish to point out to the directors of clinics, polyclinics and similar establishments that medical interventions for purposes other than diagnosis, therapy and immunization are absolutely prohibited, even though all other legal and ethical requirements for performing such interventions are fulfilled if:
1. The person in question is a minor or is not fully competent on other grounds;
2. The person concerned has not declared unequivocally that he consents to the intervention;
3. The declaration has not been made on the basis of a proper explanation of the adverse consequences that may result from the intervention.
II. In addition, I prescribe that:
1. Interventions of this nature may be performed only by the director of the institution himself or with his special authorization;
2. In every intervention of this nature, an entry must be made in the medical case-record book, certifying that the requirements laid down in Items 1–3 of Section I and Item 1 of Section II have been fulfilled, specifying details of the case.
III. This directive shall not apply to medical interventions intended for the purpose of diagnosis, therapy, or immunization.[24]

The 1900 Prussian directive was issued, at least in part, in response to a public debate in the German daily press, Parliament, and the courts about the permissibility of human experimentation. Much of the debate focused on the "Case of Neisser." Albert Neisser, a professor of dermatology and venereology in Breslau, had conducted experiments in 1892 on the possibility of immunizing healthy persons against syphilis by inoculating them with serum from known syphilis patients. Four children served as healthy controls and were inoculated with syphilis serum. Three adolescent female prostitutes were similarly injected and contracted syphilis. Consent was not obtained from any of the subjects or their legal guardians. Legal and legislative debate ultimately led to the 1900 "Instructions to the Directors of Clinics, Out-Patient Clinics and Other Medical Facilities."[25]

The Prussian directive explicitly prohibits nontherapeutic research on minors or incompetents. This may be the first document dealing with the ethics of human experimentation that specifically recognizes the need for the protection of uniquely vulnerable populations such as minors or incompetents. The document further demands unequivocal consent and a proper explanation of the possible adverse consequences of the research. This recognition of voluntary informed consent as fundamental to ethically sound experimentation is a much more refined notion of the protection of human subjects than is seen in earlier documents. If research is to be carried out according to the directive, then it can only be done by the director of the institute or with special supervision. Furthermore, all experiments must be entered into a medical record book, along with documentation of how the requirements for human experimentation were met. This 1900 Prussian document is critical in the history of the development of human experimentation guidelines in that it not only states the substantive standards for the ethical conduct of research, but also contains specific procedural mechanisms to ensure responsibility for the experimentation.

One of the defenses raised at the Nuremberg trial by the Nazi physicians was the relativism of codes of ethics, especially in regard to human experimentation. The Nazi physicians claimed that standards of ethics of earlier times or other locales could not be considered the standard for Germany, and thus they could not be held accountable to these codes of ethics (see Chapter 13 for a discussion of ethical relativism). It is thus most important to look at German regulations from the 1930s on to see what the standards of research ethics were during that period.

Medicine in prewar Germany was a showcase of academic, scholarly, and analytical pursuits (see Chapters 2 and 3). The prewar German Medical Association was a democratic forum with such progressive concerns as hygiene and public health. Germany had legislated compulsory health insurance for workers. Questions of medical ethics and malpractice were handled through the German Medical Association and the Reich Chamber of Physicians. Physicians were licensed by the Ministry of Education and the Reich Health Office in the Minister of Interior, which had been established in 1876 by the German Imperial Reich and was responsible for drafting legislation and policy, compiling health statistics, carrying out research, and publishing information.

Criticism of the German medical profession for alleged unethical conduct became widespread in the 1920s. Such criticism was unparalleled in other countries at that time, especially as the German criticism appeared in the daily press.[26] A paper appearing in 1931 written by Alfons Stauder, a member of the Reich Health Office, described the state of medical research as

> naked cynicism; placing the lives of small children on the same level as those of experimental animals (rats), dubious experiments having no therapeutic purpose; science sailing under false colors; crimes against the health of defenseless children; lack of sensibility; mental and physical torture; martyrization of children in hospitals; the worst forms of charlatanism; disgustingly shameful abominations in the name of science run mad; horrors of the darkest middle ages, outstripping the infamous deeds of the inquisition and the hangman; social injustice; discrimination between the rich and the poor.[27]

Further criticisms were lodged by Friedrich Müller in 1930 in referring to the increased number of medical pharmaceuticals being "thrown onto the market and advertised." Müller accused hospitals of working for the chemical industry and big business.[28]

On March 14, 1930, the Reich Health Council held a session to discuss "the permissibility of medical experiments on healthy and sick subjects." The two speakers were Friedrich Müller of Munich and Alfons Stauder of Nuremberg. Müller postulated several principles that should guide human experimentation. Müller's principles included the agreement of the patient, the weighing of consequences, planning, and competent and responsible investigation. Stauder, while acknowledging that abuses existed, suggested that it was the physician's duty to cure patients and that without human experimentation, medical progress would cease.[29]

An important and interesting regulation was promulgated in Germany in 1931 by the Reich Minister of the Interior. It consisted of guidelines for medical experimentation with humans that were probably set down by the Reich Health Council at the urging of Dr. Julius Moses. Moses practiced general medicine in Berlin from 1920 to 1932 and was a member of Parliament for the Social Democratic Party. In 1930, Dr. Moses alerted the public to the deaths of 75 children caused by pediatricians in Lübeck in the course of experiments with tuberculosis vaccinations.[30] In his role as physician/legislator, Moses was in a unique position to respond to these abuses. The 1931 Reich Minister's guidelines are also important because they were recognized and cited during the Nuremberg tribunal as a standard of ethics for the practice of human experimentation during the Nazi period.[31]

There was a great deal of controversy at the trial and in subsequent writings regarding the legal force of the 1931 document. This controversy surfaced during the trial, where Ivy cited the 1931 regulations and the defense counsel claimed that they had no force of law.[32] The International Office of Public Hygiene in Paris, which had the task of monitoring national and international laws and regulations on health under the Rome Arrangement of 1907, did not cite the 1931 guidelines as part of their monitoring of legislation, and there is no mention of the 1931 guidelines in the Bulletin of the Office between 1931 and 1932.[33] This is of particular interest in that there are numerous reports of items on legislation relating to the quality of milk, standards for bread, and hygienic standards for housing, but not on the German guidelines for experimentation. Several authors have claimed that the 1931 Reich Guidelines constituted a valid, enforceable law up to 1945.[34] Others have claimed that the Reich guidelines were only recommendations and did not have legal force.[35] Independent of their legal standing, however, they are useful in understanding prewar German principles concerning the acceptable limits of human experimentation.

These guidelines were issued in a Reich Circular on February 28, 1931, and were entitled, "Regulations on New Therapy and Human Experimentation." This German document contains almost all of the points subsequently cited in the Nuremberg Code. Some would even argue that the guidelines are even more inclusive and formalistic than the Nuremberg Code in that they demand complete responsibility of the medical profession for carrying out human experimentation. The document explicitly states that it is the individual physician and the chief physician who are responsible for the well-being of the patient or subject. The 1931 Reich Circular states:[36]

> The Reich Health Council [*Reichsgesundheitsrat*] has set great store on ensuring that all physicians receive information with regard to the following guidelines. The Council has agreed that all physicians in open or closed health care institutions should sign a commitment to these guidelines when entering their employment.

The final draft of the Circular continues with 14 points:

1. In order that medical science may continue to advance, the initiation in appropriate cases of therapy involving new and as yet insufficiently tested means and procedures cannot be avoided. Similarly, scientific experimentation involving human subjects cannot be completely excluded as such, as this would hinder or even prevent progress in the diagnosis, treatment, and prevention of diseases.

    The freedom to be granted to the physician accordingly shall be weighed against his special duty to remain aware at all times of his major responsibility for the life and health of any person on whom he undertakes innovative therapy or perform an experiment.
2. For the purposes of these Guidelines, "innovative therapy" means interventions and treatment methods that involve humans and serve a therapeutic purpose, in other words, that are carried out in a particular, individual case in order to diagnose, treat, or prevent a disease or suffering or to eliminate a physical defect, although their effects and consequences cannot be sufficiently evaluated on the basis of existing experience.
3. For the purposes of these Guidelines, "scientific experimentation" means interventions and treatment methods that involve humans and are undertaken for research purposes without serving a therapeutic purpose in an individual case, and whose effects and consequences cannot be sufficiently evaluated on the basis of existing experience.
4. Any innovative therapy must be justified and performed in accordance with the principles of medical ethics and the rules of medical practice and theory.

    In all cases, the question of whether any adverse effects that may occur are proportionate to the anticipated benefits shall be examined and accessed.

    Innovative therapy may be carried out only if it has been tested in advance in animal trials (where these are possible).
5. Innovative therapy may be carried out only after the subject or his legal representative has unambiguously consented to the procedure in the light of relevant information provided in advance.

    Where consent is refused, innovative therapy may be initiated only if it constitutes an urgent procedure to preserve life or prevent serious damage to health and prior consent could not be obtained under the circumstances.
6. The question of whether to use innovative therapy must be examined with particular care where the subject is a child or a person under 18 years of age.
7. Exploitation of social hardship in order to undertake innovative therapy is incompatible with the principles of medical ethics.
8. Extreme caution shall be exercised in connection with innovative therapy

involving live microorganisms, especially live pathogens. Such therapy shall be considered permissible only if the procedure can be assumed to be relatively safe and similar benefits are unlikely to be achieved under the circumstances by any other method.

9. In clinics, polyclinics, hospitals, or other treatment and care establishments, innovative therapy may be carried out only by the physician in charge or by another physician acting in accordance with his express instructions and subject to his complete responsibility.

10. A report shall be made in respect of any innovative therapy, indicating the purpose of the procedure, the justification for it, and the manner in which it is carried out. In particular, the report shall include a statement that the subject or, where appropriate, his legal representative has been provided in advance with relevant information and has given his consent.

    Where therapy has been carried out without consent, under the conditions referred to in the second paragraph of Section 5, the statement shall give full details of these conditions.

11. The results of any innovative therapy may be published only in a manner whereby the patient's dignity and the dictates of humanity are fully respected.

12. Section 4–11 of these Guidelines shall be applicable, *mutatis mutandis*, to scientific experimentation (cf. Section 3).

    The following additional requirement shall apply to such experimentation:
    (a) Experimentation shall be prohibited in all cases where consent has not been given;
    (b) Experimentation involving human subjects shall be avoided if it can be replaced by animal studies. Experimentation involving human subjects may be carried out only after all data that can be collected by means of those biological methods (laboratory testing and animal studies) that are available to medical science for purposes of clarification and confirmation of the validity of the experiment have been obtained. Under these circumstances, motiveless and unplanned experimentation involving human subjects shall obviously be prohibited;
    (c) Experimentation involving children or young persons under 18 years of age shall be prohibited if it in any way endangers the child or young person;
    (d) Experimentation involving dying subjects is incompatible with the principles of medical ethics and shall therefore be prohibited.

13. While physicians and, more particularly, those in charge of hospital establishments may thus be expected to be guided by a strong sense of responsibility toward their patients, they should at the same time not be denied the satisfying responsibility [*verantwortungsfreudigkeit*] of seeking new ways to protect or treat patients or alleviate or remedy their suffering where they are convinced, in the light of their medical experience, that known methods are likely to fail.

14. Academic training courses should take every suitable opportunity to stress the physician's special duties when carrying out a new form of therapy or a scientific experiment, as well as when publishing his results.

These guidelines on human experimentation were visionary in their depth and scope. The Reich Circular enumerates clear directives concerning the general, technical, and ethical standards of medicine, informed consent, documented justification of any deviation from protocol, a risk-benefit analysis, justification for the study of especially vulnerable populations (such as children), and the necessity to maintain written records. In many ways, these guidelines are more extensive than either the subsequent Nuremberg Code or the later Declaration of Helsinki recommendations (see Chapter 8).

One final piece of German legislation concerning the ethics and limits of scientific experimentation is relevant. On November 24, 1933, the Nazis passed a law to prevent cruelty and indifference of humans toward animals.[37] The law stated that all operations or treatments that were associated with pain or injury, especially experiments involving the use of cold, heat, or infection, were prohibited and could be permitted only under exceptional circumstances. This law, of course, would prevent the use of animals as an alternative to human experimentation. If the 1931 Reich Circular did have any force of law, the guidelines' stipulation that animal experimentation precede any human experimental trials would have been revoked by this 1933 Nazi legislation. Ironically, if this law for the protection of animals were seen as including human beings as a type of animal, most, if not, all Nazi human experimentation would also have been outlawed.[38]

THE NUREMBERG TRIAL AND JUDGMENT

The Doctors' Trial, Military Tribunal I, Case 1, United States of America v. Karl Brandt et al., began on December 9, 1946, at the Palace of Justice in Nuremberg. Twenty-three defendant Nazi physicians were indicted for war crimes and crimes against humanity (see Chapter 5). The charges included human experimentation involving unconsenting prisoners. The experiments included military-related studies to test the limits of human endurance to high altitudes and freezing temperatures. Medically related experiments included inoculation of prisoners with infectious disease pathogens and tests of new antibiotics. Various mutilating bone, muscle, and nerve experiments were also performed on unconsenting prisoner subjects. (Chapter 5 includes a complete description of the medical experiments conducted on concentration camp prisoners.)

The question of what were or should be the universal standards for justifying human experimentation recurred throughout the trial. The lack of universally accepted principles for carrying out human experimentation was an issue pressed by the defendant physicians throughout their testimony. The ethical arguments presented by the defendants during the trial as justification for their participation in human experimentation with concentration camp prisoners can be summarized as follows:

1. Research is necessary in times of war and national emergency. Military and civilian survival may depend on the scientific and medical knowledge derived from human experimentation. Extreme circumstances demand extreme action.[39]

2. The use of prisoners as research subjects is a universally accepted practice. The defense counsel cited examples of human experimentation on prisoners throughout the world, with particular emphasis on research conducted in U.S. penitentiaries.[40]

3. The prisoners utilized for human experimentation were already condemned to death. Thus, prisoner involvement in human experimentation actually served the prisoners' best interests by keeping them alive and preventing their certain execution.[41]

4. Experimental subjects were selected by the military leaders or the prisoners themselves. An individual physician thus could not be held responsible for the selections.[42]

5. In times of war, all members of society must contribute to the war effort. This includes the military, civilians, and those who are incarcerated.[43]

6. The Germans physicians involved in human experimentation were only following the German law.[44]

7. There are no universal standards of research ethics. Standards have varied according to time and place. (For further discussion of this argument of ethical relativism, see Chapter 13.) The defense counsel cited 60 published papers involving human experimentation carried out throughout the world. Many of these experiments involved questionable informed consent, serious consequences, and repeated justification of the research based on the necessity of the data for scientific progress.[45]

8. If the physicians did not participate in the research, they would be putting their own lives at risk and might be killed. Furthermore, if the physicians did not carry out the medical experiments themselves, less skilled nonmedical technicians would perform surgery and medical tests, producing even greater harm.[46]

9. The state determined the necessity for human experimentation. The physicians were just following orders.[47]

10. Sometimes it is necessary to tolerate a lesser evil, the killing of some, to achieve a greater good, the saving of many. That the experiments were useful, the defense claimed, was evident by the use of the data derived from Nazi human experimentation by the United States and Britain in the war against Japan.[48]

11. The prisoners' consent to participation in human experimentation was tacit. Since there were no statements stating that the subjects did not consent, it should be assumed that a valid consent existed.[49]

12. Without human experimentation, there would be no way to advance the progress of science and medicine.[50]

In countering these defenses, the prosecution focused its arguments concerning ethical standards for the conduct of human experimentation on the testimony of the prosecution's two chief medical expert witnesses. It was these witnesses and their testimony that served as the substance for the ethical principles for human experimentation that appear in the final judgment and constitute the Nuremberg Code.

Andrew Ivy's testimony during the trial focused primarily on the ethical standards for the conduct of human experimentation. As a noted physiologist and research scientist, Dr. Ivy cited the Hippocratic tradition as central to his views. In his testimony, he also noted that the United States had specific standards for the ethics of research that were embodied in the American Medical Association guidelines.[51] The archives of the American Medical Association reveal no evidence of such explicit principles on the ethics of human experimentation prior to December 28, 1946. The guidelines that Dr. Ivy cites in his testimony on June 12–14, 1947, were published 19 days after the prosecution's opening arguments were presented at trial. It appears that Ivy studied the tribunal prosecution's pretrial records and exhibits and then reported his views on the ethics of human experimentation to the American Medical Association's trustees, who subsequently incorporated his guidelines into the *Journal of the American Medical Association.*

These "Principles of Ethics Concerning Experimentation on Human Beings" included three points:

1. The voluntary consent of the individual upon whom the experiment is to be performed *must* be obtained.
2. The danger of each experiment *must* be previously investigated by animal experiments.
3. The experiment *must* be performed under proper medical protection and management.[52]

In cross-examination, the defense readily discovered the lack of universally held or published substantive standards on human experimentation in the United States prior to the published 1946 American Medical Association principles. Thus, the principles of ethics concerning human experimentation could not be held to be relevant prior to 1946.

As the trial was drawing to a close, Dr. Alexander, in consultation with Dr. Ivy, attempted to pull together their testimony into a set of ethical principles that could be utilized by the judges in their final decision. These principles served as the basis for the Nuremberg Code. There remains controversy as to who was the primary author of the final 10-point code. Some writers claim that "the primary compiler of the ten principles of the Nuremberg Code was the physician A. C. Ivy."[53] Still other writers note that "no one knows for sure who formulated those ten points" but conclude that Alexander is the primary author.[54]

Dr. Alexander did prepare a memorandum entitled "Ethical and Non-Ethical Experimentation on Human Beings," which he submitted to the United States Chief of Counsel for War Crimes and the court on April 15, 1947.[55] It is not clear if this memorandum was also given to the defense.[56] Alexander proposed six essential requirements for ethically and legally permissible experiments on human beings:

1. Legally valid voluntary consent of the experimental subject is essential. This requires specifically
   a. The absence of duress;
   b. Sufficient disclosure on the part of the experimenter and sufficient understanding on the part of the experimental subject of the exact nature and consequences of the experiment for which he volunteers to permit an enlightened consent.
   In the case of mentally ill patients, for the purpose of experiments concerning the nature and treatment of nervous and mental illness, or related subjects, such consent of the next of kin or legal guardian is required; whenever the mental state of the patient permits (that is, in those mentally ill patients who are not delirious or confused), his own consent should be obtained in addition.
2. The nature and purpose of the experiment must be humanitarian, with the ultimate aim to cure, treat, or prevent illness, and not concerned with methods of killing or sterilization (kienology). The motive and purpose of the experiment shall also not be personal or otherwise ulterior.
3. No experiment is permissible if the foregone conclusion exists, or the probability or the *a priori* reason to believe that death or disabling injury of the experimental subject will occur.
4. Adequate preparations must be made and proper facilities be provided to aid the experimental subject against any remote chance of injury, disability, or death. This provision specifically requires that the degree of skill of all those who are taking an active part as experimenters, and the degree of care which they exercise during the experiment, must be significantly higher than the skill which is considered qualifying and the care which is considered adequate for the performance of standardized medical or surgical procedures, and for the administration of well-established drugs. American courts are very stringent in requiring for the permissible use of any new or unusual technique or drug, irrespective of whether this use is experimental or purely therapeutic, a degree of skill and care on the part of the responsible physician, which is higher than that required for the purpose of routine medical or surgical procedures.
5. The degree of risk taken should never exceed that determined by the humanitarian importance of the problem to be solved by the experiment. It is ethically permissible for an experimenter to perform experiments involving significant risks only if the solution, after thorough exploration along all other lines of scientific investigation, is not accessible by any other means, and if he considers the solution of the problem important enough to risk his own life along with the lives of his non-scientific colleagues, such as was done in the case of Walter Reed's yellow fever experiments.
6. The experiment to be performed must be so designed and based upon the results of thorough thinking-through, investigation of simple physico-chemical systems and of animal experimentation that the anticipated results will justify the performance of the experiment. That is, the experiment must be such as to yield decisive results for the good of society and should not be random and unnecessary in nature.[57]

This memorandum contains almost all of the principles that appear in the final 10-point Nuremberg Code. Point 1 is concerned with free, voluntary, and informed consent, as well as proxy consent. It is of interest that the first point of the Nuremberg Code also deals with free, voluntary, and informed consent. (For a discussion of the centrality of informed consent for the Nuremberg Code, see Chapter 12.) The first, point 1 of the Code expands on the substance and procedure of informed consent and suggests the duty and responsibility of the physician to ascertain the quality of the consent. The Code does not address the problem of proxy consent for incompetent subjects. (Chapter 8 points out the problems that the Code's absence of provision for proxy consent caused for later international codes such as the Declaration of Helsinki.) Point 2 of the memorandum is concerned with the nature, motive, and purpose of experimentation. This point is subsumed in points 2 and 6 of the Code. Point 3 of the memorandum forbids experiments in which death or disabling injury might occur. This subject is covered in point 5 of the Code. It is interesting that the code qualifies this absolute prohibition by "those experiments where the experimental physicians also serve as subjects." Point 4 of the memorandum is concerned with proper facilities, qualified investigators, and the avoidance of unnecessary injury. These principles are covered in points 4, 7, and 8 of the Code. Point 5 of the memorandum is concerned with risk-benefit analysis. This principle is found in point 6 of the Code. Point 6 of the memorandum deals with the scientific merits and experimental design of research. This principle is covered in points 2 and 3 of the Code. Finally, the Code covers two principles that do not appear in the memorandum. These principles, covered in points 9 and 10 of the Code, are concerned with the interruption of the experiment at any time if either the subject or the scientist deems termination necessary.

Dr. Alexander, in a commentary on his own memorandum, notes:

> The judges enlarged these criteria to ten points by dividing my point No. 4 into three separate points, and by adding two provisions for prompt termination of an experiment at the discretion of the investigator or at the request of an experimental subject. These were incorporated in their final judgment as the basic principles which must be observed in order to satisfy moral, ethical and legal concepts with regard to medical experiments. However, they omitted from my original point No. 1 provisions for valid consent in the case of mentally sick subjects to be obtained from the next of kin and from the patient whenever possible, probably because they did not apply to the specific cases under trial.[58]

The closing arguments for the United States were delivered on July 14, 1947, by James McHaney, the chief prosecutor for the Medical Case. This final statement incorporates Alexander's memorandum and Ivy's testimony, foreshadowing the final text of the Code. The statement does not, however, focus on informed consent as a critical prerequisite. Prosecutor McHaney closes:

> It will be seen from this review of the indictment and from the evidence submitted by the prosecution that these defendants are, for the most part, on trial for the crime of murder. As in all criminal cases, two simple issues are presented: Were crimes committed and, if so, were these defendants connected with their commission in any of the ways specified by Law No. 10? It is only the fact that these crimes were committed in part as a result of medical experiments on human

beings that makes this case somewhat unique. And while considerable evidence of a technical nature has been submitted, one should not lose sight of the true simplicity of this case. The defendant Rose, who was permitted to cross-examine the prosecution's witness, Dr. A. C. Ivy of the Medical School of the University of Illinois, became exasperated at his reiteration of the basic principle *that human experimental subjects must be volunteers*, that, of course, is the cornerstone of this case. There are, indeed, other prerequisites to a permissible medical experiment on human beings. *The experiment must be based on the results of animal experimentation and a knowledge of the natural history of the disease under study and designed in such a way that the anticipated results will justify the performance of the experiment. This is to say that the experiment must be such as to yield results for the good of society unprocurable by other methods of study and must not be random and unnecessary in nature. Moreover, the experiment must be conducted by scientifically qualified persons in such a manner as to avoid all unnecessary physical and mental suffering and injury. If there is a priori reason to believe that death or disabling injury might occur, the experimenters must serve as subjects themselves, along with the nonscientific personnel. These are all important principles, and they were consistently violated by these defendants and their collaborators. For example, we have yet to find one defendant who subjected himself to the experiments which killed and tortured their victims in concentration camps. But important as these other considerations are, it is the most fundamental tenet of medical ethics and human decency that the subjects volunteer for the experiment after being informed of its nature and hazards. This is the clear dividing line between the criminal and what may be noncriminal. If the experimental subjects cannot be said to have volunteered, then the inquiry need proceed no further. Such is the simplicity of this case.*[59]

The final judgment was delivered after the conclusion of the trial on July 19, 1947, by Judge Beals. Although Judge Beals was the presiding judge, the chief prosecutor, Brigadier General Telford Taylor, noted that "the moving spirit on legal and evidentiary problems on the court was Judge Harold Siebring." Taylor also believed that the "10 point code was primarily his work."[60] Of the 23 physicians on trial, 16 were convicted of war crimes and crimes against humanity and 7 were condemned to death. The judgment reviews the evidence of criminal action and, in the final section, addresses the question of the permissibility of medical experimentation and enumerates the 10 principles later to be known as the Nuremberg Code. (Page 2 of this volume contains the final form of the Nuremberg Code.)

CONCLUSIONS

It is impossible to analyze the origins of the Nuremberg Code apart from the historical setting of the atrocities and murders committed in Nazi Germany. It is not surprising that, in the context of a criminal judgment, the judges found the need to go beyond the guilty verdict and to speak to the broader norms of medical ethics. The Nuremberg Code is an attempt to provide a natural law based universal set of ethical principles.

The Code was written in direct response to the criminal human experimentation detailed during the Medical Trial. As such, the Code specifically addresses the scope and limits of acceptable, nontherapeutic human experimentation conducted on adult prisoners. Because of the unique characteristics of such a competent yet confined population, the Code is particularly concerned with elements of coercion and duress. Informed consent becomes a fundamental method for ensuring the protection of this special population. The ethical limits of human experimentation on an incarcerated adult population probably remain the same today. The United States federal regulations, however, have added the further restriction that prisoners, because of their particular vulnerability, should be used only if the study cannot be carried out scientifically on a nonprison population. This restriction essentially limits experimentation on prisoners to the study of problems found uniquely in prisoners and can thus be achieved only in the prison setting. Consent remains the hallmark of protection in this population.

It is not known if the judges at Nuremberg actually held the defendant physicians accountable to the standards articulated in the Nuremberg Code. Because the defendants were adjudicated as guilty of murder and crimes against humanity, the subtler stipulations for ethical human experimentation did not need to be invoked. If the judges had held the Nazi physicians to the standards enumerated in the Code, however, it would have been necessary to condemn many other physicians and scientists throughout the world for violations of the ethical limits of human experimentation.

The evidence of widespread, ethically suspect medical research in countries other than Germany must have been most disturbing to the judges at Nuremberg. Throughout the trial, the debate surrounding the historical and existing standards of medical ethics surfaced. The judges soon realized that while there was a significant number of codes and regulations dealing with the standards of human experimentation prior to the Tribunal, there was also significant disparity among them. The Nuremberg Code embodies many of the principles enumerated in the 1931 Reich Circular Guidelines. Despite the existence of these Guidelines, the Nazi physicians were either unaware of their existence or their force of law, or simply chose to disregard them. Whether the status of any of the prewar standards was embodied in medical ethics, statutory, or administrative law, all of these codes were violated. It is possible that the judges at Nuremberg incorporated the Nuremberg Code as part of their legal judgment to ensure its place in common law. It was their hope and vision that, once established in international criminal law, this Code would be widely disseminated and, if followed, would guard against future atrocities. Furthermore, while punishment for violation of ethical codes and principles might be unclear, punishment for violation of international law would have clarity and force. (See chapter 10 for a discussion of the use of the Nuremberg Code in U.S. common law and Chapter 11 for a discussion of the Nuremberg Code in international law.)

If the Nuremberg Code was to be viewed solely as just another ethical framework to guide human experimentation, it would have no greater force than the earlier ethical codes. The Code, as an ethical document, would take its historical place as yet another new code created in response to violations and abuses of medical researchers. Once the Code was established in law, however, it might serve to enforce ethical standards by holding researchers accountable.

As medical research and human experimentation since World War II have become increasingly sophisticated, the specific application of the Nuremberg Code has become problematic. (See Chapter 16 for an overview of modern medical research.) Most modern research is therapeutic, involving either competent or incompetent patients as subjects. Even during the Nuremberg trial, however, it was hoped that the ethos and spirit of this international tribunal would establish a universal sense of human experimentation ethics. The judges at the trial probably did not envision the use of the Code for this broader application, as the Nuremberg Tribunal focused solely on competent, unconsenting prisoners. Therefore, the judges had edited out of Leo Alexander's memorandum the recommendation to include incompetent patients and the provision for proxy consent. Alexander, however, clearly believed that the Code would have a broader audience:

> These ten points constitute what is now known as the Nuremberg Code, a useful guide setting the limits for experimental research on human beings. It is evident, of course, that the crimes to which this Code owes its formulation could not have occurred in any country in which the ordinary laws concerning murder, manslaughter, mayhem, assault, and battery had not been suspended in regard to all or certain groups of its citizens and inhabitants. This Code is also unlikely to prevent another dictatorial government from repeating the crimes of the National Socialist Government. Nevertheless, it is a useful measure by which to prevent in less blatant settings the consequences of more subtle degrees of contempt for the rights and dignity of certain classes of human beings, such as mental defectives, people presumably dying from incurable illnesses, and people otherwise disenfranchised, such as prisoners or other inarticulate public charges whose rights might be easily disregarded for the apparently compelling reason of an urgent purpose.[61]

The Nuremberg Code articulates a set of principles that must be considered in any ethical use of humans as experimental subjects. These principles set the framework for United States federal regulations as well as the international guidelines. The concerns outlined in the Nuremberg Code include the research setting, the integrity of the investigator, the specifics of voluntary informed consent, the balancing of risks and benefits, and the unique problems of special vulnerable populations.

The exact origin of the Nuremberg Code will probably remain a historical mystery. It appears to have been derived from multiple sources, including the writings of Percival, Beaumont, and Bernard. Early German guidelines on human experimentation were also considered by the framers. Andrew Ivy and Leo Alexander were the primary compilers, who together formulated the points that Alexander ultimately cited in his memorandum to the judges. The judges, in turn, incorporated much, but not all, of the memorandum, added some points of their own, and formalized the final Nuremberg Code in their judgment. The legal judgment delivered at the Nuremberg trial went beyond the simple charges and convictions for war crimes and crimes against humanity. Medical ethics would be forever changed after the Holocaust. The Nuremberg Tribunal attempted to pave the way for a reconstituted moral vision. The source of that vision need not lie solely in a legal framework derived from the criminal law. The Nuremberg Code is prefaced by the judges' statement:

> *All agree*, however, that certain basic principles must be observed in order to satisfy moral, ethical and legal concepts.[62]

It is this vision that makes the Nuremberg Code the cornerstone of modern human experimentation ethics.

In 1949, in their official history of the Medical Trial, two German Medical Commission observers, Mitscherlich and Mielke, quoted the chief U.S. prosecutor, Telford Taylor. General Taylor's statement remains a challenge for those who are interested in the Nuremberg Code, its origin, its source, and its present standing:

> The tribunal judgment will be of profound and enduring value in the field of medical jurisprudence; and the trial as a whole is an epochal step in the evolution of forensic medicine. The trial illustrates, furthermore, how rapidly the focus of activity in international law has moved from the academic lecture hall and toward the courtroom. The Nuremberg proceedings are among the outstanding examples of modern international law in action.[63]

N O T E S

1. *Trials of War Criminals Before the Nuremberg Military Tribunals Under Control Council Law 10* (Washington, D.C.: Superintendent of Documents, U.S. Government Printing Office, 1950). *Military Tribunal 1, Case 1, United States v. Karl Brandt et al.*, October 1946–April 1949, Vol. I, pp. 1–1004; Vol. II, pp. 1–352 (1949).

2. Ibid., *Military Tribunal*, Vol. II, Section VIII, I, Medical Ethics, pp. 70–93.

3. Andrew Conway Ivy, M.D., Ph.D., was a professor of physiology and pharmacology. From 1946 to 1953, Dr. Ivy was vice president of the University of Illinois in charge of the Chicago Professional Colleges. He was a consultant to the U.S. Secretary of War and the U.S. Chief Counsel for War Crimes of the Nuremberg Tribunal at the request of the American Medical Association. Leo Alexander, M.D., was a professor of psychiatry and neurology and a colonel, U.S. Army Reserves. Dr. Alexander served as a consultant to the U.S. Secretary of War and the U.S. Chief Counsel for War Crimes during the Doctors' Trial, and he examined many of the survivors of the Nazi medical experiments.

4. See A. C. Ivy, "The History and Ethics of the Use of Human Subjects in Medical Experiments," *Science* 108 (1948): 1–5; L. Alexander, "Ethics of Human Experimentation," *Psychiatric Journal of the University of Ottawa* 1 (1976): 40–46;

L. Alexander, "Limitations in Experimental Research on Human Beings," *Lex et Scientia* 3 (1966): 8–24.

5. *Military Tribunal*, Vol. II, Direct Examination; Trial transcript, pp. 9029–9324; Ivy, "History and Ethics."

6. Alexander, "Ethics of Human Experimentation," 41. Dr. Alexander cites the Hippocratic oath in a section entitled "Medical-Ethical (Hippocratic) Requirements." This paper was written to republish his original memoranda to the U.S. Chief of Counsel for War Crimes at Nuremberg in December 1946.

7. See P. Carrick, *Medical Ethics in Antiquity* (Hingham, Mass.: D. Reidel/ Klüwer, 1985); pp. 69–94, for a discussion of the Hippocratic tradition. The Hippocratic oath is reprinted in O. Temkin and C. Temkin, eds., *Ancient Medicine: Selected Papers of Ludwig Edelstein* (Baltimore: Johns Hopkins University Press, 1967).

8. Ibid.

9. There is a certain irony in even discussing the Hippocratic tradition in the context of Nazi medical experimentation. The Jews of Cos, the city in Crete where Hippocrates was born and where he taught his beliefs on medicine, were assembled in 1944, perhaps at the very site where Hippocrates had once sat, and shipped to the Auschwitz and Buchenwald concentration camps. They arrived at the train station in Germany in 1944 and were divided into groups to be killed and others to be interned for concentration camp work. It was the very heirs of Hippocrates, Nazi *physicians*, who made those selections. Many of these same physicians probably took the Hippocratic oath on graduation from medical school. This poignant irony was pointed out by Prof. William Seidelman of McMaster University, Ontario, Canada, in his unpublished manuscript "An Inquiry Into the Spiritual Death of Dr. Hippocrates."

10. For a complete discussion of the historical aspects of human experimentation, see N. Howard-Jones, "Human Experimentation in Historical and Ethical Perspectives," in *Human Experimentation and Medical Ethics*, F. Bankowski and N. Howard-Jones, eds., (Geneva: XVth CIOMS Council for International Organization of Medical Sciences Round Table Conference, 1982), pp. 453–495.

11. Ibid.; see also C. Bernard, *Principes de la medecine experimentale* (Paris: Presses Universitaires de France, 1947), and John Scarborough, "Celsus on Human Vivisection at Ptolemaic, Alexandria," *Clio Medica* 11 (1976): 25–38.

12. James Johnston, *Abraham Lettson, His Life, Times, Friends and Descendants* (London: Heinemann, 1933), pp. 186–188.

13. E. Jenner, *An Inquiry Into the Cause and Effects of the Variolae Vaccine.* (London: S. Low, 1789).

14. See H. Beecher, *Research and the Individual Human Subject* (Boston: Little, Brown, 1970), pp. 219–225, for a discussion of the American Medical Association codes of 1846, 1847, 1946, 1949, 1958, 1966, and 1967. Also see the *Archives of the American Medical Association Proceedings* of the National Medical Conventions held in New York in May 1846 and in Philadelphia in May 1847, printed for the American Medical Association by T. K. and D. G. Collins Printers, Philadelphia (1847). The first American Medical Association code to deal specifically with human experimentation was promulgated in 1946.

15. Percival's code is cited in Beecher, *Research*, p. 218 (emphasis added). Also see S. Reiser, A. Dyck, and W. Curran, eds., *Ethics in Medicine: Historical Perspectives and Contemporary Concerns* (Cambridge, Mass.: Massachusetts Institute of Technology Press, 1977), pp. 18–25, and T. Percival, *Medical Ethics*, 3rd ed. (Oxford: John Henry Parker, 1949), pp. 27–68.

16. See Beecher, *Research*, pp. 219–220. Also see K. Wiggers, "Human Experimentation as Exemplified by the Career of Dr. William Beaumont," *Alumni Bulletin*, School of Medicine and Affiliated Hospitals, Western Reserve University (September 1950), pp. 60–65, where other authors and scientists have noted that "the ethical principles . . . of William Beaumont gradually grew into an unwritten code consonant with the moral dictates and laws of all civilized countries." Also see R. Numbers, "William Beaumont and the Ethics of Human Experimentation," *Journal of the History of Biology* 12 (1979): 113–135, which questions Beaumont as the source for the ethics of human experimentation in the United States as well as the ethics of Beaumont's human experimentation with patient Alexis St. Martin.

17. The text of Beaumont's code as found in Beecher, *Research*, p. 219 (selections by the author).

18. See note 4.

19. See C. Bernard, *An Introduction to the Study of Experimental Medicine*, trans. Henry Copley (New York: Macmillan, 1927), pp. 101–102. The original volume was published in Paris in 1865 and was entitled *Introduction à l'Étude de la Médicine Expérimentale* (emphasis added).

20. See Howard-Jones, "Human Experimentation," p. 458.

21. See Alexander, "Limitations in Experimental Research with Human Beings," 15.

22. See *Pratt v. Davis*, 79 NE 562 (1906); Consent as Condition of Right to Perform Surgical Operations; *American Law Reports* 76 (1942): 562–571; E. H. Smith, "Antecedent Grounds of Liability in the Practice of Surgery," *Rocky Mountain Law Review* 14 (1942): 233–293; and W. R. Arthur, "Some Liability of Physicians in the Use of Drugs," *Rocky Mountain Law Review* 17 (1945): 131–162.

23. L. Ebermayer, *Der Arzt in Recht* (Leipzig: Georg Thieme, 1930), pp. 1–287. As cited in 4 Alexander, "Limitations in Experimental Research with Human Beings."

24. *Centralblatt der gesamten Unterrichtsverwaltung in Preussen* pp. 188–189 (1901). This informal translation was prepared by the Health Legislation Unit of the World Health Organization.

25. See B. Elkeles, "Medizinishe Menschenversuche gegen Ende des 19. Jahrhunderte und der Fall Neisser," *Medizin Historisches Journal* 20 (1985): 135–148.

26. An extensive discussion regarding public concern about human experimentation in prewar Germany is found in Howard-Jones, "Human Experimentation," pp. 470–473.

27. See A. Stader, *Die Zülassigkeit ärtzlieber Versuche an gesunden und Kranken Menschen Münchener Medizinische Wochenschrift* 78 (1931): 107–112, as it appears in Howard-Jones, "Human Experimentation."

28. See F. Müller, *Die Zülassigkeit ärtzlicher Versuche an gesunden und Kranken Menschen Münschner Medizinische Wochenschrift* 78 (1931): 104–107, as cited and discussed in Howard-Jones, "Human Experimentation," pp. 471–472.

29. See Howard-Jones, "Human Experimentation," p. 472.

30. See further discussion in C. Pross and A. Götz, eds., *Der Wert des Menschen-Medizin in Deutschland 1918–1945* (Berlin: Hentrich, 1989), pp. 92–93. I would like to thank Professor Ezraim Kohack, Boston University Department of Philosophy, for translation of this German document. Dr. Moses perceptively warned in 1932: "Thus in the name of the National Socialist 'Third Reich Empire,' a medical doctor would have the following mission, in order to create a 'new noble humanity': only those who can recover would be healed. The sick who cannot recover, however, are dead weight existences, human refuse, unworthy of living and unproductive. They

must be destroyed and eliminated. So in a word, the physician would become an executioner!"

31. See *Military Tribunal*, Vol. II, p. 83.

32. See Trial Transcript testimony and cross examination of Dr. Andrew Ivy, June 13, 1947, pp. 9141–9145 and 9170–9171.

33. Personal communication, Mr. Sev Fluss, chief of the Health Legislation Unit of the World Health Organization.

34. See S. Fluss, "The Proposed Guidelines as Reflected in Legislation and Codes of Ethics," in Seidelman, "An Inquiry," where Fluss states that the 1931 guidelines "appear to have remained in force until 1945." Also see F. Fischer and H. Breuer, German Research Society, Federal Republic of Germany, "Influence of Ethical Guidance Committees on Medical Research. A Critical Appraisal," in *Medical Experiments and the Protection of Human Rights* (Geneva: XIIth CIOMS Round Table, 1989), which states that the 1931 guidelines were "valid up to 1945." Also see H. Sass, "Reichsrundschreiben 1931: Pre-Nuremberg German Regulation Concerning New Therapy and Human Experimentation," *Journal of Medicine and Philosophy* 8 (1983): 99–111. Sass states that the guidelines "remained binding in Germany even during the period of the Third Reich."

35. See Howard-Jones, "Human Experimentation," which notes that "These guidelines were recommendations not having legal force."

36. *Reichsgesundheitblatt* 11, No. 10, (March 1931), 174–175. This is believed to be the first English translation of the 1931 regulations. Published in the *International Digest of Health Legislation* 31 (1980): 408–411.

37. See *Military Tribunal*, Vol. I, p. 71. It is of interest that Hitler himself was a vegetarian.

38. A parallel irony existed in the United States, where the first laws for the prevention of cruelty to children were enacted only after the Society for the Prevention of Cruelty to Animals had succeeded in securing the protection of animals by law. The first case brought on behalf of a child, on April 19, 1874, stated explicitly that the child, being an animal, should be protected. This led to legislation for the protection of children. The American Society for the Prevention of Cruelty to Children was organized in December 1874. See T. Cone, *History of American Pediatrics* (Boston: Little, Brown, 1979), p. 100.

39. See *Military Tribunal*, Vol. II, pp. 1–9.

40. See *Military Tribunal*, Vol. I, pp. 983–987; Vol. II, pp. 90–93. For a defense of the ethically appropriate use of prisoners for medical research see R. Strong, "The Service of Prisoners," *Journal of the American Medical Association* 136 (1948): 457. Also see M. H. Pappworth, *Human Guinea Pigs: Experimentation on Man* (Boston: Beacon Press, 1967), pp. 61–63. Also see *"Ethics Governing the Service of Prisoners as Subjects in Medical Experiments*, Report of a Committee Appointed by Governor Dwight H. Greene of Illinois," *Journal of the American Medical Association* 136 (1948): 457–458.

41. See *Military Tribunal*, Vol. II, pp. 9–12.

42. See *Military Tribunal*, Vol. I, pp. 983–984; Transcript, p. 2567.

43. See *Military Tribunal*, Vol. I, pp. 989–992.

44. See *Military Tribunal*, Vol. II, pp. 10–16.

45. See *Military Tribunal*, Vol. I, pp. 991; Vol. II, pp. 72–73, 94–110, 149.

46. There is no evidence that any physician was executed for refusing to participate in Nazi human experimentation. Many unskilled technicians were directly involved in performing human experiments.

47. This "only following orders" claim is a variation on the "Fuerher defense" used by many of the military defendants during the military trials at Nuremberg. See *Military Tribunal*, Vol. I, pp. 980–982; Vol. II, pp. 5–10, 29–30, 50; Transcript, pp. 2566–2571.

48. For this utilitarian argument, see *Military Tribunal*, Vol. I, pp. 64–66, 74–77.

49. See *Military Tribunal*, Vol. II, pp. 53–56.

50. See *Military Tribunal*, Vol. II, pp. 61–70; Transcript, p. 11186.

51. See Dr. Ivy's testimony of June 13, 1947, in Transcript, pp. 9141–9145, 9168; *Military Tribunal*, Vol. II, pp. 82–86.

52. *Journal of the American Medical Association* 132 (1946): 1090 (emphasis added).

53. W. Curran, "Subject Consent Requirement in Clinical Research: An International Perspective for Industrial and Developing Nations," in Seidelman, "An Inquiry," pp. 35–79. Curran is the Francis Glessner Lee Professor of Health Law at Harvard University's School of Public Health.

54. E. Deutsch, "Die Zehn Punkte des Nürnberger Ärzteprozesses Über die Klinische Forshung am Menschen: der sog. Nürnberger Codex," *Festschrift für Wasserman*, trans. by Jennifer Cizick and Deborah Banford of Boston University. (1985), pp. 69–79. Professor Dr. Erwin Deutsch is the director of the Abteilung für Internationales und Auslandisches Privatrecht Juristisches Seminar of Göttingen University.

55. See Alexander, "Limitations on Experimental Research with Human Beings," and Alexander, "Ethics of Human Experimentation." Also see F. Bayle, *Croix Gammée Contre Caducée: Les Expériences Humaines en Allemange pendant la deuxième guerre mondiale* (Berlin and Neustadt: Palatinat, 1950), I–XXCII, pp. 1430–1432.

56. See *Die Zehn Punkte*, where Professor Deutsch claims that no published proof exists that any counsel for the defense knew of or utilized this memorandum.

57. See note 55, where the memorandum is reproduced.

58. See note 54 and Alexander, "Limitations in Experimental Research on Human Beings," pp. 15–16.

59. See *Trials of War Criminals*, Closing Argument for the United States of America by James M. McHaney, July 14, 1947, transcript pp. 10718–10796 (emphasis added).

60. Personal communication in letter dated March 6, 1989, signed by Telford Taylor.

61. See L. Alexander, "Limitations of Experimentation on Human Beings with Special Reference to Psychiatric Patients," *Diseases of the Nervous System* 27 (1966): 61–65, at 62.

62. See *Military Tribunal*, Vol. II, pp. 181–185 (emphasis added).

63. A Mitscherlich and F. Mielk, *Doctors of Infamy* (New York: Henry Schuman, 1949), p. XXVI.

III

THE ROLE OF CODES IN INTERNATIONAL AND U.S. LAW

This part of the book explores the legal aspects of the Nuremberg Code. Two basic perspectives are developed. First, the Code is viewed in its international context, with the aim of understanding both its position as a statement of international law and its influence on international law and human rights. Second, the Code is viewed from the perspective of the United States. The U.S. perspective is used for two basic reasons: the Code was promulgated by U.S. judges, and the United States does more human experimentation than any other country in the world.

This part opens with an exploration of the uses of the Nuremberg Code in international law by four coauthors at the World Health Organization. In Chapter 8, they make a powerful case for the proposition that although the Declaration of Helsinki has surpassed the Code as a primary statement of research ethics, and although peer review has eclipsed informed consent as a *sine qua non* of ethical research throughout the world, the Nuremberg Code remains the foundational document, and retreat from it can come only at the expense of the experimental subject's human rights.

In Chapter 9, Robert Drinan, law professor and former U.S. congressman, distinguishes the Nuremberg Code from the Nuremberg Principles, which were developed at the International War Crimes Trial at Nuremberg, the only trial that involved the British, French, and Russians, as well as the Americans as judges and the one that immediately preceded the Doctors' Trial. Drinan makes it clear that although the Nuremberg Principles have become part of international law, the Nuremberg Code itself has no such independent status. He also makes an eloquent plea for a "World Nuremberg," an international tribunal that could actually hear cases of individuals accused of crimes against humanity. Such a tribunal is also, of course, required if the Nuremberg Code itself is to be more than simply a code of ethics.

In Chapter 10, attorney Leonard Glantz explores how the Nuremberg Code has been used as a basis for federal regulations and state statutes regulating human experimentation. The Code is widely cited as the source for most of these documents, but exceptions for therapeutic experimentation and for minimal-risk experimentation are the rule. On the other hand, the Code has had a profound effect on the regulation of research on prisoners and on fetuses. Almost no prisoner research is currently done in the United States because of its inherently coercive nature, and many states have criminalized research on human fetuses because of their inability to give consent and the absence of a caring person to speak on their behalf.

Finally, in Chapter 11, George Annas traces the ways in which the Nuremberg Code has (and has not) been used in U.S. courts since World War II. Throughout this period the Code has seldom been cited, and when it has, it is often in the context of dissenting opinions. It has never been used as the basis for awarding monetary damages to a victim of human experimentation and has never been used as a basis for a criminal charge in the United States. In short, the Nuremberg Code remains more a statement of ethics than of law in the United States.

8

The Nuremberg Code:
An International Overview

SHARON PERLEY
SEV S. FLUSS
ZBIGNIEW BANKOWSKI
FRANÇOISE SIMON

> If any single negative image is associated with [human experimentation] in the minds of most people, it is the experiments carried out on unconsenting prisoners in the Nazi death camps during World War II; and if any single document is taken as central to the process of asserting legal control over research on human beings, it is the judgment rendered by the tribunal of the Nazi camp physicians after the war.[1]

The Nuremberg Code has often been cited as one of the leading influences on the subsequent development of international and national codes governing the ethical aspects of research involving human subjects.[2] Indeed, the *Encyclopedia of Bioethics*, in the appendices presenting "Directives for Human Experimentation," starts with the Nuremberg Code, as do most compilations of codes of conduct in this area.[3] Many regulations or guidelines governing human experimentation refer to the Nuremberg Code as one of their sources. Countless articles and books written about the ethics of biomedical research note the Code's importance in the development of the field.

And yet, some critics have argued that current codes or regulations for the protection of human subjects of medical research would not have been any different had the Nuremberg Doctors' Trial (*United States v. Karl Brandt et al.*) never taken place.[4] They argue that professional codes, such as the successive versions of the World Medical Association's Declaration of Helsinki, and legislative and regulatory actions, such as the revision of the drug-testing regulations of the U.S. Food and Drug Administration in response to the thalidomide tragedy, have had a much greater impact on the development of research ethics. It has been asserted that, at most, the Nuremberg Code provides a starting point for an examination of the ethical issues related to biomedical research on human subjects. For all intents and purposes, however, the Code, in their view, is a historical document created in response to the atrocities committed during the Nazi era, a document that has little to do with the current field of human experimentation.[5]

This chapter disputes that argument. As there appears to be a significant gap in the literature regarding the actual relationship between the Nuremberg Code and the development of international codes and regulations, we shall document this relationship and demonstrate that, more than being merely a catalyst for discussion, the Nuremberg Code has been influential in the development of such texts. Moreover, we shall demonstrate that, even though the Declaration of Helsinki, as amended, has for the most part technically superseded the Nuremberg Code, the latter remains a viable force, influencing the regulation of human experimentation more than 40 years after its promulgation.[6]

A HISTORICAL PERSPECTIVE

It is sometimes asserted that the Nuremberg Code was the first code to establish ethical standards for human experimentation.[7] While it is almost certainly the first *international* code, the 10 principles enumerated by the Nuremberg Tribunal have many antecedents. Celsus, practicing in Alexandria in the third century BCE, spoke out against the dissection of living persons, and the Hippocratic oath has been viewed as giving implicit advice on experimental diagnosis and therapy.[8] As early as 1830, English law was interpreted as providing that the physician had to obtain the informed consent of the research subject when conducting therapeutic experiments; otherwise, the physician would be obliged to provide compensation for any injury that might arise from adopting a new method of treatment.[9] In 1865, Claude Bernard stated that the "'principle of medical and surgical morality' was never to perform on a human subject an experiment whose outcome could only be harmful in some degree, even though the result could be very interesting scientifically, and therefore of interest for the health of others."[10]

The first known regulatory action relating specifically to the field of human experimentation was promulgated at the turn of this century. In December 1900, the Prussian Minister of Religious, Educational, and Medical Affairs issued a directive establishing basic criteria for medical interventions other than for diagnostic, therapeutic, or prophylactic purposes.[11] This directive provided that such interventions should not be performed on minors, on persons incompetent for other reasons, or on other persons unless they had given their unequivocal consent in the knowledge of any possible detrimental consequences. Further, such interventions could be carried out only by the heads of clinics or other medical institutions.[12] An

English translation of this directive appears on p. 127. (As far as the authors are aware, it has never previously been published in English.)

The issue of informed consent was examined in greater detail in the writings of Paul Ehrlich 10 years after the Prussian directive was issued. Ehrlich compared the duty of the experimental "pharmacotherapist" to that of the surgeon, arguing that just as a surgeon must inform his patient fully of the statistical risks of an operation compared to those of nonintervention, the pharmacotherapist must tell his patient what possibilities of risk exist and how frequently they occur.[13]

However, the most significant instrument promulgated prior to the Nuremberg Code was undoubtedly the Circular of February 28, 1931, of the (German) Reich Minister of the Interior.[14] The "Guidelines on Innovative Therapy and Scientific Experimentation" established by this Circular resulted from an ongoing polemic between the German press and the medical profession regarding the ethics of human experimentation (for a translation, see pp. 130–131).[15] It is interesting, and rather ironic, to note that there appears to have been no parallel for such concern, or for governmental action, in any other country[16] (and yet, the ethics of animal experimentation were the subject of animated debate in the British Parliament prior to the enactment of the Cruelty to Animals Act of 1876).

The 1931 Guidelines have been described as being "clearer, more concrete, and more far-reaching than both the Nuremberg Code and the [Declaration of Helsinki] recommendations."[17] In the words of a preeminent historian of human experimentation, Norman Howard-Jones:

> [The Guidelines provided that] the planning and execution of new treatments must be compatible with medical ethics and the rule of the art and science of medicine. Risks should be carefully weighed against expected benefits, and the treatment should previously have been tested by animal experiments. New treatments should not be undertaken without the patient's consent after receiving an unequivocal explanation, except in life-threatening situations where it was impossible to obtain the patient's consent. . . . In all institutions for the care of the sick, new treatments should be carried out only by the chief physician, or with his express authorization and under his full responsibility. . . .[18]

Indeed, these Guidelines greatly resemble present-day codes and regulations. However, as Hans-Martin Sass has noted, "the fact that such a governmental regulation actually existed, at a time when the Nazis were carrying out human experiments in an irresponsible manner in concentration camps, underlines the irrelevance of legal regulations if they are not enforced by the authorities."[19]

DEVELOPMENT OF THE NUREMBERG CODE

As has been amply documented elsewhere in this book, the Nuremberg Code was enumerated as part of the judgment against Karl Brandt and his co-defendants. The Code was based on the testimony of two U.S. physicians, Drs. Leo Alexander and Andrew Ivy, who served as expert medical witnesses for the prosecution. Indeed, "the Code was not the outcome of an attempt to frame new principles of medical ethics, but rather a formulation, in the course of a trial for war crimes, of criteria said to be widely accepted by the medical procession against which the acts of certain physicians carried out on prisoners might be judged."[20]

Some have argued that the Code is, in essence, a natural-law document in the sense that it is derived from "the principles of the law of nations as they result from the usages established among civilized peoples, from the laws of humanity, and from the dictates of public conscience."[21]

However, the principles are also based on customary law, for the U.S. physicians' testimony represented what they perceived to be common principles of practice and understanding. Ivy argued that "these experiments were all performed contrary to the ethics under which legitimate human experimentation is performed and has been performed throughout the world even in Germany before and during the war."[22] Indeed, Alexander relied in part on the prewar German standards when he testified at the trial.[23]

Ivy's testimony is often cited as providing the actual framework for the Nuremberg Code.[24] During his testimony, he articulated three principles that, if human experimentation is to be justified, must be followed, as they are designed to protect the rights and welfare of the research subject. First, the freely informed consent of the subject must be obtained. All subjects must be volunteers, in the absence of coercion of any form. The subjects must be informed of any risks. Second, the experiment must be designed and based on the results of animal experimentation and on the knowledge of the natural history of the disease. Moreover, the experiment must be such as to yield the results for the good of society, unprocurable by other methods of study, and must not be random and unnecessary in nature. Finally, the experiment must be conducted only by scientifically qualified persons.[25]

These are the principles by which the Nazi physicians in this trial were judged, and which they were found to have violated. In the judgment, the principles were expanded into 10 principles—which have now become known as the Nuremberg Code. The actual text of the Code has been discussed in other chapters and can be found on page 2 of this book. For the purposes of this chapter, it is important to note that the principles enumerated in the Nuremberg Code have been embodied in many, if not all, subsequent ethical codes governing biomedical research involving the use of human subjects.

EARLY INFLUENCE OF THE NUREMBERG CODE

Thus, while the Nuremberg Code had historical antecedents, their impact was clearly circumscribed. The Code raised the consciousness of the global community; it succeeded in bringing the issue of human experimentation to the forefront of public debate. A series of international documents were thereafter created whose genesis can be traced to the Nuremberg Code.

Perhaps one of the most significant documents influenced by the Nuremberg Code is the International Covenant on Civil and Political Rights.[26] Article 7 of this Covenant provides that "No one shall be subjected to torture or to cruel, inhuman, or degrading treatment or punishment. In particular, no one shall be subjected without his free consent to medical or scientific experimentation." Though the Covenant was not adopted by the United Nations General Assembly until 1966 and did not take legal effect until 1976, its origins date back to 1947 and the earliest sessions of the United Nations Commission on Human Rights.[27]

The first reference to human experimentation can be found in the Proposals Submitted by the United Kingdom Representative on the Drafting Commission for the International Bill of Human Rights. Proposal 1 stated that no person shall be subjected to, *inter alia*, "any form of physical mutilation or medical or scientific experimentation against his will."[28] It must be noted that these proposals were submitted on June 18, 1947, two months before the judgment in the Nuremberg Medical Trial was issued. However, as the trial commenced on December 8, 1946,[29] one may well assume that representatives from the United Kingdom had heard Ivy's testimony and were greatly influenced by it.

Similarly, on May 6, 1948, after the promulgation of the Nuremberg Code, the French government submitted a Draft Declaration on Human Rights to the Commission, which stated in Article V that "It shall be unlawful to subject any person to any form of physical mutilation or medical or scientific experimentation against his will."[30] In 1949, when the proposed article regarding human experimentation was discussed, the Israeli delegate recalled that "it was mainly on account of the Nazi activities that the need had been felt for the conclusion of a Covenant ensuring the enforcement of human rights."[31] During the sixth session of the Commission, chaired by Eleanor Roosevelt, in 1950, it was pointed out that the article (by this time, Article 7 of the Draft International Covenant on Human Rights) had been introduced so as to prevent any return of the abuses and atrocities committed in Germany during the war."[32] And in 1952, the words "against his will" were replaced by "without his free consent," words that are more consistent with those found in principle 1 of the Nuremberg Code.[33]

Another international document in which the Nuremberg Code's influence can be discerned is the four Geneva Conventions of August 12, 1949.[34] The main thrust of these Conventions is to "establish a humanitarian law of armed conflict which aims at protection of noncombatant military personnel and civilians not involved in the hostilities."[35] In doing so, the Conventions provide the basic protection against unlawful human experimentation during wartime. Thus, Article 12 of both the First and Second Conventions provides that members of the armed forces and other persons (as specified) shall, *inter alia*, "not be subjected to biological experiments." Article 13 of the Third Convention provides that "no prisoner of war may be subjected to physical mutilation or to medical or scientific experiments of any kind which are not justified by the medical, dental or hospital treatment of the prisoner concerned and carried out in his interest." Finally, Article 32 of the

Fourth Convention prohibits medical or scientific experiments not necessitated by the medical treatment of a protected person. As the commentary to the Conventions explains:

> By prohibiting the carrying out of biological experiments on persons who are wounded or ill, the intent was to prohibit forever the criminal practices of which certain prisoners had been victims. In addition, the intent was to avoid the possibility of captive wounded or ill persons from serving as "guinea-pigs" in medical experimentation.[36]

Finally, the early influence of the Nuremberg Code can be seen in the activities of the World Medical Association (WMA), which was founded in 1947, soon after the Code was promulgated. In light of the Code and the horrors that had been revealed at the Medical Trial, the founding physicians determined that professional ethical codes and guidelines were urgently needed.[37] This is perhaps best seen by examining statements published in the first issue of the WMA's journal, then known as the *World Medical Association Bulletin*.

An article entitled "The Dedication of the Physician" asserted that "among the most important of the actions taken by the WMA in its assembly in Geneva in September 1948 was the adoption of a form of dedication by the physician to his profession of medicine."[38] This dedication has become known as the Declaration of Geneva, a modern restatement of the Hippocratic oath.

The General Assembly adopted a statement entitled "War Crimes and Medicine: The German Betrayal and a Restatement of the Ethics of Medicine." It explains that "The first meeting of the General Assembly was held in September, 1947, soon after the passing of judgment by the International Military Tribunal sitting at Nuremberg, on 23 Nazi doctors found guilty, as German major war criminals, of horrible crimes against human beings, many of them committed in the name of medical science."[39] The statement condemns the crimes committed by the German medical practitioners and then "endorses the judicial punishment of such crimes." It concludes that "in view of the recent war crimes and the continued troubled state of the world," the recital of the Declaration of Geneva by every newly qualified doctor should have a beneficial effect on his attitude toward medical practice and its obligations.[40]

It is important to note that the Declaration of Geneva was published, for the first time, as part of this statement. Thus, while there is no reference to human experimentation per se, one can argue that the Declaration is based, at least in part, on the Nuremberg Code. Indeed, this interpretation is supported by the current Executive Director of the WMA.[41] Furthermore, a WMA report issued in 1954 on human experimentation noted that the principles from which those involved in biomedical research must not deviate are condensed in the Declaration of Geneva.[42]

A year later, the WMA's General Assembly adopted the International

Code of Medical Ethics. This Code provides, *inter alia*, that "A physician shall act only in the patient's interest when providing medical care which might have the effect of weakening the physical and mental condition of the patient." Again, while there is no reference to human experimentation, one can discern the underlying principles of the Nuremberg Code restated in the WMA documents.

Finally, in 1953, the WMA began to consider the need for professional guidelines with respect to experiments on human beings.[43] While its 1954 Resolution on Human Experimentation goes further than the Nuremberg Code in establishing principles for biomedical research, the Code's influence can once again be seen.[44]

Thus, within the first 10 years of its promulgation, the Code influenced the development of codes and guidelines, both in the general field of medical ethics and, more specifically, in the field of human experimentation. The principles enumerated in the Nuremberg Code (informed consent, responsibility of the physician, welfare of the research subject, risk-benefit analysis) were adopted, interpreted, and applied on an international scale.

THE NUREMBERG CODE: AN IMPERFECT DOCUMENT

This is not to say, however, that the Code is faultless. Indeed, it has been criticized on a number of levels. Arguments have been put forth that suggest that "the Code, in an attempt to provide for all contingencies, unduly restricts the investigator by requiring him to anticipate and provide for every situation and by demanding the impossible in some instances."[45]

Perhaps the most important contribution of the Code is principle 1, which provides that consent must be voluntary, uncoerced, and informed. The notion of informed consent of human subjects in clinical medical investigations has received strong support in both international and national codes. In some respects, it has become the *sine qua non* for human experimentation.

And yet, this principle has also received the most criticism. It is phrased in absolute terms, stating that "voluntary consent . . . is absolutely essential."[46] By making the requirement absolute, the Code limits the populations upon which experimentation may be conducted. Indeed, the U.S. researcher Henry K. Beecher, as well as many others, have asserted that adherence to this provision would effectively curtail the study of mental illness and children's diseases, as neither population (the mentally ill or children) has the legal capacity to give consent.[47] Similarly, although the Code is especially applicable to people in captivity, it has been asserted that prisoners are never able to give actual voluntary consent, as they may be enticed by financial rewards, special treatment, and the hope of early release in exchange for good behavior.[48] Finally, it has been argued that there are other groups who may also be unable to provide truly voluntary consent; research assistants and charity patients in hospitals are two examples.[49]

The absolute requirement of the subject's consent was also challenged by the British biostatistician Sir Austin Bradford Hill. Hill questioned whether the consent of the patient-subject is always necessary for his inclusion in a controlled trial. Specifically, he questioned the necessity of informing patient-subjects when two equally beneficial treatments are being evaluated and the patient's response is important. Similarly, he challenged the requirement for informed consent with respect to placebo trials. Must a research subject be informed that he is receiving a placebo, or is informing him that he is part of a drug trial and may or may not receive a placebo sufficient?[50]

The word *informed* has also been criticized on two separate grounds. First, it is often impossible for the researcher to provide comprehensive information on every possible risk, for often these risks are unknown until the experiment is actually conducted.[51] Second, many of the procedures and drugs used in experiments are too technical for research subjects to understand, either as to the effects of the treatment or the risks involved.[52] Thus, Beecher suggested that the investigator should *strive to achieve* adequate understanding by the subject, even if this can rarely be fully accomplished.[53] "The principle [then] becomes a duty to disclose adequate information; not a duty to achieve full understanding in every subject."[54]

Other principles of the Code have been criticized as well. Principle 3, which concerns the justification for the experiment, has been questioned, for the investigator is not always able to guarantee success.[55] Principle 5 asserts that willingness of the experimenter to expose himself to serious and possibly fatal consequences may justify recourse to other human subjects, exposing them to serious and possibly fatal consequences as well. This principle has been almost universally rejected. As the 1964 U.S. National Conference on the Legal Environment of Medical Science's Committee on the Re-evaluation of the Nuremberg Experimental Principles found, "if an experiment is morally contraindicated, under basic human considerations, as wrong, the participation of the investigator would not morally rectify it."[56] Finally, principle 6 (the degree of risk must be weighed against the humanitarian importance of the problem) has been criticized as "presumptuously evaluating the ultimate significance of one's own research."[57]

The Code has also been criticized not merely with respect to what it includes, but also in regard to what it does not include. The Nuremberg Medical Tribunal attempted to create a "decalogue of universal principles to be adhered to by all ethical investigators throughout the world."[58] The Code, however, deals with investigations on healthy subjects, not sick people, and thus fails to differentiate between clinical research on healthy subjects for the advancement of scientific knowledge and clinical research with therapeutic objectives.

It has also been argued that by placing the burden of responsibilities on the individual initiating, directing, or engaging in the experiment, the Code provides no mechanism for review of the researcher's actions. It is assumed that the clinical investigator is capable of making all necessary ethical deliberations.[59]

Finally, the Code has been criticized merely because it has been ignored. Even after its promulgation, blatant breaches of the principles enumerated in the Code still occurred. One only has to recall the Tuskegee syphilis study (initiated in the 1920s but not terminated until the 1970s) or experiments conducted at the Jewish Chronic Disease Hospital in Brooklyn, New York. The writings of Beecher in the United States and of M. H. Pappworth in the United Kingdom further highlight the abuses committed by researchers conducting experiments on human subjects.[60] A set of "universal principles," with no legal or professional authority, is successful only if researchers choose to abide by them.

PROFESSIONAL GUIDELINES: THE DECLARATION OF HELSINKI

Far from being a perfect document, the Nuremberg Code thus highlighted the need for more extensive and comprehensive guidelines. In an article submitted to the March 1960 issue of the *World Medical Journal*, Beecher cited the adoption of the Nuremberg Code by the U.S. Public Health Service and then suggested that a general code by an international organization "might be developed which would serve the best interests of science and mankind in the realm of human experimentation."[61]

Indeed, the WMA's Committee on Medical Ethics had begun grappling with the issue of human experimentation in 1953. At that time, it was recognized that there was a need for *professional* guidelines designed by physicians for physicians (as opposed to the Nuremberg Code, which was formed by jurists for use in a legal trial). Moreover, it was recognized that experiments must be classified into two groups: "experiments in new diagnostic and therapeutic methods" and "experiments undertaken to serve other purposes than simply to cure an individual."[62]

In 1954, the 8th General Assembly of the WMA adopted a "Resolution on Human Experimentation: Principles for Those in Research and Experimentation." The Resolution contained five basic principles. In essence, it provided the following: (1) Experiments must always be conducted by qualified scientists who adhere to the general rules of respect for the individual. (2) The first results of medical experimentation must be published with prudence and discretion. (3) The researcher bears primary responsibility when conducting human experimentation. (4) In experimentation on healthy subjects, the researcher must take every step to obtain fully informed, free consent. In experimentation on ill subjects, the researcher must obtain the consent of the subject or his next of kin. The researcher must inform the subject or the person who is legally responsible for the subject of the nature of, the reason for, and the risks entailed by the proposed experiment. (5) Operations or treatment of a daring nature may be conducted only in desperate cases.[63]

Between 1954 and 1960, the Committee on Medical Ethics continued to study the issue. Indeed, the March 1960 issue of the *World Medical Journal* is devoted to the subject of human experimentation. In September 1961, the Committee submitted its provisional conclusions regarding a code of ethics for human experimentation to the WMA's 15th General Assembly.[64] The draft code went through a number of revisions and was finally adopted by the 18th World Medical Assembly in Helsinki in 1964.[65]

It must be noted that the words "Nuremberg Code" are nowhere mentioned in either the 1954 Resolution or any of the successive drafts of the Declaration of Helsinki. There appears to be no recorded explanation for this omission. However, the current Executive Director of the WMA affirms that the drafters of the Declaration *did* consult the text of the Code. Moreover, he recalls the Code's being discussed in meetings of the World Medical Assembly.[66]

Indeed, when one looks at the origins of earlier WMA Declarations (see the discussion above), the fact that the Nuremberg Code was mentioned in two of the articles in the March 1960 issue of the *World Medical Journal*, and the principles contained in the actual Declaration, one cannot help but conclude that the Declaration was greatly influenced by the Nuremberg Code. Although nowhere documented, this very conclusion has been reached by almost all commentators who have written about medical research ethics.

Like the Nuremberg Code, the 1964 Declaration of Helsinki (Helsinki I) requires that research on human subjects be based on laboratory and animal experiments or other scientifically established facts. Both documents require that research be conducted only by scientifically qualified persons. Similarly, both mandate that the foreseeable benefits of the research must be balanced against the inherent risks to the research subject. Both provide that at any time during the experiment, the research subject should be free to withdraw. Also, both provide that at any time during the experiment, the investigator should discontinue the research if, in his judgment, its continuation would be harmful to the subject. In the 1964 Declaration of Helsinki, these two principles apply only to nontherapeutic clinical research. Finally, both the Nuremberg Code and Helsinki I require that the researcher obtain informed consent.

Unlike the Nuremberg Code, however, Helsinki I provides that in cases where the research subject is legally or physically unable to provide consent, the consent of the legal guardian is sufficient. Indeed, the requirement of informed consent is much less stringently worded in Helsinki I than in the Nuremberg Code; it is not even listed as a basic principle. And yet, Helsinki I states that, as a rule, consent should be given in writing, a provision that does not appear in the Nuremberg Code.

Perhaps the greatest difference between the Nuremberg Code and Helsinki I is the Declaration's differentiation between "clinical research combined with professional care" and "nontherapeutic clinical research." The Declaration thus recognizes that ethical principles that must be followed when experimenting on healthy volunteers must also be followed when experimentation is combined with therapeutic care.

The Declaration remained untouched from 1964 to 1975, although it was suggested on several occasions that it be revised to take account of the rapid advances in medical technology. It was finally revised at the 29th World Medical Assembly in Tokyo in 1975, following consultation with the World Health Organization (and no doubt other organizations) and recommendations made by a special committee appointed especially for that purpose.[67]

Helsinki II, which was further revised in 1983 and 1989, is recognized by most as providing the fundamental guiding principles for the conduct of biomedical research involving human subjects.[68] It has been adopted, in modified but similar forms, in international texts and national legislation and by many professional medical organizations throughout the world.[69] In many respects, the revised Declaration corrects the problems noted in the Nuremberg Code (and thus, for the most part, also in Helsinki I).

Perhaps the greatest change from Helsinki I to Helsinki II is the inclusion of ethical review committees. The Declaration requires that the protocol for each experimental procedure "be transmitted to a specially appointed independent committee for consideration, comment, and guidance."*

Helsinki II also places greater emphasis on the notion of informed consent. Principle I.9 of the basic principles (rather than just those applying to clinical and nonclinical biomedical research) requires that the researcher obtain the "freely given informed consent" of the research subject (after he has been informed of the aims of the research, the methods to be employed, and any potential risks). Principle I.10 cautions that great care should be taken if the subject is in either a dependent relationship to the researcher or may consent under duress. However, unlike the Nuremberg Code, Principle I.11 provides that in the case of legal incompetence, or physical or mental incapacity, the consent of the legal guardian is sufficient. Moreover, Principle II.5 provides that if the physician considers it essential not to obtain the informed consent of the patient when the research is combined with therapeutic care, he may not do so, provided that the specific reasons for this are explained to (and presumably approved by) the independent review committee.

Like Helsinki I, Helsinki II differentiates between research with potential therapeutic value and research merely for the advancement of scientific knowledge. In Helsinki II, however, the terminology is changed to "medical research combined with professional care (clinical research)" and "nonthera-

---

*Principle I.2 of the 1989 revision of the Declaration (Helsinki IV) provides that the experimental protocol "should be transmitted for consideration, comment and guidance to a specially appointed committee independent of the investigator and the sponsor, provided that this independent committee is in conformity with the laws and regulations of the country in which the research experiment is performed". Ethical review committees serve two important functions. First, "they provide a mechanism for specific application of general ethical principles to proposed research projects." Second, they operate to review projects *before* they begin rather than after some problem arises and a complaint is made." This practice is preventive in nature, protecting the research subject rather than merely punishing the investigator.[70] Thus, while the Declaration still places great weight on the integrity and judgment of the researcher, principle 2 provides a mechanism for review, a system of checks and balances.

peutic biomedical research involving human subjects (nonclinical biomedi-cal research)." This terminology, although not universally accepted, is now generally used in the literature of human experimentation.

It must also be noted that Helsinki II largely eliminated the differences in regulation of these two types of activity. "Neither the interests of science nor the desire for successful completion of research should be allowed to prevail over the health or life of the research subject."[71]

Finally, unlike both the Nuremberg Code and Helsinki I (but reminiscent of the WMA's 1954 Resolution), Helsinki II mandates that reports of experi-mentation not in accordance with the principles laid down in the Declara-tion should not be accepted for publication.

It has been suggested that the two sets of principles, the Nuremberg Code and the revised Declaration of Helsinki, constitute the basis of universality in the field of ethical-moral standards in human experimentation.[72] And indeed, although the revised Declaration of Helsinki goes much further in establishing guidelines to protect the research subject, the underlying princi-ples are the same. Both place emphasis on obtaining freely informed con-sent. Both call for a balancing of risks and benefits. Both mandate that experimentation on human subjects must be based on laboratory and ani-mal experimentation. Finally, both place great weight on the integrity and judgment of the medical investigator.

However, even if they constitute the basis of universality, the two sets of principles are just that: sets of ethical principles. Although they are highly influential, neither the Nuremberg Code nor the Declaration of Helsinki has any legally binding authority. The rules they set out are tenuous, unaccom-panied by any real controls, traditional sanctions, or other means of en-forcement. Moreover, as a series of general statements, they are ambiguous with respect to both the principles themselves and their practical applica-tion.[73] As one commentator has noted, "the various declarations and codes defining ethical aspects of research on human subjects [are] really no more than pious hopes that doctors [will] behave ethically."[74]

It has been suggested that, "by their very nature, international declara-tions can only be general."[75] Adequate protection of human research sub-jects is therefore not guaranteed by the existence of international codes alone. The general nature of these codes has dramatized the need for nation-al legislation and/or international documents with binding authority.[76]

ETHICS IN PRACTICE: PROPOSED INTERNATIONAL GUIDELINES

One of the most recent significant developments in the international sphere of medical research ethics is the issuance in 1982 of the WHO/CIOMS "Proposed International Guidelines for Biomedical Research Involving Hu-man Subjects." It should be noted that the word *Proposed* does not mean that the Guidelines are in draft form, pending further comment and revi-sion, but rather, that they have been proposed to countries as guidelines worthy of consideration and adoption under national standards and mores. Thus, the Guidelines suggest means for actually implementing ethical principles on a national level, remedying the problems endemic to international codes.

The origins of the Guidelines can be traced back to March 1976, when a conference co-sponsored by WHO, the WMA, the Council for International Organizations of Medical Sciences (CIOMS), the International Association of Biological Standardization, and the U.S. Centers for Disease Control was held in Geneva.[77] The conference examined "the role of the individual and the community in the research, development, and use of biologicals." During the conference, a series of recommendations were made, including the recommendation that CIOMS continue its work on the protection of human rights in relation to scientific progress in biology and medicine, with particular focus on community-based research and research conducted in the developing countries. Moreover, criteria for guidelines regarding human involvement in biologicals research were formulated by the participants at the conference.[78]

In 1978, CIOMS and WHO joined together to "develop guidelines to assist developing countries in evolving mechanisms that would ensure observance of the principles of medical ethics in biomedical research."[79] Specifically, the objective of the study was to "develop guidelines for the establishment of ethical review procedures for research involving human subjects [so as to] enable countries" to

   a. define a national policy on the ethics of medical and health research and to adopt ethical standards appropriate to their specific local needs; and
   b. establish adequate mechanisms for ethical review of research activities involving human subjects.[80]

In 1979, a questionnaire was distributed to health ministries and medical schools in over 100 developing countries. Replies were received from over 60 countries (from 45 health ministries and 91 medical schools). A working group was formed, and three CIOMS Round Table Conferences related to the ethics of human experimentation (including, but not limited to, human experimentation in developing countries) were held.[81]

A number of problems were highlighted in the course of this project. As discussed earlier, problems exist with the notion of voluntary informed consent. Particular reference was also made to certain vulnerable groups, including children, the mentally incompetent, those in a dependent and/or subordinate relationship to the investigator, prisoners, and pregnant and nursing women.

Attention was also paid to the problems associated with informed consent when research is conducted at the community level. Examples of such research include studies in compulsory vaccination programs, addition of fluoride to public water supplies, and addition of vitamins to staple foods — public health policies that require study and evaluation. Often, however, large communities or whole populations may be involved. Obtaining the free, informed consent of each individual is difficult, impractical, and often impossible.

The problems associated with informed consent in developing countries were also studied. Subjects who are members of developing communities are often not sufficiently aware of the implications of participating in an experiment to give adequately informed consent directly to the investigator.[82] Moreover, as one commentator noted,

> seeking informed consent to research from individuals may tend to weaken the social fabric of a nonindividualist society, forcing it to deal with values it does not hold and possibly sowing disorder that the community will have to reap long after the investigators may have gone home.[83]

Indeed, it was noted that the Nuremberg Code and the Declaration of Helsinki were designed by Westerners and are based on Western ethical principles not necessarily applicable to other cultures.

Finally, problems related specifically to externally funded research were considered. It was noted that investigators may serve external rather than internal interests. Moreover, foreign investigators and sponsors may not possess adequate insight into local mores, customs, and legal systems. Absence of a long-term commitment to research subjects and withdrawal of personnel on completion of their task often result in local disillusionment, while lack of accountability often deprives subjects of any form of compensation for injury. Most disturbing, it was recognized that standards applied when conducting research in developing countries are often less stringent than those that would be applied if the research was carried out in the initiating country.[84]

From this project emerged the Guidelines, endorsed in September 1981 by the 56th Session of the CIOMS Executive Committee and in October 1981 by the 23rd Session of the WHO Advisory Committee on Medical Research. The Guidelines are based on the Tokyo revision (1975) of the Declaration of Helsinki and are intended to indicate how these principles can be effectively applied, particularly in developing countries, taking into account socioeconomic circumstances, national legal provisions, and administrative arrangements.

The Guidelines do not have (nor are they intended to have) the character, force, or specificity of a legal text. Rather, they are meant to provide an operational approach to the ethics of medical research, a framework upon which countries that have not yet formalized their regulatory requirements for the ethical review of research protocols may build.[85]

Perhaps the most significant contribution of the WHO/CIOMS Guidelines is the thorough analysis of the problems associated with informed consent. The Guidelines acknowledge that "the involvement of human subjects in biomedical research must be contingent, whenever feasible, upon freely-elicited informed consent and upon liberty to withhold or withdraw collaboration at any stage without fear or prejudice."[86] However, the Guidelines recognize that, in many instances, this is an unobtainable goal. They therefore strive to determine when research involving human subjects in such circumstances can still be vindicated, and if so, "by what mechanism their welfare can be protected and the ethical propriety of the research be assured."[87]

The Guidelines take great pains to determine when experimentation on the above-mentioned "vulnerable groups" may be justified. Particular attention is paid to children, pregnant and nursing women, and the mentally ill.[88] With respect to community-based research, the Guidelines propose that "all possible means should be used to inform the community concerned of the aims of the research, the advantages expected from it, and any possible hazards or inconveniences." Although the ultimate decision to undertake the research should rest with the responsible public health authority, "if feasible, dissenting individuals should have the option of withholding their participation."

In communal cultures, where individual members of a community often do not have the necessary awareness of the implications of participation in an experiment so as to adequately give informed consent, the Guidelines suggest that the decision on whether or not to participate should be elicited through the intermediary of a trusted community leader. Some people criticize this approach on the grounds that there should be no discrimination between one population group and another, and that the fundamental principle must remain that only a person's individual consent can properly justify involvement as a subject of biomedical research. The Guidelines mandate that the intermediary should make it clear to the research subject that participation is entirely voluntary and that he may abstain or withdraw from the experiment at any time.

In all these situations (vulnerable groups, community-based research, research conducted among communal cultures), the emphasis is no longer on obtaining the informed consent of the research subject. Instead, stress is placed on the importance of prospective ethical review. It is suggested that "the limited application of the informed consent procedure, and its vulnerability to abuse, render it inadequate as an exclusive means of protecting the human rights and welfare of research subjects." Moreover, even when valid consent is obtainable, the Guidelines suggest that both the subject and the researcher should "have assurance to proceed in the knowledge that the research is sanctioned by representative professional and, where appropriate, lay opinion."[89]

By mandating ethical review of all experimental protocols, the Guidelines strive to protect the same rights protected under principle 1 of the Nuremberg Code. However, by mandating ethical review, the Guidelines provide for exceptions to the absolute requirement of informed consent in instances where consent may not be obtainable, yet experimentation on human subjects may still be ethically and morally justified.

The General Survey that accompanies the Guidelines suggests that ethical review committees should strive to make research protocols conform to a number of principles. These are worthy of quotation, as their resemblance to the Nuremberg Code cannot be denied.

[It should be established] that:
- the objectives of the research are directed to a justifiable advancement in biomedical knowledge that is consonant with prevailing community interests and priorities;
- the interventions are justifiable in terms of these objectives; the required information cannot be obtained from animal models; and the study has been designed with a view to obtaining this information from as few subjects as possible who will be exposed to a minimum of risk and inconvenience;
- the responsible investigator is appropriately qualified and experienced, and commands facilities to ensure that all aspects of the work will be undertaken with due discretion and precaution to protect the safety of the subjects;
- adequate preliminary literature research and experimental studies have been undertaken to define, as far as practicable, the risk inherent in participation;
- every effort will be made to inform prospective subjects of the objectives and consequences of their involvement, and particularly of identifiable risks and inconvenience;
- any arrangement to delegate consent has adequate justification, and appropriate safeguards will be instituted to ensure that the rights of the subjects will be in no way abused;
- appropriate measures will be adopted to ensure the confidentiality of data generated in the course of research.[90]

Thus, even though the emphasis has shifted from informed consent to ethical review, the underlying principles, established to protect the rights and welfare of the research subject, remain basically the same.

The Guidelines depart from previous international codes in two other significant ways. They are the first international set of principles to consider the problems associated with externally funded research. According to the Guidelines, such research implies two ethical imperatives:

- the research protocol should be submitted to ethical review by the initiating agency. The ethical standards applied should be no less exacting than they would be for research carried out within the initiating country;
- after ethical approval by the initiating agency, the appropriate authorities of the host country should, by means of an ethical review committee or otherwise, satisfy themselves that the proposed research meets their own ethical requirements.[91]

The Guidelines also suggest that an important secondary objective of externally sponsored research should be the training of health personnel to carry out similar research projects independently.[92]

Finally, the Guidelines assert that any volunteer subjects involved in medical research who may suffer injury as a result of their participation are entitled to financial or other assistance so as to compensate them fully for any temporary or permanent disability. Moreover, the Guidelines suggest that the research subject must merely establish a causal relationship between the investigation and his injury, and does not have to show negligence or lack of a reasonable degree of skill on the part of the investigator. Thus, the Guidelines are also the first international code to consider the subject of compensation of research subjects for injury sustained as a result of participation.

The Guidelines (especially if one considers the General Survey to be a part of the Guidelines) are a far cry from the 10 ethical principles enumerated at the Nuremberg Medical Trial. Indeed, one could refer to the Introduction of the Guidelines ("The fundamental ethical principles that guide the conduct of biomedical research involving human subjects, and on which these guidelines are based, are embodied in the World Medical Association's Declaration of Helsinki, as revised by the 29th World Medical Assembly in Tokyo in 1975") and conclude that the Nuremberg Code served no purpose in the drafting of one of the most recent international statements on the ethics of human experimentation.

And yet, one only has to look at the original proposal for the project to conclude otherwise. The Nuremberg Code is cited, along with the Declaration of Helsinki, as an international code providing guidance to investigators, a code that had to be reviewed and evaluated as part of the preliminary study.[93] Moreover, the questionnaire sent out to developing countries asked if they used international criteria for biomedical research, specifying the Nuremberg Code (and the Declaration of Helsinki) as "International Declarations." In many of the round tables and conferences leading up to the formation of the Guidelines, the Code was often discussed.

While the Nuremberg Code may no longer be the fundamental guiding principles upon which the Guidelines are based, it certainly had an impact on their development. In some ways, the principles enumerated in both codes are fairly similar. In others, however, they are quite divergent. But even in the latter case, the point from which the Guidelines have departed is the Nuremberg Code itself. In fact, in many aspects, the Guidelines remedy the very problems raised by the Nuremberg Code that the Declaration of Helsinki was unable to solve. Most important, however, the fundamental underlying principle of the Nuremberg Code—protection of the research subject's rights and welfare—has not changed at all.

The Guidelines have been (and continue to be) distributed as a consultative document to health ministries, medical research councils, medical faculties, nongovernmental organizations, medical journals, and other interested institutions, including research-based pharmaceutical companies. A survey conducted in 1982 indicated that the Guidelines were being used throughout the world and that, for the most part, they provided useful ethical criteria for biomedical scientists engaged in research involving human subjects.[94] Responses also indicated that, while useful, certain parts of the Guidelines could be improved by review and/or amplification.

INTERNATIONAL CODES OF RESEARCH ETHICS:
WHERE DO WE GO FROM HERE?

Responses to the above survey indicate that while the WHO/CIOMS Guidelines are an important tool in the field of international research ethics, there is room for further study and yet more developed codes. One significant outcome of the Guidelines is a call for similar guidelines aimed particularly at the ethical issues related to the conduct of epidemiological research. CIOMS, in collaboration with WHO, has recently developed International Guidelines for Ethical Review of Epidemiological Studies.

Similarly, there has been a call for a revised version of the 1982 Guidelines. In particular, there have been requests for more guidance with respect to experimentation involving communities and so-called "vulnerable groups." Accordingly, CIOMS, in collaboration with WHO, is currently revising the "International Guidelines for Biomedical Research Involving Human Subjects."

It must be mentioned that one of the most eminent experts in the field of human rights law, M. Cheriff Bassiouni, has developed a draft convention for the prevention and suppression of unlawful human experimentation.[95] This convention, which was drafted so as to define unlawful human experimentation as a crime under international law, was considered in 1984 by the United Nations Sub-Commission on Prevention of Discrimination and Protection of Minorities.[96] In its work, the Sub-Commission adopted a resolution that would have authorized a Special Rapporteur to "prepare a study on the current dimensions and problems arising from unlawful human experimentation."[97] The resolution was referred to the Commission on Human Rights for action or consideration.[98] It seems, however, that no further steps were taken. Bassiouni believes that one possible explanation for this is that representatives of certain countries feared that such a convention would infringe on the practices of their pharmaceutical industries.[99]

In his article accompanying the draft convention, Bassiouni argues that "a convention for the protection of human subjects would be consonant with the attitude of the world community by guaranteeing additional rights heretofore implicit in many such documents but not yet singled out."[100] An international code with binding authority is thus "a logical progression from the strong influence of the Nuremberg and Helsinki Codes and from the broad doctrinal foundation already laid for cooperation among sovereign nations in this largely unexplored area of international law."[101]

To discuss the principles of the draft convention would be to reiterate the impressive work of its author. However, it is important to note that the draft convention is based in large part on the Nuremberg Code, more so than any other text promulgated in the past two decades. While, for the present, the Sub-Commission on Prevention of Discrimination and Protection of Minorities has chosen not to pursue the subject of human experimentation, the possibility remains that the draft convention will be reintroduced at some point in the future.

Finally, given the current state of affairs in Europe, it must be noted that, in 1990, the 23-member Council of Europe's Committee of Ministers adopted a Recommendation (No. R (90) 3) to member states concerning medical research on human beings.[102] The Recommendation is "intended to lead to legislation or other appropriate means which will introduce, for the first time in member states, a series of binding rules on medical research on human beings."[103] The Recommendation lists a series of principles that member states are invited to introduce into their national law by legislation or by other appropriate means. The aim of these principles is to protect the human rights and health of persons undergoing medical research, as well as to establish legal rules on the duties of research workers and promoters of medical research.[104]

As in the Declaration of Helsinki and the WHO/CIOMS Guidelines, there is no specific mention of the Nuremberg Code. Reference is, however, made to the Code in the Draft Explanatory Memorandum to the Recommendation, not yet published. Moreover, the Council's Deputy Director of Legal Affairs affirms that the Code was in fact influential in the development of the principles.[105]

Quite significant is the emphasis in the Recommendation on the notion of informed consent. It marks a definitive turn away from the Declaration of Helsinki and the WHO/CIOMS Guidelines, as it "underlines that it is *absolutely necessary* to obtain the informed consent of the person undergoing medical research."[106] The Recommendation asserts that it is a fundamental legal principle "that no research may be imposed on anyone without his consent. This consent should be free, informed, express and specific."[107] Although the Recommendation allows for experimentation on subjects who are unable to provide consent in limited circumstances, it resembles the Nuremberg Code much more than any other international document with respect to this issue.†

Discussion of the Recommendation in detail would prove to be repetitive of what already has been considered in this chapter in regard to other codes. Yet again, protection of the research subject is mandated by placing emphasis on the importance of individual autonomy, the interests of the person over the interests of society and science, and the integrity of both the research and the researcher. Indeed, the Recommendation is simply the latest in the chain of international documents dealing with the ethics of human experimentation, a chain that began with the promulgation of the Nuremberg Code.

This chapter has attempted to demonstrate that the Nuremberg Code is far from a historical relic. And, through the examination of primary texts, often analyzed for the first time, we believe that we have succeeded in doing

---

†It must be noted, however, that principle 7 of the Recommendation states that "Persons deprived of liberty may not undergo medical research unless it is expected to produce a direct and significant benefit to their health." Thus, unlike the Nuremberg Code, the Recommendation prohibits nontherapeutic experimentation on prisoners even with their informed consent.

so. In our attempt to document the Nuremberg Code's influence in the international field of research ethics, we have discovered links that clearly establish that the principles of the Code did, and still do, provide invaluable guidance for the protection of the rights and welfare of human research subjects.

At one point in this chapter, the Nuremberg Code was described as an "imperfect document." As the promulgation of later documents (as well as the criticisms discussed above) indicates, the Code is, in fact, imperfect. However, its imperfections do not, and should not, minimize its importance. For although the field of international research ethics has evolved greatly over the past 40 years, its origins can always be traced back to the 10 principles first enumerated at the trial of the Nazi physicians.

NOTES

1. Alexander Capron, *BioLaw*, Vol. I, "Human Experimentation," in James Childress et al., eds., (Frederick, Md.: University Publications of America, 1986), p. 227.

2. See, e.g., Hans-Martin Sass, "Reichsrundschreiben 1931: Pre-Nuremberg German Regulations Concerning New Therapy and Human Experimentation," *Journal of Medicine and Philosophy* 8 (1983): 99–111, at 99. "[The Nuremberg Code] serves as the most basic platform for further discussions on the ethics of human experimentation. The fundamental influence of the Nuremberg Code is also evident in the subsequent shaping of national and international codes and regulations."

3. Warren Reich, ed., *Encyclopedia of Bioethics*, Vol. 4 (New York: Free Press, 1978), pp. 1764–1782. See also, e.g., William Curran, Arthur Dyck, and Stanley Reiser, ed., *Ethics in Medicine: Historical Perspectives and Contemporary Concerns* (Cambridge, Mass.: MIT Press, 1977), pp. 225–331; William Curran and E. Donald Shapiro, *Law, Medicine, and Forensic Science*, 3rd ed. (Boston: Little, Brown, 1982), pp. 989–1013.

4. See, e.g., Norman Howard-Jones, "Human Experimentation in Historical and Ethical Perspectives," *Social Science and Medicine* 16 (1982): 1429–1448, at 1443.

5. Ibid.

6. See, e.g., M. Cheriff Bassiouni, Thomas G. Baffes, and John T. Evrard, "An Appraisal of Human Experimentation in International Law and Practice: The Need for International Regulation of Human Experimentation," *Journal of Criminal Law and Criminology* 72 (Winter 1981): 1587–1666. "Imperfect as the language or fundamental principles may seem, the Nuremberg Code established the first internationally accepted safeguards and guidelines for the conduct of human experimentation. The Code remains a viable force. It squarely acknowledges the scientist's responsibility for the respect of human rights" (1642).

7. See, e.g., David Frenkel, "Human Experimentation: Codes of Ethics," in Amnon Carmi, ed., *Medical Experimentation: Its Legal and Ethical Aspects* (Ramat Gan, Israel: Turtledove Publishing, 1977), pp. 127–141, at 127.

8. Bassiouni, "An Appraisal," 1601, citing Henry Beecher, "Research and the Individual," *Human Studies* 5 (1970): 10–12.

9. Howard-Jones, "Human Experimentation," 1430, citing J. W. Willcock, *The*

Laws Relating to the Medical Profession with an Account of the Rise and Progress of its Various Orders (London: J. & W. T. Clarke, 1830), pp. 109–110.

10. Ibid., 1431, citing Claude Bernard, *Principes de Médecine Expérimentale* (Paris: Presses Universitaires de France, 1947), ref. [1], pp. 141–142. See also Erwin Deutsch, "Das internationale Recht der experimentellen Humanmedizin," *Neue Juristische Wochenschrift* 31 (1978): 570–575.

11. Directive of December 29, 1900, of the Prussian Minister of Religious, Educational, and Medical Affairs addressed to the directors of clinics, polyclinics, and similar establishments (*Centralblatt der gesamten Unterrichtsverwaltung in Preussen*, 1901, pp. 188–189).

12. Howard-Jones, "Human Experimentation," 1435. See also Erwin Deutsch, "Medical Experimentation: International Rules and Practice," *Victoria University of Wellington Law Review* 19 (1989): 1–10, at 4. For a contemporary comment, see Ludwig von Bar, "Medizinische Forschung und Strafrecht," *Festgabe der Göttinger Juristen-Fakultät für Ferdinand Regelsberger* (Leipzig, 1901), pp. 229–251.

13. Howard-Jones, "Human Experimentation," 1435, citing Paul Ehrlich and S. Hata, *Die experimentelle Chemotherapie der Spirillosen (Syphilis, Ruckfallfieber, Hühnerspirillose, Frambosie)* (Berlin: Julius Springer, 1910), pp. 139–141.

14. *Reichsgesundheitsblatt*, March 11, 1931, No. 10, pp. 174–175. For an English translation, see *International Digest of Health Legislation* 31 (1980): 408–411.

15. Howard-Jones, "Human Experimentation," 1435.

16. Ibid., 1443.

17. F. W. Fischer and H. Breuer, "Influence of Ethical Guidance Committees on Medical Research—A Critical Reappraisal," in Norman Howard-Jones and Zbigniew Bankowski, ed., *Medical Experimentation and the Protection of Human Rights* (Geneva: Council for International Organizations of Medical Sciences and Sandoz Institute for Health and Socio-Economic Studies, 1979), pp. 65–71, 66. See also, Sass, "Reichsrundschreiben," 100: "Many of the requirements of the Richtlinien seem to be stricter than those of the Nuremberg Code and subsequent regulations."

18. Howard-Jones, "Human Experimentation," 1436.

19. Hans-Martin Sass, "Comparative Models and Goals for the Regulation of Human Research," in Stuart Spicker et al., ed., *The Use of Human Beings in Research* (Dordrecht, the Netherlands: Kluwer Academic Publishers, 1988), pp. 47–85, at 52.

20. Howard-Jones, "Human Experimentation," 1436.

21. *U.S. v. Karl Brandt et al., Trials of War Criminals Before the Nuremberg Military Tribunals Under Control Council Law No. 10* (October 1946–April 1949), Vol. II, p. 183.

22. Andrew C. Ivy, "Nazi War Crimes of a Medical Nature," reprinted in Curran et al., *Ethics in Medicine*, pp. 267–272, at 270.

23. Capron, "Human Experimentation," p. 231, citing Alexander, "Limitations in Experimental Research on Human Beings," *Lex et Scientia* 3 (1966): 15. See also Claire Ambroselli, *L'Ethique Médicale* (Paris: Presses Universitaires de France, 1988), pp. 97–98.

24. Kenneth Vaux and Stanley Schade, "The Search for Universality in the Ethics of Human Research: Andrew C. Ivy, Henry K. Beecher, and the Legacy of Nuremberg," in Spicker et al., *The Use of Human Beings*, pp. 3–16, at 4.

25. Ivy, "Nazi War Crimes," p. 270.

26. G. A. Res. 2200 A, 21 U.N. GAOR Supp. (No. 16) 49, U.N. Doc. A/6316 (Dec. 16, 1966).

27. See, e.g., E/CN.4/AC.1/4/Add.1, June 18, 1947, "Commission on Human Rights, Drafting Committee, International Bill of Rights, Proposals submitted by the United Kingdom representative on the drafting committee"; E/CN.4/82/Add.8, May 6, 1948, "Commission on Human Rights, Third Session, Observations of governments on the draft international declaration of human rights, the draft international covenant on human rights, and methods of application."

28. E/CN.4/AC.1/4/Add.1.

29. Telford Taylor, "Statement," *Doctors of Infamy: The Story of the Nazi Medical Crimes*, ed. Alexander Mitscherlich and Fred Mielke (New York: Henry Schuman, 1949), p. xviii.

30. E/CN.4/82/Add.8.

31. E/CN.4/SR.91, "Summary Record of the 91st Meeting of the Fifth Session of the Commission on Human Rights," May 31, 1949, p. 17.

32. E/CN/.4/SR.141, "Summary Record of the 141st Meeting of the Sixth Session of the Commission on Human Rights," April 7, 1950, p. 11.

33. E/CN.4/SR.312, "Summary Record of the 12th Meeting of the Eighth Session of the Commission on Human Rights," June 12, 1952, pp. 11–12.

34. Convention for the Amelioration of the Condition of the Wounded and Sick in Armed Forces in the Field, 75 U.N.T.S. 31; Convention for the Amelioration of the Condition of the Wounded, Sick and Shipwrecked Members of Armed Forces at Sea, 75 U.N.T.S. 85; Convention relative to the Treatment of Prisoners of War, 75 U.N.T.S. 135; Convention relative to the Protection of Civilian Persons in Times of War, 75 U.N.T.S. 287. These Conventions are reproduced in the *International Red Cross Handbook*, 12th ed. (Geneva: International Committee of the Red Cross, 1983), pp. 23–195.

35. Bassiouni, "An Appraisal," 1659.

36. Jean Pictet, *Commentaire: La Convention de Genève pour l'Amélioration du Sort des Blessés et des Malades dans les Forces Armées en Campagne*, (Geneva: International Committee of the Red Cross, 1952), p. 153 (unofficial translation).

It must be noted that Article 11, Protocol 1 of the Additional Protocols of June 8, 1977 to the Geneva Conventions of August 12, 1949, provides that it is prohibited to carry out on persons [described in the Article], even with their consent, *inter alia*, medical or scientific experiments. The commentaries indicate that the aim of Article 11 was to clarify and develop the protection of persons protected by the Conventions and the Protocol against medical procedures not indicated by their state of health, and particularly against unlawful medical experiments. Yves Sandoz, Christophe Swinarski, and Bruno Zimmerman, ed., *Commentary on the Additional Protocols* (Geneva: International Committee of the Red Cross, Martinus Nijhoff, 1987), p. 150.

37. Personal communication from Angel Orozco, Executive Director of the World Medical Association, to the senior author.

38. "The Dedication of the Physician," *World Medical Association Bulletin* 1 (April, 1949): 4–13, at 4.

39. Ibid.

40. Ibid., 4–13.

41. Unfortunately, no documents verify this interpretation, and no one who partook in the drafting of the Declaration is still alive. However, given the text of the Statement on War Crimes and the positioning of the Declaration of Geneva, the interpretation is difficult to dispute. As mentioned above, this interpretation is supported by the Executive Director of the WMA. (Personal communication to the senior author.)

42. WMA document 17.6/54, "Human Experimentation," by Dr. L. A. Hulst.

43. Ibid.

44. "Resolution on Human Experimentation: Principles for Those in Research and Experimentation," adopted by the 8th General Assembly of the WMA, Rome, Italy, 1954.

45. Bassiouni, "An Appraisal," 1611, citing Beecher, *Research*, pp. 278–279.

46. William Curran, "Subject Consent Requirements in Clinical Research: An International Perspective for Industrial and Developing Countries," in Zbigniew Bankowski and Norman Howard-Jones, eds., *Human Experimentation and Medical Ethics* (Geneva: Council for International Organizations of Medical Sciences, 1982), pp. 35–79, at 36.

47. See, e.g., Henry Beecher, "Experimentation in Man," *Journal of the American Medical Association* 169 (1959): 461–478.

48. Aileen Adams and Geoffrey Cowan, "The Human Guinea Pig: How We Test New Drugs," *World* (December 5, 1972), pp. 20–24.
See also William Curran, "Evolution of Formal Mechanisms for Ethical Review of Clinical Research," in Howard-Jones and Bankowski, *Medical Experimentation*, pp. 11–20, at 12.

49. Bernard Barber, "Experimenting with Humans," *The Public Interest* 6 (Winter 1967): 91–102, at 98.

50. Curran, "Subject Consent," p. 41, summarizing Austin Bradford Hill, "Medical Ethics and Controlled Trials," *British Medical Journal* 2 (1963): 1043–1049.

51. Bassiouni, "An Appraisal," 1611, citing Beecher, *Research*, pp. 278–279. See also World Health Organization (WHO) and the Council for International Organizations of Medical Sciences (CIOMS) Proposed International Guidelines for Biomedical Research Involving Human Subjects (Geneva: CIOMS, 1982), General Survey, p. 8.

52. Barber, "Experimenting," 98; Vaux and Shade, "The Search," p. 9.

53. Henry Beecher, "Some Guiding Principles for Clinical Investigation," *Journal of the American Medical Association* 195 (March 1966): 157–158.

54. Curran, "Subject Consent," p. 41.

55. Bassiouni, "An Appraisal," 1642.

56. Committee on the Re-evaluation of the Nuremberg Experimental Principles, *Report of the National Conference on the Legal Environment of Medical Sciences* (Chicago: National Society for Medical Research and the University of Chicago, 1959), pp. 88–90, at 89. See also Erwin Deutsch, "Die zehn Punkte des Nürnberger Ärzteprozesses uber die Klinische Forschung am Menschen: der sog. Nürnberger Codex," in Broda et al., ed., *Festschrift für Rudolf Wassermann zum sechszigsten Geburtstag* (Darmstadt: Luchterhand, 1985), pp. 69–79, at 76.

57. Bassiouni, "An Appraisal," 1642, citing Welt, "Reflections on the Problems of Human Experimentation," in I. Ladimer and R. Neuman, ed., *Clinical Investigation in Medicine: Legal, Ethical, and Moral Aspects* (Boston: Law-Medicine Research Institute, Boston University, 1963), p. 129.

58. Curran, "Evolution," in Howard-Jones and Bankowski, *Medical Experimentation*, p. 11.

59. Frank Gutteridge et al., "The Structure and Functioning of Ethical Review Committees," in Bankowski and Howard-Jones, *Human Experimentation*, pp. 200–225, at 205.

60. See, e.g., Henry Beecher, "Ethics and Clinical Research," *New England Journal of Medicine* 274 (1966): 1354–1360; M. H. Pappworth, *Human Guinea Pigs: Experimentation on Man* (Boston: Beacon Press, 1968).

61. Henry Beecher, "Human Experimentation—A World Problem from the Standpoint of a Medical Investigator," *World Medical Journal* 8 (1960): 79–80, at 80.

62. WMA document 38.3/53; also personal communication from Angel Orozco to the senior author.

63. WMA Resolution on Human Experimentation; see also, Bassiouni, "An Appraisal," 1643.

64. WMA document 17.3/61. Report of the Committee on Medical Ethics, 15th General Assembly, September 15–20, 1961.

65. Personal communication from Angel Orozco to the senior author.

66. Ibid. One of the three experts responsible for the 1975 revision of the Declaration of Helsinki, Professor Povl Riis (professor of medicine at the University of Copenhagen), has confirmed that the concepts contained in the Nuremberg Code underpinned both the 1964 and 1975 versions, although the actual wording of the Nuremberg Code did not "function as a paradigm" (personal communication to the second author).

67. Ibid.

68. See, e.g., "Introduction, WHO/CIOMS Proposed International Guidelines." See also Christian Byk, "Les Instances d'Ethique en Droit Comparé," *Cahiers Internationaux de Sociologie* 88 (1990); 215–230, at 219.

69. Bassiouni, "An Appraisal," 1611.

70. Curran, "Evolution," p. 15.

71. "Biomedical Experimentation Involving Human Subjects," Working Paper 61, Law Reform Commission of Canada, 1989, p. 9.

72. Curran, "Evolution," p. 12.

73. *Biomedical Experimentation*, p. 10.

74. Alfred Gellhorn, "Medical Ethics in the Modern World," in Bankowski and Howard-Jones, *Medical Experimentation*, p. 9.

75. "WHO/CIOMS Project Proposal for the Development of Guidelines for the Establishment of Ethical Review Procedures for Research Involving Human Subjects," March 1978, p. 4.

76. See, e.g., Session D, "Development of National Ethics Standards for Research on Human Subjects," *Towards an International Ethic for Research with Human Beings: Proceedings of the International Summit Conference on Bioethics* (Ottawa, Canada: Medical Research Council of Canada, 1987), pp. 39–41, at 39. For an extensive discussion of national legislation regarding human experimentation, see Sev Fluss, "The Proposed Guidelines as Reflected in Legislation and Codes of Ethics," in Bankowski and Howard-Jones, *Human Experimentation*, pp. 323–366. See also Zbigniew Bankowski, John Dunne, and Sev Fluss, "Ethical Standards for Research Across Nations and Cultures," document produced at the request of the Medical Research Council of Canada for the International Summit Conference on Bioethics, Ottawa, April 1987.

77. "The Role of the Individual and the Community in the Research, Development, and Use of Biologicals with Criteria for Guidelines: A Memorandum," *Bulletin of the World Health Organization* 54 (1976): 645–655.

78. Ibid., pp. 649–651.

79. "WHO/CIOMS Project for the Development of Guidelines for the Establishment of Ethical Review Procedures for Research Involving Human Subjects," Interim Report Submitted to the WHO Advisory Committee on Medical Research, November 19–22, 1979, p. 1.

80. "WHO/CIOMS Project Proposal," p. 4.

81. Bankowski and Dunne, "History," p. 445.

82. Zbigniew Bankowski and Frank Gutteridge, "Medical Ethics and Human Research," *World Health* (November, 1982): 10–13, at 13.

83. Lisa Newton, "Ethical Imperialism and Informed Consent," *IRB — A Review of Human Subjects Research* 12 (1990): 10–11, at 11.

84. WHO/CIOMS Proposed International Guidelines, General Survey, p. 5.

85. Bankowski and Dunne, "History," p. 452.

86. WHO/CIOMS Proposed International Guidelines, General Survey, p. 7.

87. Ibid., p. 9.

88. Ibid.; see General Survey, pp. 9–13, and principles 7–13.

89. Ibid.; see General Survey, p. 15.

90. General Survey, p. 16.

91. Ibid.; see also principle 28.

92. Ibid.; see also principles 27–29.

93. "WHO/CIOMS Project Proposal," pp. 7–8.

94. "Proposed International Guidelines for Biomedical Research Involving Human Subjects: Analysis of Replies to a Questionnaire and Summary of Other Comments Received by Correspondence," August 1983, p. 2.

95. Draft Convention for the prevention and suppression of unlawful human experimentation, "Etude Générale," *Revue Internationale de Droit Pénal* 51 (1980): 419–445.

96. E/CN.4/Sub.2/1984/43, "Report of the Sub-Commission on Prevention of Discrimination and Protection of Minorities," 37th Session, Geneva, August 6–31, 1984. See also E/CN.4/Sub.2/1984/SR.34, p. 7.

97. E/CN.4/Sub.2/1984/1.21, p. 2. See also E/CN.4/Sub.2/1984/SR.34, p. 7.

98. E/CN.4/Sub.2/1984/43, p. ii.

99. Personal communication from M. Cheriff Bassiouni to the senior author.

100. Bassiouni, "An Appraisal," 1656.

101. Ibid., 1618.

102. Recommendation No. R (90) 3 of the Committee of Ministers to member states concerning medical research on human beings, adopted by the Committee of Ministers on February 6, 1990, at the 433rd meeting of the Ministers' Deputies.

103. Draft Explanatory Memorandum to Recommendation No. R [(90) 3] of the Committee of Ministers to member states concerning medical research on human beings, Council of Europe document CAHBI (89) 11, p. 17.

104. Ibid.

105. Personal communication from Frits Hondius, Deputy Director of Legal Affairs of the Council of Europe, to the senior author.

106. Draft Explanatory Memorandum, p. 18; emphasis added.

107. Ibid., p. 20.

9

The Nuremberg Principles in International Law

ROBERT F. DRINAN

I lived through the Nuremberg trials years ago when Father Edmond Walsh, a distinguished Jesuit from Georgetown University, spent several months at Nuremberg investigating all of the atrocities against priests, ministers, and nuns. I learned at that time of the potential impact that Nuremberg would have on international human rights law. This chapter addresses the legal background of Nuremberg, the difference between the Nuremberg Principles and the Nuremberg Code, the impact the Nuremberg Principles have had on protecting human rights in world law, and, most importantly, what we can do to construct a permanent Nuremberg.

THE NUREMBERG PRINCIPLES

The Allied powers warned all of the warring countries of the consequences of human atrocities on January 13, 1942, when they issued a declaration at St. James Palace in London. The nine European powers said, there will be punishment of those guilty of or responsible for the crimes whether they have ordered them, perpetrated them, or participated in them. At that moment, the Allied powers made it clear that the world would punish all people, even those who would say that they were only following the orders of their superiors. Never before in the history of the world had such a group gathered to say that there would be international punishment for those who had victimized innocent individuals. And there was so much to punish! Six million Jews were murdered, out of a total of 35 million persons killed during the war.

President Roosevelt knew the historical dimensions of the massacre. This is why he persuaded Justice Robert Jackson to leave the United States Supreme Court and go to Nuremberg as the principal prosecutor. Justice Jackson justified the Nuremberg Tribunal by saying that the worldwide scope of the Nazi aggression had left very few neutrals; consequently, either the victors must judge the vanquished or the world must leave the defeated to judge themselves. Humanity learned after the first World War that the latter is never satisfactory. We should recall that, at that time, a tribunal was constructed. The Allies handed thousands of persons over to the Germans, but they failed to carry out the tribunal's mandate. They convicted only a handful of persons; the rest went free. As a result, at Nuremberg, the Allied powers argued that the Kellogg-Briand Pact of 1928 was binding, and that they intended to punish the guilty, even though the prosecution admitted the technical difficulty of the victors punishing the vanquished.

The Charter of Nuremberg stated that one who has committed criminal acts may not take refuge in the defense of "following orders" or in the doctrine that his crimes were acts of the state. Consequently, at Nuremberg, a double revolution occurred. First, "following orders" was no longer a defense. Second, individuals, and not merely states, may be held accountable under the rule of international law. There were problems, to be sure. But the fact is that everything the Nazis did was already forbidden, not merely by the law of Germany but also by international law.

The first trial at Nuremberg, the War Crimes Trial, took 216 trial days spread over 10 months. The proceedings fill 22 volumes. There were 33 witnesses for the prosecution and 204 for the defense; 19 of the 21 persons on trial took the stand. Four thousand documents were submitted. A staggering amount of evidence was collected. The Nazis were convicted by their own testimony and their own writings. When the Allied powers entered the concentration camps, they took photographs of all the heinous things the Nazis did. The evidence of Nuremberg included photographs of corpses, along with lampshades made of human skin. It is astonishing that, even now, some people say that Nuremberg never really validly prosecuted or punished defendants.

The "Nuremberg Principles" consist of the London Charter (the agreement for the prosecution and punishment of major war criminals of the European Axis, dated August 8, 1945), the War Crimes Trial indictment, and the judgment rendered by the Nuremberg Tribunal in the War Crimes Trial.[1] In 1946, the General Assembly of the United Nations unanimously adopted the "Principles of International Law Recognized by the Charter of the Nuremberg Tribunal," which state that there are international war crimes and crimes against humanity; that violators can be tried and punished by an international tribunal, even if their acts are not in violation of domestic law, and even if they are acting under orders of a superior; and that a civil court (rather than a court martial) can try such international criminal acts.[2]

Germany was divided after the War Crimes Trial. The second echelon of criminals was designated, but people became weary of prosecuting war criminals, and prosecutions were not as vigorous as they should have been.

The United States proceeded with the Doctors' Trial, and the 11 additional Nuremberg Trials, on its own. Unlike the Nuremberg Principles, the Nuremberg Code, designed to protect human rights in experimentation, is the product of judges from only one country, and thus has significantly less standing in international law than the Nuremberg Principles.

The Nuremberg Principles have been incorporated into world law and have been ratified by the world community. It is astonishing that they were ratified without difficulty by the General Assembly of the United Nations. The problem 40 years later is how to get these principles, which are universally accepted, implemented and enforced throughout the world. Looking back at Nuremberg we must wonder, for example, who will punish all of the people who were hurt in the war between Iran and Iraq. At Nuremberg it was agreed that there should be some world tribunal that would sit in judgment on the deprivations of liberty and life like those that were caused by these two nations.

The Nuremberg Principles were incorporated in the military law of the United States, England, and other countries, and accepted in the four Geneva Conventions of 1949. They were applied by the United States, feebly but with good intentions, in Vietnam.

The trial of Lt. William Calley for his acts at My Lai involved the principle of Nuremberg that we should punish even our own soldiers, even if they acted on orders from their superiors. Calley was in fact punished, but all the others involved in the operation were exonerated.[3] The Calley case was not our finest hour. But in fairness, the U.S. Army did try diligently to punish soldiers in Vietnam who had committed acts that are indefensible under U.S. law and the Military Code of Justice.

In 1969, I was in Saigon with a human rights group, and we talked to a Vietnamese lawyer. There were files all over his office. In response to our inquiry as to their nature he responded: "They are files of atrocities like My Lai. Someday when this war is over, we will have our own Nuremberg in Asia." He added, "The Americans will be convicted of being barbarians." I have often wondered what happened to those files. What is significant is that this lawyer, in a completely different part of the world, knew about Nuremberg and said that his nation would hold people accountable, including the Americans.

The Nuremberg Principles were also used in the Adolph Eichmann trial, one more example indicating the need for a world tribunal to which all people would be accountable. The people of Israel felt strongly that Eichmann had done terrible things. As a result, they kidnapped him from Argentina, took him to Israel, and gave him a fair trial; afterward, he was executed.

THE NEED FOR A PERMANENT NUREMBERG

Looking back at Nuremberg, one sees everywhere in the proceedings the dream, shared by physicians, jurists, and people throughout the world, for a permanent Nuremberg tribunal. That was the dream of Justice Robert Jackson, who sought to institutionalize Nuremberg so that if any depravity was perpetrated by leaders or their followers in any nation, there would be one tribunal to try and punish them. That dream is still alive in this new era at the end of the cold war. We should not believe that it is unobtainable. Indeed, we must dream again of a permanent Nuremberg because the United States, the Soviet Union, and all of the other Allied powers that came together in Nuremberg are closer at this moment then at any time in the past 40 years.

The concept of a permanent Nuremberg assumes that when there are "crimes against humanity"—and that very phrase was invented at Nuremberg—there should be just punishment. The League of Nations urged the establishment of a permanent international court in 1920; jurists and scholars examined this possibility throughout the 1920s and 1930s. After Nuremberg, unfortunately, there was apathy. But the great idea remains. Every time new atrocities occur, jurists look to the possibility of creating a permanent world Nuremberg tribunal.

Recently, I visited Argentina, witnessing the trials of those who were accused of atrocities during the dark night of this country from 1976 to 1985. The generals, the colonels, and the admirals went to jail. The people of Argentina would have been more satisfied if this had been done by an international tribunal. Why? Because the situation in Argentina involved one administration sitting in judgment on a previous one. Nonetheless, these trials are a lesson for all the dictators of the world.

I dream of a tribunal where Ferdinand Marcos could have been punished and where the Shah of Iran could have been called to justice, as could the Quadaffis and Husseins of the world. This is not an impossible dream. Lawyers will wonder how we can ever make this dream a reality. Would there be a World Attorney General? Would the death penalty apply? Would the tribunal use the principles of American or European law? There are many difficulties. But these do not change the fact that a permanent Nuremberg is desperately needed. It is needed so that people will know that if they deprive others of their rights, or of their liberties, or of their lives, they will be punished.

Think of the potential that a permanent world Nuremberg would have in settling the dreadful problems of El Salvador. The United States would be charged with wrongdoing for its actions in that nation. Over the last 10 years, the United States has sent more than $4 billion dollars to that tiny country. Over 71,000 people have been killed and up to one-fourth of the population has been displaced. Nonetheless, the murderers of Archbishop Oscar Romero have not been identified, nor has there been accountability for the murder of six Jesuit priests.

One thing we could do before a permanent Nuremberg is established is to establish the role of a United Nations Commissioner for Human Rights. We are familiar with and admire the United Nations Commission on Refugees, which has received the Nobel Peace Prize. This agency, based in New York and Geneva, predicts the number of refugees and orchestrates world efforts to alleviate their plight. The United Nations Commissioner for Human

Rights would do the same things on behalf of human rights throughout the world. It is my hope that this position will be established in the not too distant future.

THE INFLUENCE OF NUREMBERG

The impact of Nuremberg is almost incalculable. That tribunal gave the first impetus to the worldwide movement for international human rights. The United Nations Charter mentions human rights five times, a development totally new in world law. The idea of human rights was not even mentioned in the Charter of the League of Nations. The Universal Declaration of Human Rights, agreed to on December 10, 1948, is quoted and used in the constitutions of the more than 100 new nations that rose from the ashes of colonialism after World War II. All of the essential parts of the United Nations Charter and the Universal Declaration of Human Rights are a part of world law.

Twenty-two covenants on human rights have emerged from the United Nations, at least partially due to Nuremberg. There are covenants against racism, sexism, torture, and genocide. I note with shame, as an American, that the United States has ratified only 6 of the least important of them. High on my agenda for the present administration is the ratification of all of these important documents. President Carter is the only president since Nuremberg who recommended that the Senate ratify all of the major covenants on human rights.

The Convention Against Torture and other Cruel, Inhumane or Degrading Treatment or Punishment, approved by the United Nations in 1984, has special applicability to physicians and lawyers. I hope that the U.S. Senate will soon ratify it. This document states that doctors may not even be present when any torture is carried out. Amnesty International is working diligently for the fulfillment of its promise to the world that torture will be eliminated by the year 2000. In this area, physicians and lawyers have a clear responsibility.[4]

At the United Nations, various commissions are now carrying out the work of the conventions, such as the Convention for the Elimination of Discrimination Against Women and the Convention on the Elimination of All Forms of Racial Discrimination (1969). Some will ask whether these world monitoring bodies are important. The organizations are relatively new. They collect data from all nations on the treatment of women and minorities. These commissions are educating the world and sometime, hopefully soon, they will add new enforcement powers so that if a nation oppresses its minorities or its women, the world will know this and levy appropriate punishments. The rights of children are echoed every day by the United Nations International Children's Emergency Fund (UNICEF). This worldwide organization was the first auxiliary of the United Nations. The Food and Agricultural Organization (FAO) asserts every day the right of all people to have food. The United Nations Educational, Scientific, and Cultural Organization (UNESCO) administers the right to literacy. Consequently, the impact of Nuremberg goes on.

Nuremberg has had a special impact on Europe. In 1952, determined never to allow another group like the Nazis to come to power, the 21 nations of Europe established a European Court on Human Rights. That tribunal has now issued 40 volumes of decisions. What an extraordinary development! These nations now have a place where all citizens' grievances can be heard. The European Declaration on Human Rights and the tribunal that defines and implements it constitute one of the most advanced safeguards of human rights in the history of the world. In addition, Latin America now has a court and a commission on human rights, which hands down rulings that help protect human rights in Latin America. This process has now started in Africa as well. The declarations and guarantees set forth in the African Convention on Human Rights are now part of the law of the 51 nations of Africa.

In the United States, Congress in 1974 enacted section 502B of the International Foreign Assistance Act, stipulating that the United States may not give aid, either economic or military, to any nation that denies internationally recognized human rights. It was signed by President Ford. A unit was set up in the State Department that, every year in February, issues a 1200-page book describing the state of human rights in every nation. The United States has become, in effect, the monitor of the implementation of the Nuremberg Principles. Unfortunately, not every administration's State Department is as thorough as that of President Carter. But at least the United States is now saying that every violation of these internationally recognized human rights is a violation of world law.[5]

I also think we owe indemnification to the people of Vietnam. History will show that the United States violated many of the rules of Nuremberg in its conduct of the war in Vietnam. U.S. soldiers are now being indemnified if they breathed Agent Orange during that war. If we indemnify Americans, why do we not also repay the people of Vietnam, whom this chemical has also harmed? Are we simply going to walk away? In Vietnam we acted in violation of the rules of war for which we punished people in Nuremberg. Gorbachev has admitted that the Soviet Union should never have invaded Afghanistan. Could not the United States declare that Vietnam was a mistake and give some indemnification for all of the damage that was done in that nation? We had a moment of grace in the recent past when finally we recognized that the internment of Japanese-Americans in World War II was a mistake. We are now giving $20,000 to every Japanese survivor out of the 130,000 people who were imprisoned.

CONCLUSION

In this new era, in which we rejoice every day because the cold war is over, we should recognize, together with all the nations of the earth, that the rights of the individual should now have top priority in our thinking. The human rights that are guaranteed by world law should be available to all people in the global village. If the physicians and lawyers of the world agreed that violations of human rights must be punished, a permanent Nuremberg tribunal for every offense in violation of international law would be created.

Everyone associated with this project and this book on the Nuremberg Code is to be commended.[6] These efforts show how much has been done, but also how much more remains to be done.

In this new era, both sides should recognize that they were together at Nuremberg and that, at this new high point in world history, they should be allied again. This is a moment when the dream of Nuremberg and the aspirations of the United States can come together. A permanent Nuremberg could punish physicians and scientists guilty of crimes under the Nuremberg Principles and, hopefully, deter criminal experimentation on human subjects.[7]

Let me conclude with the wonderful words of Archibald MacLeish, who summed up the dream and vision of Nuremberg and of the United States:

> There are those who will say that the liberation of humanity, the freedom of man and mind are nothing but a dream. They are right. It is a dream. It is the American dream.

NOTES

1. Gerhard O. W. Mueller, "Four Decades After Nuremberg: The Prospect of an International Criminal Code," *Connecticut Journal of International Law* 2 (1987): 499, 499–500.

2. Ibid. In 1947 the General Assembly's Committee on the Progressive Development of International Law and Its Codification recommended that the International Law Commission prepare a draft code incorporating the Nuremberg Principles, as well as a general plan for the codification of offenses against the peace and security of mankind. In 1950, the Commission presented its first formal report. The text of that report is the first attempt to codify Nuremberg:

> *Principle I.* Any person who commits or is an accomplice in the commission of an act which constitutes a crime under international law is responsible therefore and liable for punishment.

> *Principle II.* The fact that domestic law does not punish an act which is an international crime does not free the perpetrator of such crime from responsibility under international law.

> *Principle III.* The fact that a person who committed an international crime acted as Head of State or public official does not free him from responsibility under international law or mitigate punishment.

> *Principle IV.* The fact that a person acted pursuant to an order of his government or of a superior does not free him from responsibility under international law. It may, however, be considered in mitigation of punishment, if justice so requires.

Principle V. Any person charged with a crime under international law has the right to a fair trial on the facts and law.

Principle VI. The crimes hereafter set out are punishable as crimes under international law:

  a. Crimes against Peace:
     (1) Planning, preparation, initiation or waging of a war of aggression, or a war in violation of international treaties, agreements or assurances;
     (2) Participation in a common plan or conspiracy for the accomplishment of any of the acts mentioned under (1).
  b. War Crimes: namely, violations of the laws or customs of war. Such violations shall include, but not be limited to, murder, ill-treatment or deportation to slave labour or for any other purpose of civilian population of or in occupied territory, murder or ill-treatment of prisoners of war or persons on the seas, killing of hostages, plunder of public or private property, wanton destruction of cities, towns or villages, or devastation not justified by military necessity.
  c. Crimes against Humanity: namely, murder, extermination, enslavement, deportation and other inhuman acts done against a civilian population, or persecutions on political, racial or religious grounds, when such acts are done or such persecutions are carried on in execution of or in connection with any crime against peace or any war crime.

Principle VII. Complicity in the commission of a crime against peace, a war crime or a crime against humanity, as set forth in *Principle VI*, is a crime under international law.

In 1954 attempts first began to go beyond the Nuremberg Principles and establish an international criminal code that would be administered both nationally and internationally by an international criminal court. Work on this project stalled almost immediately and was not revived until 1981. Currently, the attempt is not simply to restate the 1954 aims but to move beyond the "three basic crime categories, namely crimes against peace, war crimes, and crimes against humanity. Rather, it should extend to more recent international crimes such as colonialism, apartheid, serious environmental offenses, economic aggression, mercenarism, hostage taking, violence against persons enjoying diplomatic privilege and immunities, the hijacking of aircraft, international terrorism, and piracy." Ibid., pp. 501–502.

3. *United States v. Calley*, 22 C.M.A. 534, 46 C.M.R. 1131 (1973); *Calley v. Callaway*, 519 F.2d 184 (5th Cir. 1975). See also R. J. Falk and J. H. E. Fried, *Vietnam and International Law* (Northampton, Mass.: Aletheia Press, 1990), and G. D. Solis, *Marines and Military Law in Vietnam: Trial by Fire* (Washington, D.C.: U.S. Marine Corps, 1989).

4. The Convention Against Torture is probably the convention most directly related to human experimentation, although no existing convention deals directly with the subject of the Doctors' Trial. Article One's definition of torture provides:

  1. For the purposes of this Convention, the term "torture" means any act by which severe pain or suffering, whether physical or mental, is intentionally inflicted on a person for such purposes as obtaining from him or a third person information or a confession, punishing him for an act he or a third person has committed or is suspected of having committed, or intimidating

or coercing him or a third person, or for any reason based on discrimination of any kind, when such pain or suffering is inflicted by or at the instigation of or with the consent or acquiescence of a public official or other person acting in an official capacity. It does not include pain or suffering arising only from, inherent in or incidental to lawful sanctions.

2. This article is without prejudice to any international instrument or national legislation which does or may contain provisions of wider application.

A few years ago in Chile, I felt proud when I learned that the physicians of Chile had censured one physician who had been present and who had aided in the torture of the enemies of General Pinochet, then president of that country. The moral revolution of Nuremberg means that all violations of the treaties, and of the Nuremberg Principles, are now violations of world law.

5. We also ought to recognize that the Helsinki Treaty, signed on August 1, 1975, had a tremendous impact on the events that have been developing in the Soviet Union and Eastern Europe. Nonetheless, the need to monitor human rights principles and to obtain their enforcement is urgent.

6. I am familiar with the work of the Physicians for Social Responsibility; we were all thrilled when the international unit of that group received the Nobel Peace Prize. I am similarly thrilled that a new organization based in Boston, Physicians for Human Rights, has been organized by Dr. Jonathan Fine. It seems to me that this project on the Nuremberg Code, and on human rights in medicine, is a landmark, bringing together the JDs and MDs of the world. I often dream of a world federation of physicians and lawyers implementing the principles of Nuremberg.

7. Making the Nuremberg Code formally part of international law would require a new Convention on Human Experimentation.

10

The Influence of the Nuremberg Code on U.S. Statutes and Regulations

LEONARD H. GLANTZ

This chapter discusses whether the principles of the Nuremberg Code have been adopted by the regulatory and legislative bodies in the United States. I am not so much interested in if or how the *words* of the Code have been adopted, but rather whether or not its *principles* have been transformed into statutory or regulatory requirements in the United States by our usual policymaking bodies. By conducting this type of analysis, one can hope to learn various lessons. First, were the principles enunciated in the Code enduring ethical statements, or were they narrowly focused on assessing the activities of specific defendants? Second, have the Code's principles had an impact on contemporary research methods and on the regulation of research? Finally, by looking at written codes, laws, or regulations, one can hope to discover how the formal expression of societal opinions views a certain activity: Is it something we wish to encourage, something we will tolerate, or something viewed with deep distrust? An examination of the evolution of research codes provides us with a view of how research has come to be regarded in an evolving cultural context.

It is worth remembering that the Code was not promulgated by a policy-making body like a legislature or an administrative agency, but rather was "enacted" by judges as a step in deciding a criminal case. Unlike other codes of conduct, which might be drafted in consultation with a number of interested groups or individuals, this Code was essentially dictated by judges.

The Code's principles can be divided into two areas that provide quite differing approaches to the protection of human subjects. The first area provides for the protection of the subject's right to decide whether or not to become a research subject. Thus, the first provision of the Code states that the informed consent of the human subject is "absolutely essential" and specifies that such consent must be rendered in an entirely voluntary manner. Furthermore, before the subject can render a valid consent, he must be informed of "all inconveniences and hazards" reasonably to be expected and the effects upon his health or person "which may possibly come from his participation in the experiment." The ninth provision requires that the "human subject should be at liberty to bring the experiment to an end if he has reached the physical or mental state where continuation of the experiment seems to him to be impossible." While the provision could have been written in more absolute terms, it seems to give human subjects the unequivocal authority to end their participation in research.

Taken together, these provisions protect the rights of the individual as an autonomous human being. Individuals are given the absolute right to refuse to be subjects and the absolute right to terminate their participation at any time. In a sense, human subjects as a group are given "veto power" over research, since the research to be conducted must be such that people will volunteer to participate, and will decide to continue to participate once they are actually exposed to the burdens of the particular research endeavor.

The remaining eight provisions of the Code do not deal directly with the subject's decision to participate. Rather, they are directed at the researchers, and either prohibit them from conducting certain types of research or require them to protect the human beings who have consented to be subjects. For example, provision 5 prohibits research where there is an "*a priori* reason to believe that death or disabling injury will occur" (although this may be permissible if the researcher also acts as a subject). Provision 4 requires investigators to avoid "all unnecessary physical and mental suffering and injury." Provision 8 limits the conduct of research to "scientifically qualified persons," who must use the "highest degree of skill and care" while performing experiments. Provision 10 requires the researcher to terminate the experiment at any stage if he has "probable cause" to believe, based on his "good faith, superior skill, and careful judgment," that continuing the experiment is likely to result in the subject's injury, disability, or death.

Thus, 8 of the Code's 10 provisions are directed not at protecting the rights of subjects, but rather at protecting their welfare. These provisions focus on researchers, and instruct them what things may not be done and what things must be done regardless of the subject's consent. Their overall message is that the researcher's primary concern must be the well-being of the research subject, not the research endeavor. Furthermore, it should be noted that the Code's requirements are directed at the researcher, and not at the institution that sponsors the research or in which the research is conducted. The rules embodied in the Code are self-executing and do not require the involvement of any review board or similar bureaucratic entity. In this sense, the Code resembles a criminal statute designed to control the behavior of those to whom it is directed.

It is also worth noting that no attempt was made to define what activities the Code covers. The Code uses the terms *human subjects* and *experiment* but does not define them. The question, then, is, precisely what activities was the Code meant to regulate?

Based on the factual background, which largely encompasses the types of research abuses confronting the judges at Nuremberg, it would appear that the Code is directed at regulating nontherapeutic research, i.e., research that offers the subject no possible direct benefit. This conclusion is also supported by the fact that *none* of the Code's provisions refer to balancing the risks of the research against the benefits the subject might be expected to obtain from participation. Indeed, the Code requires a balancing of values, but benefit to the subject is never an element. Provision 6 states that the degree of risk to the subject "should never exceed that determined by the humanitarian importance of the problem to be solved by the experiment." Provision 2 requires the experiment to "yield fruitful results for the good of society." These are the only provisions of the Code that deal with the outcome of the experiment. Both involve expressions of larger societal benefit and contain no mention of any benefit to the individual subject.

One can conclude from this that the Code was not designed to regulate therapeutic research that may benefit the subject. Rather, its purpose is to regulate pure research, which is designed to provide new knowledge but is in no way intended to benefit the subject. If this is so, then the Code is directed at a relatively simple problem and has only limited relevance to the complexities of research with human subjects as it is conducted today.

THE CODIFICATION OF THE CODE

The most extensive codification of the regulation of research has occurred at the federal level. Some states have also enacted research rules that are usually designed to deal with local concerns or pressures — in particular, the protection of fetuses.

In the mid-1950s, the Clinical Center of the National Institutes of Health (NIH) adopted guidelines that applied to the use of normal volunteers. In a pamphlet explaining the role of normal volunteers to potential research subjects, the NIH stated:

> The rigid safeguards observed at NIH are based on the so-called "ten commandments" of human medical research which were adopted at the Nuremberg War Crime trials after the atrocities performed by Nazi doctors had been exposed.
>
> Every volunteer must give his full consent to any test, and he must be told exactly what it involves so that he goes into it with his eyes open. Among other things, the experiment must be designed to yield "fruitful results for the good of society," unnecessary "physical and mental suffering and injury" must be avoided, the test must be conducted by "scientifically qualified" persons, and the subject must be free to end it at any time he feels unable to go on. And at NIH, a special board of scientists also studies every projected experiment before it is okayed.[1]

As can be readily observed, these stated safeguards are taken directly from the Nuremberg Code. It should also be noted that these guidelines are directed at "healthy volunteers," the same group to which the Nuremberg Code was meant to apply. In addition, it is interesting that the NIH referred to the Nuremberg Code as the "ten commandments" of human research, since this characterization portrays the Code as a powerful set of *ethical* principles that one should strive to follow. However, it does not describe the Code in terms of *legal* requirements.

Before normal volunteers could be used at the Clinical Center, approval had to be sought from various individuals and committees. The Clinical Center's 1961 handbook regarding normal volunteers listed the following as "applicable broad principles" the reviewers should use in evaluating proposed research:

> 3.06   In considering the approvability of projects in which it is proposed that normal volunteers be used, reviewers are guided by both moral and scientific principles. The principal guides followed are the Nuremberg Code and that of the American Medical Association. The possibility of hazard to the individual is always of primary concern. Some of the factors other than safety which concern reviewers are: (a) Need for such observations in man; (b) Potential fruitfulness of the project; (c) Biological soundness of the research design; and (d) Skill of the investigator.[2]

Starting in 1962, the federal government became more formally involved in the regulation of research. Professor William Curran has described the development of research regulations at the Food and Drug Administration (FDA) and at NIH in the 1960s.[3] The FDA's entry into the regulation of research came as a result of the Drug Amendments Act of 1962. The primary purpose of the law was to keep unsafe or useless drugs off the market by requiring proof of safety and efficacy from the drug companies. In the wake of the thalidomide experience, Congress noted that no state required physicians to inform patients that an experimental drug was being used on them. As a result, the final version of the 1962 law contained a provision that required "experts using such drugs for investigational purposes" to inform persons to whom they are to be administered that they are being given drugs for investigational purposes and to obtain the consent of these individuals or their representatives, except "where they deem it not feasible or, in their professional judgment, contrary to the best interests of such human beings."[4] It was not until 1966 that the FDA promulgated patient consent regulations, at least partially in recognition of the widespread failure of the industry to obtain patient consent.

In 1966, the NIH promulgated the policy of not approving new or continuing grants involving research with human beings unless the grantee institution provided prior review of the judgment of the principal investigator by a committee of his institutional associates regarding the "rights and welfare [of subjects], the appropriateness of the methods used to secure informed consent, and the risks and potential medical benefits of the investigation."[5]

In the application, the grantee was to describe the "Committee of Associates" who would provide the review. On July 1, 1966, the Surgeon General of the United States revised the policy statement to permit grantee institutions to file an institutionwide assurance and to set up a standing institutional committee to review research applications. In commenting on this approach, Professor Curran notes:

> It applies a philosophy of encouraging academic freedom and imagination in the research it supports in the interest of achieving the best possible scientific results. Instead of a substantive, regulatory program uniformly applied across the nation, it has installed a system of decentralized, institutional review committees and generalized ethical guidelines to protect patients and subjects in the projects it supports.[6]

Indeed, the approaches of the FDA and NIH set the tone for future federal involvement in regulating research. Both sets of rules view research in a positive light and try to protect subjects, but not at the expense of hindering research. Also, the regulations are directed not at researchers but at institutions — either drug companies or research institutions. Violation of these rules could lead to lack of funding or the nonacceptance of research data to support a new drug application, but there were no other penalties.

The federal government became more involved in the regulation of research with human subjects in 1974 when it adopted a basic set of regulations governing the protection of human subjects involved in research that was supported or conducted by the Department of Health, Education and Welfare (DHEW).[7] On July 12, 1974, the National Research Act[8] created the National Commission for the Protection of Human Subjects of Biomedical and Behavioral Research, with the specific charge of studying the nature of research conducted with fetuses. The Commission was also given the more general charge of identifying "the basic ethical principles which should underlie the conduct of biomedical and behavioral research involving human subjects" and of developing guidelines and recommendations for the Secretary of DHEW. By August 8, 1975, there was a comprehensive set of federal regulations governing government-conducted or -sponsored research with human subjects and special regulations governing research with fetuses, pregnant women, and *in vitro* fertilization.[9] These regulations were applicable to all DHEW grants and contracts in which human subjects were involved. Accordingly, the regulations were not applicable to research funded by other sources. This was not because DHEW was not concerned about other research populations, but because this was the only body of research over which it had jurisdiction.

Unlike the Nuremberg Code, which set forth rules that were applicable to researchers, the federal regulations, like previous federal rules, were directed at the *institution* that received research funds. Thus, Section 46.102 (a) states: "safeguarding the rights and welfare of subjects at risk . . . is primarily the responsibility of *the institution* which receives or is accountable to DHEW for the funds awarded for the support of the activity." No research activity would be funded by DHEW unless a potential grant recipient had an Institutional Review Board (IRB) that reviewed and approved the activity. The IRB must be composed of no fewer than five persons with varying backgrounds to ensure complete and adequate review of all potential research activities. The IRB must also include members who, with their maturity, experience, and expertise, could review proposals from both a scientific and an ethical perspective. Furthermore, the IRB must be able to ascertain that the proposed project complied with institutional commitments and regulations, applicable law, standards of professional conduct, and community attitudes.[10]

In reviewing proposed research involving human subjects, the IRB was to determine whether these subjects would be placed at risk, and if risk is involved, whether:

(1) The risks to the subject are so outweighed by the sum of the benefits to the subject and the importance of the knowledge to be gained as to warrant a decision to allow the subject to accept these risks;

(2) The rights and welfare of any such subjects will be adequately protected; and

(3) Legally effective informed consent will be obtained by adequate and appropriate methods in accordance with the provisions of this part.[11]

The determination that subjects will or will not be at risk is critical because it is the subject at risk who is protected under these regulations. Although, surprisingly, the term *research* is never defined, the term *subject at risk* is defined at length:

"Subject at risk" means any individual who may be exposed to the possibility of injury, including physical, psychological, or social injury, as a consequence of participation as a subject in any research, development, or related activity which departs from the application of those established and accepted methods necessary to meet his needs, or which increases the ordinary risks of daily life, including the recognized risks inherent in a chosen occupation or field of service.[12]

If individuals will be subjects at risk, then their informed consent, or the informed consent of their "legally authorized representative," must be obtained before the research takes place.[13] *Informed consent* is defined as follows:

"Informed consent" means the knowing consent of an individual or his legally authorized representative, so situated as to be able to exercise free power of choice without undue inducement or any element of force, fraud, deceit, duress, or other form of constraint or coercion.[14]

The basic elements of informed consent are then listed, including a fair explanation of the procedures to be followed; specific identification of those procedures that are experimental; a description of the discomforts, benefits, and risks reasonably to be expected; a disclosure of alternative procedures that might be beneficial to the subject; and an instruction that the subject is "free to withdraw his consent and discontinue participation in the project or activity at any time without prejudice to the subject."[15]

These regulations depart from the Nuremberg Code in a number of significant ways. As discussed earlier, they place responsibility for the protection of human subjects on the institution in which the research is conducted, not on the investigator who conducts the research. If research is conducted in violation of these regulations, the sanction is loss of funding, not criminal penalties.[16] Furthermore, while the "rights and welfare" of subjects are to be protected, the emphasis is far more on subjects' rights than on their welfare. In this regard, the regulations emphasize the role of informed consent and the right of the subject to withdraw at any time, which is similar to the Code's provisions 1 and 9. Indeed, the regulation's definition of informed consent is taken almost verbatim from the Code. But unlike the Code, which states that the "voluntary consent of the human subject is absolutely essential," the regulations permit consent from a "legally authorized representative." This discrepancy is likely due to the fact that the regulations deal with research that may be beneficial to the subject, a scenario not anticipated by the Code. While the Code appears to have been drafted to govern nonbeneficial research, the regulations apply to any "research, development, or related activity which departs from those accepted methods necessary to meet [the subject's] needs." Thus, any novel approach that may be used to treat a person's condition is covered by the regulations, which makes their reach much longer than the Code's. However, the Code's detailed rules for protecting subjects, such as requiring prior animal experimentation, requiring that the beneficial results be "improcurable by other methods or means of study," requiring that the experiment should be conducted so "as to avoid all unnecessary physical and mental suffering," and prohibiting experiments "where there is reason to believe that death or disabling injury will occur," are absent.

Interestingly, the 1975 regulations regarding fetal research *do* adopt these Nuremberg Code provisions. Under these regulations, research on fetuses will not be supported by DHEW unless appropriate studies on animals and nonpregnant individuals have been completed; and where the purpose of the activity is to meet the health needs of the individual fetus, the risk to the fetus is minimal, and the risk is the "least possible risk for achieving the objectives of the activity."[17] Nontherapeutic research can be conducted on fetuses *in utero* where the risk to the fetus is minimal and the purpose of the activity is the development of "important biomedical knowledge which cannot be obtained by other means."[18] Similar restrictions are also placed on research with *ex utero* fetuses.[19]

Why were more stringent requirements enacted to protect the welfare of fetuses than to protect other subjects? There seem to be two reasons. First, these regulations came on the heels of *Roe v. Wade*,[20] which legalized abortions throughout the United States. While one concern may have been that more fetuses would become available for research, numerous abortions had already been performed prior to *Roe*. Indeed, in 1972, one year prior to *Roe*, there were 586,760 legal abortions in the United States.[21] However, protecting fetuses from research abuses was a symbolic way for those who opposed abortion to express their concern for fetal life. Second, unlike research with adults, informed consent was not perceived as a way to protect fetuses, who obviously could not consent on their own behalf. These stringent fetal research regulations were designed to protect fetuses from presumably uncaring pregnant women, especially those who were contemplating abortion, and overzealous researchers. In the absence of the subject's ability to give informed consent and protect his own interest, the fetal research regulations were designed to protect the subject's welfare along the lines of the Nuremberg Code.

REVISED FEDERAL REGULATIONS

As a result of the work of the National Commission, the general rules applicable to research were revised in 1981,[22] and new rules were adopted to protect prisoners[23] and children[24] as research subjects. While similar in their general institutional approach to the previous rules, they are more explicit in a number of ways. Once again, the rules apply specifically only to research conducted or funded by the Department of Health and Human Services (DHHS), the successor agency to DHEW. However, in their general assurances to the DHHS, institutions must provide a statement of "principles governing the institution in the discharge of its responsibilities for protecting the rights and welfare of human subjects of research conducted at or sponsored by the institution, *regardless of source of funding*."[25] [Emphasis added.] This requirement expands the populations who are protected by these regulations.

Unlike either the Code or previous regulations, the new regulations define the term *research* to mean "a systematic investigation designed to develop or contribute to generalizable knowledge."[26] This means that novel therapies are not covered by these rules unless they are used in a protocol designed to contribute to generalizable knowledge. While research is defined, various types of research are exempted from the regulations' purview.[27] What is exempted are classes of research that do not put subjects at risk and do not require any physical contact with subjects. Included in this category is research involving surveys or observation, or research with pathological specimens.

These rules also adopt some Nuremberg Code-like guidelines for protecting the welfare of subjects. Thus, IRBs are to ensure that subjects are not "unnecessarily" exposed to risks, and that the risks are "reasonable in relation to anticipated benefits" to both the subjects (if any) and the importance of the knowledge that may reasonably be expected to result. These provisions are similar to provision 4 of the Code, which states that the experiment should be so conducted as to avoid "all unnecessary physical and mental suffering and injury," and provision 6, which states that the degree of risk to be taken "should never exceed that determined by the humanitarian importance of the problem to be solved by the experiment."

The revised regulations have a detailed informed consent provision. However, unlike the Code and previous regulations, which require the subject to be "so situated as to be able to exercise free power of choice without undue inducement or any element of force, fraud, deceit, duress or other form on constraint or coercion,"[28] the revised rules only require the investigator to seek consent under circumstances "that minimize the possibility of coercion or undue influence."[29] After elaborately setting out the elements of informed consent, the revised rules provide that the IRB can waive the requirement for obtaining informed consent if it finds and documents that all the following apply:

(1) The research involves no more than minimal risk to the subjects;
(2) The waiver or alteration will not adversely affect the rights and welfare of the subjects;
(3) The research could not practicably be carried out without the waiver or alteration; and
(4) Whenever appropriate, the subjects will be provided with additional pertinent information after participation.[30]

The waiver of the informed consent provision is a stark departure from the Code, which begins: "The voluntary consent of the human subject is absolutely essential." Indeed, if this Code provision is true, then the second waiver provision becomes impossible to apply because research without the subject's consent would always "adversely affect" the subject's right to give informed consent. While the waiver provision only includes research that involves no more than minimal risks, it does not limit the waiver to research that offers the prospect of benefit to the subject. As a result, it would seem that nonbeneficial research could be conducted on a nonconsenting subject, precisely the behavior the Nuremberg Code explicitly prohibits.

RESEARCH ON PRISONERS

The regulations specifically address the issue of prisoners as research subjects.[31] Because they are a captive population, prisoners present both the perceived and real problems of possible exploitation. Indeed, the Nuremberg "subjects" were obviously also a captive population. In many ways, the prisoner regulations are the most directive and prescriptive of all the research regulations. A majority of the IRB members reviewing prison research must have no association with the prison, and at least one member of the IRB must be a prisoner or a prisoners' representative. Prisoners may not be offered advantages, such as better food, living conditions, or medical care that would be of such magnitude that his or her ability to weigh the risks of participation in research would be impaired. Selection of prisoners as research subjects must be fair and immune from arbitrary intervention by prison authorities, and the prisoner must be informed that parole boards may not take into account a prisoner's participation in research when making parole decisions.

Only four classes of research involving prisoners are permitted: (1) the study of the possible causes, effects, and processes of incarceration and of criminal behavior; (2) the study of prisons as institutions or of prisoners as incarcerated persons; (3) research on conditions particularly affecting prisoners as a class (such as vaccine trials for diseases that are much more prevalent in prisons than elsewhere); and (4) research on innovative and accepted practices that have the "intent and reasonable probability" of improving the health or well-being of the subject.[32] All research in category 3 must be approved by the Secretary of DHHS and the intent to approve such research published in the *Federal Register*. This same approval and publication requirement applies to category 4 when some prisoners will act as controls in the study and, therefore, will not benefit. All research in categories 1 and 2 must present no more than minimal risk and no more than inconvenience to the subjects. No other research using prisoners as subjects is permissible under the regulations.

These prisoner regulations are even more stringent than the Code. They explicitly prohibit risky, nonbeneficial research, even with consent. They also require that there be a good reason for choosing prisoners as subjects. They are, therefore, very protective of the welfare of prisoner-subjects, while at the same time protecting their rights by removing the elements of coercion that might cause a prisoner to participate in a research project.

RESEARCH ON CHILDREN

The regulations that govern research with children were among the most difficult for the policymakers to draft and adopt. The first "draft working document" on research with children was published in 1973,[33] and it was not until 1983 that final regulations were adopted.[34] Adopting research regulations regarding children as subjects is complicated because arguments for and against such research are compelling. Children have been exploited as research subjects and indeed were particularly sought out for some of the Nazi experiments. On the other hand, children have benefited enormously from the biomedical and behavioral knowledge that has been acquired through properly conducted research. Many children, because of their immaturity, cannot give informed consent to research. On the other hand, unlike prisoners, children have advocates for and protectors of their health and well-being—their parents. However, the protective role of parents of sick children may be compromised because they will consent to almost any procedure that might preserve their child's life or health. There also may be limits on a parent's legal authority to consent to nonbeneficial, at-risk research. Because the term *children* encompasses everyone from newborns to 17-year-olds, the subjects themselves will have various levels of understanding and capacity. Furthermore, if the Nuremberg Code's categorical statement that the informed consent of the human *subject* is "essential" is true, then research on young children cannot be conducted.

The research rules governing children are a series of compromises that reflect these concerns. These rules divide research on children into four classes: (1) research not involving greater than minimal risk; (2) research involving greater than minimal risk but presenting the prospect of direct benefit to the subject; (3) research involving greater than minimal risk and no prospect of direct benefit to the subject, but likely to yield generalizable knowledge about the subject's disorder or condition; and (4) research not otherwise approvable which presents an opportunity to understand, prevent, or alleviate a serious problem affecting the health or welfare of children. This categorization constitutes a spectrum of risk and benefit to the child. Thus, research in category 1 has the fewest requirements. When the risk is minimal, even in the absence of benefit, research is permissible if adequate provisions are made for soliciting the "assent" of the child and permission from one parent. In category 2, an additional requirement is that the risk is justified by the anticipated benefit, and the risk-benefit ratio is at least as favorable as that presented by available alternative approaches. For category 3, which involves research that will not benefit the individual child, the risk must represent a minor increase over minimal risk, and the intervention or procedure must be commensurate with those inherent in the child's medical, psychological, social or educational situation. In addition, the intervention or procedure must be likely to yield generalizable knowledge about the subject's condition that is of "vital importance" for the understanding or amelioration of the subject's condition. Consent of both parents is required if they are both available. Category 4 includes all other research, and it requires the Secretary of DHHS's approval after consultation with experts. Such research may be approved if it presents a reasonable opportunity to further understand, prevent, or alleviate a serious problem affecting the health or welfare of children and will be conducted in accordance with sound, ethical principles. Again, both parents must consent if they are available. While the assent of the child is supposed to be solicited, it is up to each individual IRB to decide how and when this is to be required. The assent of the child is never required when research holds out the prospect of direct benefit to the child.

The child research regulations are the most vague and least prescriptive of the regulations protecting special populations. For example, while the fetal research regulations require appropriate research on animals and nonpregnant individuals to have been *completed* before conducting research on fetuses, no such limitation appears in the child research regulations. The prisoner research regulations permit only four types of research. By contrast, if the risks are minimal, any type of research can be conducted with children, even nonbeneficial research.

There are at least two possible reasons for the more liberal child research rules. First, unlike prisoners or fetuses (particularly fetuses subject to abortion), children are perceived as having natural protectors of their welfare — their parents. In a sense, these regulations make parents, as a class, the ultimate IRB for research with children. However, one may well question the parents' ability to perform this role in certain circumstances, such as when their child is very ill and an experimental procedure provides the only hope for survival.

Second, unlike prisoners, who are a subclass of adults, children are a unique research class. Children differ from adults in a variety of physiological, biological, and developmental ways, and some diseases and conditions are found only in children. Therefore, from a purely utilitarian point of view, children, unlike prisoners, are *needed* as research subjects, and the regulations are written so as not to block what is perceived as necessary research. However, fetuses are also a unique research population, and policymakers decided to make fetal research much more difficult to conduct than research with children.

STATE REGULATION OF RESEARCH

Little can be said about state regulation of research because so few states have such regulations. This may be because it is widely perceived that research is regulated by the federal government. As a practical matter, since so much human research is done using federal funds, or in institutions that receive federal funds, a great deal of such research is in fact federally regulated. It is not known how much research with human subjects is conducted that is not federally connected in some way, but however much it is, it is unregulated absent state law.

Three states have passed statutes that regulate human studies research: California,[35] New York,[36] and Virginia.[37] Their laws regulating human research have many similarities, and they all apply only to research that is not covered by federal regulations.[38] The California law contains legislative findings justifying the law, one of which is that "neither the Nuremberg Code nor the Declaration of Helsinki are codified under law and are, therefore, unenforceable."[39]

Each state defines experimentation or research somewhat differently. California defines *medical experiment* to mean:

   (a) The severance or penetration of damaging of tissues of a human subject or the use of a drug or device, as defined in Section 26009 or 26010, electromagnetic radiation, heat or cold, or a biological substance or organism, in or upon a human subject in the practice of research of medicine in a manner not reasonably related to maintaining or improving the health of such subject or otherwise directly benefiting such subject.

(b) The investigational use of a drug or device as provided in Sections 26678 and 26679.
(c) Withholding medical treatment from a human subject for any purpose other than maintenance or improvement of the health of such subject.[40]

New York law defines the term *human research* as follows:

"Human research" means any medical experiments, research, or scientific or psychological investigation, which utilizes human subjects and which involves physical or psychological intervention by the researcher upon the body of the subject and which is not required for the purposes of obtaining information for the diagnosis, prevention, or treatment of disease or the assessment of medical condition for the direct benefit of the subject. Human research shall not, however be construed to mean the conduct of biological studies exclusively utilizing tissue or fluids after their removal or withdrawal from a human subject in the course of standard medical practice, or to include epidemiological investigations.[41]

Virginia defines *human research* as follows:

"Human research" means any medical or psychological research which utilizes human subjects who may be exposed to the possibility of physical or psychological injury as a consequence of participation as subjects and which departs from the application of those established and accepted methods appropriate to meet the subject's or subjects' needs but does not include (i) the conduct of biological studies exclusively utilizing tissue or fluids after their removal or withdrawal from human subject in the course of standard medical practice, (ii) epidemiological investigations or (iii) medical treatment of an experimental nature intended to save or prolong the life of the subject in danger of death, to prevent the subject from becoming disfigured or physically or mentally incapacitated or to improve the quality of the subject's life.[42]

These definitions are largely directed at pure or nonbeneficial research. The Virginia definition explicitly excludes "medical treatment of an experimental nature" from its coverage. The California law covers only those research or medical interventions not "reasonably related" to maintaining or improving the health of the subject or directly benefiting the subject. By including the withholding of medical treatment in its definition of *medical experiment*, the California law clearly covers the use of placebos and subjects in the control arm of a research project. The New York definition would include even possibly beneficial research if it was not "required" for the direct benefit of the subject. This interpretation of the New York law is bolstered by its definition of the term *human subject*, which means an individual exposed to the "possibility of injury," including physical, psychological, or social injury, as a result of participation in research or a related activity "which departs from the application of those established and accepted methods necessary to meet his needs."[43]

All three state statutes have extensive sections regarding informed consent that are similar to the federal rules; and all use the language from the Nuremberg Code regarding the voluntary nature of the consent and the absence of force, fraud, deceit, or other undue inducements.

New York law authorizes parents and guardians to consent to all research. In Virginia, "legally authorized representatives" may *not* consent to non-therapeutic research that presents a "hazardous risk" to the subject.[44] In California, informed consent given on behalf of an incompetent subject shall "only be for medical experiments related to maintaining or improving the health of the human subject or related to obtaining information about a pathological condition of the human subject,"[45] although it is unclear if this limitation applies to parents of minor children.

The statutes in Virginia and New York also require proposed research to be reviewed by a "human research review committee" established by the institution in which the research is to be performed. The tasks of these committees are similar to those of IRBs, such as reviewing the adequacy of consent and weighing the risks and benefits of the proposed research. In New York, a board must determine "the necessity" for the research, and in both states the committee must determine if the person proposing the research is "appropriately competent and qualified."

Neither the Virginia nor the New York statutes specify a sanction for their violation. The California law contains both civil and criminal sanctions. A researcher who negligently or willfully fails to obtain a subject's informed consent is liable to the subject in amounts ranging from $50 to $5,000. A researcher who willfully fails to obtain a subject's informed consent and thereby exposes the subject to a known substantial risk of either bodily or psychological harm is guilty of a misdemeanor punishable by imprisonment of up to 1 year and/or a fine of $10,000. By adopting criminal penalties, the California legislature mirrored the actions of the Nuremberg judges.

Fetal experimentation is the one exception to the rule that states tend not to regulate human research by statute. At least 25 states have laws that regulate research with fetuses.[46] There is a wide array of approaches, varying from merely requiring the mother's consent, to the prohibition of the sale or distribution of fetal remains, to the banning of all fetal research not designed to benefit the individual fetus.[47] Unlike other human research laws, fetal research laws are often criminal statutes. For example, in Massachusetts, violation of the fetal research statute is punishable by imprisonment of 1 to 5 years and a fine of up to $10,000.

CONCLUSION

Has the Nuremberg Code been adopted through statutes and regulations in the United States? The answer to this question varies depending on how one views the Code and current statutes and regulations. In terms of overall philosophy, the Code itself does not take a position on the issue of the propriety of human research. The judges pointed out that "protagonists of the practice of human experimentation justify their views" on the basis that society secures substantial benefits from the practice. The judges themselves never said if they agree with this argument. The best they could do was to find that the weight of evidence indicates that when human experimentation is "kept within reasonably well-defined bounds," it "conforms to the ethics of the medical profession generally."[48] This is a rather lukewarm acceptance of human experimentation. Thus, the judges concluded that even if research is good, it is an optional good that must be balanced against respect for human beings, which is not optional but mandatory. Where the welfare of human beings is threatened by research, the research must not be done.

This approach is largely due to the context in which the Code was adopted. While we currently struggle to understand terms like *therapeutic research* or *nontherapeutic research*, or to define the exact scope of *informed consent*, these matters were of no concern to the Nazi doctors. From their perspective, what the Nazi doctors were doing was more akin to animal research than human research. Indeed, the practices of the Nazi doctors and the conditions their victims were forced to live in would violate current animal research regulations, let alone human research regulations. Frankly, it is insulting to legitimate researchers to compare what they do with anything the Nazi doctors did. While the Nazi doctors may have been performing "research" in the sense that they were answering "scientific questions" they posed, their tools were torture and murder.

Given this, the Nuremberg Code was devised to resolve a straightforward, though horrifying, situation. One even wonders why a code of conduct was needed to prohibit future "experimentation" of the type the Nazis conducted; the laws prohibiting murder, mayhem, and maiming should have been sufficient. The judges' adoption of a "Code" is probably indicative of their shock in finding that there were essentially no written standards for human experimentation that had been adopted by an authoritative institution. The Code itself is simply 10 universal standards of human decency. One would require no special training in law, ethics, or medicine to create such a Code if it did not now exist. By explicitly setting forth these minimal standards on paper, the judges ensured that no future researcher could attempt to argue that he was not aware of them.

Because of the monstrous nature of the acts committed by the defendants, the subtle nuances of the ethics of human experimentation were not an issue. The judges were not required to consider, and did not consider, for example, the issues that arise when research is proposed on children whose parents are available to consent or research that has inherent dangers but might offer direct benefit to individual subjects. In this respect, the Nuremberg Code offers little to guide us other than its general regard for the well-being of human subjects in dealing with these more complicated issues. Indeed, these shortcomings of the Nuremberg Code were well recognized by the drafters of the Declaration of Helsinki, who suggested the differences between nontherapeutic research and clinical research combined with professional care, and explicitly recognized the validity of proxy consent in certain circumstances.

The closest we have come to adopting the principles of the Nuremberg Code in the United States is in the area of fetal research. The federal regulations do not permit such research unless animal research and research on nonpregnant individuals is first completed; the research itself must not put the fetus at added risk; the purpose of the research must be to develop important biomedical knowledge unobtainable by other means; and the experimental activities must not themselves terminate the fetal heartbeat or respiration. Only research that is designed to meet the health needs of the fetus or its mother is permissible, but the risk must be the least possible for achieving its objectives. State laws tend to prohibit nontherapeutic research on fetuses altogether. Unlike most other areas of human research, the emphasis is on the protection and welfare of the subject, not on the subject's consent. This is because the supporters of fetal research restrictions perceive the fetus as extraordinarily vulnerable to misuse, particularly fetuses who are the subject of planned abortions. They also see such fetuses as having no concerned person available to protect them. The balance that has been drawn in fetal research is that the creation of new knowledge will have to give way to protective concerns. The other aspect of the state fetal research statutes that makes them similar to the Nuremberg Code is that the individual investigator is subject to criminal penalties for their violation.

The strict limitation on prisoner research also reflects the Nuremberg Code's concern for captive, and therefore exploitable, populations. These regulations can be summarized by stating that unless an investigator can prove that there is a good reason for conducting research in prisons, it presumptively cannot be done in that setting.

The rest of the population, including children, is covered by a much more general and permissive set of guidelines. Unlike the federal fetal research regulations or the Nuremberg Code, there is no requirement that animal testing be completed or even attempted. In children's regulations, unlike prisoner regulations, there is no explicit requirement that only children would be acceptable research subjects. Probably the greatest departure from the Nuremberg Code is the federal regulations' approval of some minimal-risk research without the consent of the subject or a surrogate, even where the research will not benefit the subject. A final significant way in which the federal regulations depart from the Code is that the Code focuses on the responsibility of the individual investigator, whereas the federal regulations focus on the institution receiving the research funds. The few applicable state statutes, however, continue to focus on the investigator.

In general, current federal regulations express much more enthusiasm for human research than the Code does. While these regulations place certain restrictions on researchers, they also are generally more permissive than the Nuremberg Code and contain language ensuring that research can be performed even on nonconsenting subjects. There are several reasons for this. First, the federal regulations were adopted by an arm of the government that itself fosters and believes in research. Second, unlike the Code, the regulations apply to therapeutic research, which may benefit the individual research subject. Therefore, failure to perform such research might be viewed as depriving subjects of a benefit. Finally, the current regulations were not written in response to terrible research abuses.

The Nuremberg Code is an exclusively substantive document, whereas the federal regulations contain procedural safeguards. These safeguards are embodied primarily in IRB review and public scrutiny by requiring at least one member of the IRB to be from the community. The mere fact of such scrutiny and the risk of exposure deter unethical research. However, such review acts as a safeguard only when the values of the reviewers are directed at protecting human well-being. It is unlikely that IRB review in Nazi Germany would have led to more humane treatment of subjects.

In regard to pure or nontherapeutic research, the Nuremberg Code is as vital a document today as it was when it was created. It also presents us with a starting point when discussing the regulation of human research. While it should not be seen as a magic talisman, which must be complied with in all circumstances, those who propose exceptions to the Code's restrictions must be able to justify them. However, the ultimate enduring value of the Code is not in its detailed provisions but in its approach to human dignity. As one commentator put it, the Code "squarely acknowledges the scientist's responsibility for the respect of human rights."[49] This overriding philosophy must guide all research, now and in the future. Scientific progress is important, but the human subject comes first.

NOTES

1. U.S. Department of Health, Education and Welfare, *Healthy Volunteers Help Scientist Conquer Disease*, PHS Pub. No. 714 (Washington, D.C.: Public Health Service, NIH, 1959), p. 14.

2. NIH, *Handbook on the Utilization of Normal Volunteers in the Clinical Center*, Section 3.06, (1961), p. 10.

3. W. Curran, "Governmental Regulation of the Use of Human Subjects in Medical Research: The Approach of Two Federal Agencies," *Daedalus: Ethical Aspect of Experimentation with Human Subjects* 98(2) (Spring 1969): 542.

4. Ibid., 554, citing sec. 505 (i) of the Federal Food, Drug and Cosmetic Act.

5. Ibid., 577.

6. Ibid., 589.

7. 39 Federal Register 18914 (May 30, 1974).

8. Public Law 93-348.

9. 45 CFR part 46; 40 Federal Regulations 33526 (August 8, 1975).

10. 45 CFR 46.106(b) (1) (1975).

11. 45 CFR 46.102(b) (1975).

12. 45 CFR 46.103(b) (1975).

13. 45 CFR 46.109, 46.110 (1975).

14. 45 CFR 46.103(c) (1975).

15. 45 CFR 46.103(c) (6) (1975).

16. 45 CFR 46.121 (1975).

17. 45 CFR 46.206(1) (2) (1975).

18. 45 CFR 46.208(a) (1975).

19. 45 CFR 209 (1975).

20. *Roe v. Wade*, 410 U.S. 113 (1973).

21. 38 MMWR 663 (September 29, 1989).

22. 46 Fed. Reg. 8386 (January 26, 1981).

23. 42 Fed. Reg. 53655 (November 16, 1978).

24. Fed. Reg. 9818 (March 8, 1983).

25. 45 CFR 46.103 (1983).

26. 45 CFR 46.102(e) (1983).

27. 45 CFR 46.101 b(1)–(6) (1983).

28. 45 CFR 46.103(c) (1975), Nuremberg Code, Provision 1.

29. 45 CFR 46.116 (1983).

30. 45 CFR 46.117(d) (1983).

31. 45 CFR 46.301 *et. seq.* (1983).

32. 45 CFR 46.306(a) (2) (A)–(D) (1983).

33. 38 Fed. Reg. 3176 (November 16, 1973).

34. 48 Fed. Reg. 9818 (March 8, 1983).

35. Ann. Cal. Code ch. 1.3, sec. 24170 *et. seq.*

36. New York Public Health Law, Art. 24A, sec. 2440 *et. seq.* (hereafter, New York Law).

37. Code of Virginia, ch. 11, sec. 37 1-234 *et. seq.* (hereafter, Virginia Law).

38. California Law, sec. 24178; New York Law, sec. 2445; Virginia Law, sec. 37.1.237.

39. California Law at 24171(b).

40. California Law, sec. 24174.

41. New York Law, sec. 2441(2).

42. Virginia Law, sec. 37.1.234(1).

43. New York Law, sec. 2441(1).

44. Virginia Law, sec. 37.1-235(b).

45. California Law, sec. 24.75(e).

46. C. Baron, "Legislative Regulation of Fetal Experimentation: On Negotiating Compromise in Situation of Ethical Pluralism," in A. Milunsky and G. J. Annas, eds., *Genetics and the Law*, Vol. III (New York: Plenum Press, 1985), p. 431.

47. See e.g. Minnesota Statutes, sec. 145.422; Ill. Rev. St. ch. 38, sec. 81-26(7) and sec. 81-32; South Dakota Compiled Laws sec. 34-23A-17.

48. J. Katz, *Experimentation with Human Beings* (New York: Russell Saga Foundation, 1972), p. 305.

49. M. C. Bassiouni, T. Baffes and J. Evrard, "An Appraisal of Human Experimentation in International Law and Practice: The Need for International Regulation of Human Experimentation," *Journal of Criminal Law and Criminology* 72 (1981): 1597, 1642.

11

The Nuremberg Code in U.S. Courts: Ethics versus Expediency

GEORGE J. ANNAS

"The most complete and authoritative statement of the law of informed consent to human experimentation is the Nuremberg Code."[1] That was the conclusion Leonard Glantz, Barbara Katz, and I reached 15 years ago in our study of informed consent to human experimentation for the National Commission for the Protection of Subjects of Biomedical and Behavioral Research. We went on to say, "This Code is part of international common law and may be applied in both civil and criminal cases, by state, federal and municipal courts in the United States."[2] I still believe these two statements are true, but viewing the Nuremberg Code from an early 1990s' perspective leads to the conclusion that these observations are less meaningful than might be supposed. Although courts in the United States *may* use the Nuremberg Code to set criminal and civil standards of conduct, none have used it in a criminal case and only a handful have even cited it in the civil context. Even where the Nuremberg Code has been cited as authoritative, it has usually been in dissent, and no U.S. court has ever awarded damages to an injured experimental subject, or punished an experimenter, on the basis of a violation of the Code.

This chapter explores the paradox that the most "complete and authoritative statement of the law of informed consent to human experimentation" has almost never been cited by U.S. courts in its more than four decades of existence. The goal is to clarify the Code's legal status in the United States. This seems a reasonable study, since the Doctors' Trial was conducted by U.S. judges under the authority of the U.S. military, U.S. procedures were followed, and U.S. lawyers acted as the prosecutors. Thus, if any country should feel itself bound by the legal precepts of the Nuremberg Code, it is the United States.

It should be stressed at the outset, however, that there have been very few court decisions involving human experimentation. This means that it is difficult for a "common law" of human experimentation to develop. But it also makes codes, especially judicially crafted codes like the Nuremberg Code, all the more important. Moreover, throughout World War II and since then, American governmental officials have evidenced a profound ambivalence with regard to human experimentation. On the one hand, we punished the Nazi physicians and scientists and publicized their brutality to deter future violations of human rights in medical experimentation, thus evidencing a sincere and serious desire to protect human rights in human experimentation. On the other hand, at the Tokyo War Crime Trials, we made a deal with the Japanese military medical officers who conducted lethal biological warfare experiments on U.S. prisoners of war in China during World War II. The deal was that we would not prosecute them if they disclosed the results of their experiments to the U.S. military.[3] This action was based on an expedient, utilitarian ethic that accepted whatever information was available to protect the national security in a world that was viewed as hostile to the United States. The tension between protecting individual rights and protecting national security had often been decided in favor of the national security during the cold war.

Any meaningful study of the role of the Nuremberg Code in U.S. law requires an examination of pre-Nuremberg litigation involving human experimentation, reaction to the Nuremberg Code as a legal document, and a discussion of the handful of U.S. cases that have cited the Nuremberg Code, directly or indirectly, since World War II.

PRE-NUREMBERG APPELLATE DECISIONS

Although we commonly make a distinction between therapeutic and non-therapeutic research today, before World War II no such distinction was made in the U.S. courts.[4] Court cases alleging experimentation all involved novel treatments for illnesses. Experimentation was often defined as a deviation from standard medical practice that could only be justified by its results.

A Missouri court, for example, said in 1926 of a physician who used an injection for hemorrhoids: "A failure to employ the methods followed or approved by his school of practice evidences either ignorance or experimentation on his part. The law tolerates neither."[5] It was not until the Depression that a Michigan court first mentioned the role of consent in experimentation:

> We recognize the fact that, if the general practice of medicine and surgery is to progress, there must be a certain amount of experimentation carried on; but such experiments must be done with the *knowledge and consent of the patient* or those responsible for him, and *must not vary too radically from the accepted method* of procedure.[6]

Two cases decided at the beginning of World War II demonstrate both a new appreciation for the role of experimentation in medical progress by U.S. courts and a new insistence on the consent of the patient or subject. In the first case, a physician's license was suspended for fraud and deceit for using a topical medication for face cancer. The medication had been developed by another patient of the physician and was used only after he had tired it on himself to be sure that there were no side effects. The physician had informed the patient that the treatment was experimental, and that it might do some good and couldn't do any harm. A complete cure was affected. In reversing the licensing board's decision to suspend his license for fraud, a New York court said:

> It is not fraud or deceit for one already skilled in the medical art, *with the consent of his patient*, to attempt new methods when all other known methods of treatment had proved futile and least of all when the patient's very life has been despaired of. *Initiative and originality should not be thus effectively stifled*, especially when undertaken with the patient's full knowledge and consent, and as a last resort.[7]

The second case is the only *nontherapeutic* experimentation case decided by a U.S. court before the articulation of the Nuremberg Code. It involved a 15-year-old junior high school student, John M. Bonner, whose cousin had been severely burned and was in a charity clinic in Washington, D.C.[8] After several attempts to find a skin graft donor failed, his aunt persuaded the boy to go to the hospital. A surgeon, Robert Moran, eventually cut a "tube of flesh" from his armpit to his waist and attached it surgically to his cousin, forming a literal flesh and blood bond between them. The attempt to nurture the skin transplant with the boy's blood was unsuccessful, and the tube itself was severed when young Bonner lost so much blood that he required transfusions. He was in the hospital for 2 months. The trial court found that Bonner was sufficiently mature to consent to the experiment and had in fact done so. The appeals court agreed that there were times when a minor was emancipated or mature enough to consent to beneficial medical treatment, but it held that these exceptions to the requirement of informed consent of a parent did not apply in the nontherapeutic context:

> *Here the operation was entirely for the benefit of another* and involved sacrifice on the part of the infant of fully two months of schooling, in addition to serious pain and possible results affecting his future life. This immature colored boy was subjected several times to treatment involving anesthesia, blood letting, and the removal of skin from his body, with at least some permanent marks of disfigurement.[9]

Accordingly, this pre-Nuremberg Code case held that if both the mature minor *and* the parent consent to nonbeneficial or nontherapeutic experimentation of this kind, it can legally be performed.

REACTION TO THE NUREMBERG CODE

The first U.S. court cited the Nuremberg Code in 1973, more than 25 years after the Code had been promulgated. This is striking because, as previously noted, all of the judges at the Doctors' Trial were Americans, the prosecutors were American, the procedural rules followed were American, and the case itself was brought under the authority of the military governor of the American Zone. Why wasn't the Nuremberg Code immediately adopted by U.S. courts as setting the minimum standard of care for human experimentation?

One reason, perhaps, is that there was little opportunity. As remains true today, almost no experiments resulted in lawsuits in the 1940s, 1950s, and 1960s. A second reason may be that the Nazi experiments were considered so extreme as to be irrelevant to the United States. This may explain why our own use of prisoners, the institutionalized retarded, and the mentally ill to test malaria treatments during World War II was generally hailed as positive, making the war "everyone's war."[10] Likewise, in the late 1940s and early 1950s, it was seen as perfectly appropriate to test new polio vaccines on institutionalized, mentally retarded children.[11] Utilitarianism was the ethic of the day.

Denial of any link to the Nazi atrocities also characterized the reaction of the medical community to the Nuremberg Code. Noting that the Code applied primarily to the outrageous nontherapeutic experiments conducted during the war, physician groups tended to find the Code too legalistic and irrelevant to their therapeutic experiments, and set about to develop an alternative code to guide medical researchers. The most successful and influential such code has been the World Medical Association's Declaration of Helsinki, adopted in 1964 and amended three times since. The World Medical Association (WMA) was formed in 1946 at the headquarters of the British Medical Association in London, where physicians from Western Europe had been meeting informally during World War II. The hope was that should war ever come again, "the action of the World Medical Association in this field will act as a brake upon medical war crimes."[12]

In 1954, the WMA's 8th General Assembly, meeting in Rome, adopted five general "Principles for Those in Research and Experimentation," including:

3. *Experimentation on Healthy Subjects.*
   Subjects . . . [should be] fully informed. The paramount factor in experimentation on human beings is the responsibility of the research worker and not the willingness of the person submitting to the experiment.
4. *Experimentation on Sick Subjects.*
   . . . one may attempt an operation or a treatment of a rather daring nature. Such exceptions will be rare and require the approval either of the person or his next of kin. In such a situation it is the doctor's conscience which will make the decision.

> 5. *Necessity of Informing the Person.* . . . It should be required that each person who submits to experimentation be informed of the nature and the reason for the risk of the proposed experiment. If the patient is irresponsible, consent should be obtained from the individual who is legally responsible for the individual. In both instances, consent should be obtained in writing.[13]

The differentiation between healthy subjects and sick subjects and the general approval of proxy consent are evident and mark a departure from the Nuremberg Code's sole emphasis on nontherapeutic experiments. Hugh Clegg, editor of the *British Medical Journal*, was given the task of drafting a new code. In a 1960 article, Clegg reviewed the Nuremberg Code with general approval but concluded that Hippocrates was the real guide: "So long as the research worker is imbued with the Hippocratic ideal, this and his conscience should be a sufficient guide."[14]

Perhaps the most important single event that helped push final adoption of the 1964 Declaration of Helsinki was the U.S. Food and Drug Administration's (FDA) proposal to standardize research on experimental drugs in the United States following the thalidomide tragedy. The advent of large-scale drug trials in the United States and throughout the world made it necessary to address the issue of human experimentation in a far different context than either the Nazi concentration camp model or the simple Hippocratic doctor–patient relationship model. Subtitled "Recommendations Guiding Doctors in Clinical Research," the Helsinki Declaration of 1964 was simply this: recommendations to physicians by physicians.

By the early 1970s, the Helsinki Declaration was widely admired by physicians as an advance over the Nuremberg Code. Perhaps Henry Beecher expressed the physician view best when he said in 1970:

> The Nuremberg Code presents a rigid act of legalistic demands. . . . *The Declaration of Helsinki*, on the other hand, presents a set of guides. It *is an ethical as opposed to a legalistic document* and is thus a more broadly useful instrument than the one formulated at Nuremberg. . . . *Until recently the Western world was threatened with the imposition of the Nuremberg Code as a Western credo.* With the Declaration of Helsinki, this danger is apparently now past.[15]

Similarly, the president of the Council for International Organizations of Medical Sciences (CIOMS) stated in 1967 that "On the whole [the Declaration of Helsinki] corrects what in the Nuremberg Rules was circumstantial, related to Nazi crimes, and places those Rules more correctly in the context of generally accepted medical traditions."[16]

On the other hand, Jay Katz argued insightfully in 1973 at an international CIOMS conference:

> Do not place too much reliance on codes of ethics, such as the Declaration of Helsinki. That would be dangerous. Codes are deceptive documents to which all of us probably could subscribe in principle; but if you study them carefully, you

will find that they are painfully vague. They do not inform us well about actual decisions which investigators have to make day after day. The Declaration of Helsinki, analogous to a legal statute, requires opportunities for interpretation; only then could it become a viable document.[17]

The only authoritative forum for interpretation of a code is the courtroom. Such interpretation began, coincidentally, the same year Professor Katz called for it: 1973.

THE NUREMBERG CODE IN LOWER U.S. COURTS

Before 1973 the Nazi doctors were alluded to only in a dissenting opinion in *Strunk v. Strunk*,[18] a Kentucky case decided by a vote of 4 to 3, in which the removal of a kidney from a mentally retarded and institutionalized adult was authorized for transplantation into his brother, justified on the basis that the "donation" would be "beneficial" to the donor. Doctors testified that had the mentally retarded brother suffered kidney failure, he would not have been eligible for either dialysis or a transplant. In dissent, Justice Samuel Steinfeld wrote:

> Apparently because of my indelible recollection of a government which, to the everlasting shame of its citizens, embarked on a program of genocide and experimentation with human bodies I have been more troubled in reaching a decision in this case than in any other. My sympathies and emotions are torn between a compassion to aid an ailing young man and a duty to fully protect unfortunate members of society.[19]

The lawyer for the widow of the recipient of the world's first artificial heart, Haskell Karp, tried to introduce the Nuremberg Code into evidence in a malpractice case following the 1969 implant. He failed when the trial judge, John V. Singleton, ruled that the Nuremberg Code was irrelevant since the implant was done to try to save Karp's life, and was therefore not experimental but therapeutic.[20]

The first U.S. case to actually make use of the Nuremberg Code involved a three-judge lower court panel in Detroit, Michigan, in a 1973 case involving psychosurgery.[21] Although not precedent anywhere outside Detroit, the case was followed nationally because of the political debate about psychosurgery (the destruction of histologically normal brain tissue for the purpose of modifying undesirable behavior) at the time. In 1972, two psychiatrists had obtained state funds to study the effects of amygdalotomy (the destruction of a portion of the brain's limbic system) and cyproterone acetate (an antiandrogen) on male aggression in prisons and mental health facilities. The goal was to modify antisocial behavior so that inmates could be safely released to the community. The study protocol was approved by both a scientific review committee and a human rights committee. Twenty-four candidates were sought for the study, but only one, Louis Smith, was considered suitable. He had been confined in a Michigan state hospital as a criminal sexual psychopath for 17 years, having been charged with (but never tried for) murder and rape. He and his parents had signed a detailed consent form when a lawsuit was commenced by a public interest group to halt the proposed experiment.

In considering the challenge, the panel of judges focused on whether involuntarily confined individuals could legally consent to experimental brain surgery designed to alter aggressive behavior. In deciding how to answer this question, the court reprinted the entire text of the Nuremberg Code for "guidance," saying:

> In the Nuremberg Judgment, the elements of what must guide us in decision are found. The involuntarily detained mental patient must have legal capacity to give consent. He must be so situated as to be able to exercise free power of choice, without any element of force, fraud, deceit, duress, overreaching, or other ulterior form of restraint or coercion. He must have sufficient knowledge and comprehension of the subject matter to enable him to make an understanding decision. The decision must be a totally voluntary one on his part.[22]

Applying these standards, the court concluded that Smith could not give voluntary, competent, informed, or understanding consent; consequently, the procedure could not be done. The court went further: It determined that given the current state of knowledge, *no one* could give an understanding consent to this procedure, effectively outlawing it in Detroit. This opinion has been justifiably criticized on a number of grounds, but its use of the Nuremberg Code as a standard for judgment has not been one of them. Shortly after this case was decided, a California appeals court ruled that portions of a statute regulating psychosurgery were unconstitutional because they were "impermissibly vague."[23] The Nuremberg Code was not mentioned.

The next U.S. judge to mention the Nuremberg Code was Justice Morris Pashman of the New Jersey Supreme Court in dissent in a 1980 employment case involving allegedly wrongful discharge.[24] A physician, Grace Pierce, had been employed as Director of Medical Research/Therapeutics at Ortho Pharmaceuticals. Her primary responsibility was to oversee the development of new drugs. In 1975 she was the only physician on a team developing loperamide, a liquid drug for treating diarrhea that contained saccharin. An Investigational New Drug (IND) application was being prepared for the FDA. Pierce objected to continued development of the drug because she believed saccharin was a risk to children and the elderly, and therefore it would violate her interpretation of the Hippocratic oath to test it on them. She was removed from the loperamide project and subsequently resigned. In her lawsuit against Ortho, she alleged that the company had required her to act contrary to the Hippocratic oath, specifically the part that states, "I will prescribe regimen for the good of my patients according to my ability and my judgment and never do harm to anyone."

The New Jersey Supreme Court found her reliance on an ethical code too vague because the FDA had yet to approve the IND application. Until it did so, no one would be given the drug, and no harm could be done. In the court's words:

> The case would be far different if Ortho had filed the IND, the FDA had disapproved it, and Ortho insisted on testing the drug on humans. The actual facts are that Dr. Pierce could not have harmed anyone by continuing to work on loperamide.[25]

The court characterized a disagreement at this point of the IND process as a "difference in medical opinions" at Ortho, and concluded that upholding Pierce's claim would lead to chaos in drug development and would harm research:

> Dr. Pierce espouses a doctrine that would lead to disorder in drug research. Under her theory, a professional employee could redetermine the propriety of a research project even if the research did not involve a violation of a clear mandate of public policy. *Chaos would result if a single doctor engaged in research were allowed to determine, according to his or her individual conscience, whether a project should continue.*[26]

In dissent, Justice Pashman argued that codes more specific than the Hippocratic oath provided Pierce with a "clear public policy" mandate, and that she should at least have the opportunity to present to a jury these "recognized codes of medical ethics that proscribe participation in clinical experimentation when a doctor perceives an unreasonable threat to human health." Justice Pashman then quoted the Helsinki Declaration, the AMA ethical guidelines for clinical investigation, and the Nuremberg Code. Of the Code he said, "A final source of ethical guidelines in what is now called the 'Nuremberg Code.' . . . The Judicial Council of the American Medical Association has adopted the Nuremberg Code as an expression of ethical principles governing human experimentation." He then set forth the text of principles 5, 6, 7, and 10, and concluded by noting that the Nuremberg Code "conditions a doctor's participation [in experimentation] on his 'good faith, superior skill and careful judgment' that the experiment is safe."[27]

THE COLD WAR MENTALITY AND HUMAN EXPERIMENTATION

The Michigan psychosurgery case and the New Jersey wrongful discharge dissent both cite and reprint all or part of the text of the Nuremberg Code itself. The next case deals with an "experiment" that might be considered uncivilized by any code. It is included because of its relevance to military experiments even though the "Nuremberg Code" the court refers to is actually the Nuremberg Principles derived from the first war crimes trial.[28] It is also the first of a series of cases that seems to justify brutal experimentation if needed to fight the cold war.

A suit was brought by a former U.S. soldier alleging that in 1953, only 6 years after the Nuremberg Code was promulgated, he and other members of his unit were ordered to stand in a field without any protection against radiation while a nuclear device was exploded in the Nevada desert.[29] As a result of this exposure, the plaintiff, Stanley Jaffee, died of cancer in November 1977. The U.S. Court of Appeals decided that Jaffee's claim for compensation for an intentional and unconstitutional tort was barred by the *Feres* doctrine, which had been interpreted by the U.S. Supreme Court to mean that soldiers "injured in the course of activity incident to service" may not sue the government for compensation. Responding to an argument by the minority that the actions of the U.S. military in this case were a violation of many international standards, including the Nuremberg Code, the court said, "The majority neither endorses nor sanctions a concentration camp mentality . . . what we are called upon to decide is simply whether the plaintiffs are entitled to money damages."[30]

The dissenting judges thought that requiring soldiers to stand near the explosion of a nuclear device without protection against radiation was "a violation of human rights on a massive scale." They noted that the allegation is that "civilian and military officials of the government, acting without legal authority and with no sufficient legitimate military or other purpose, conducted a human experiment upon soldiers subject to their control, without their knowledge, permission or consent, by exposing them to radiation which those officials knew to be dangerous."[31] The dissenters further argued that no law should place the plaintiffs beyond its protection because this conduct went "beyond the bounds of social acceptability." In their words:

> the complaint alleges conduct which would violate the Universal Declaration of Human Rights, the International Covenant on Civil and Political Rights, the Geneva Convention, the Declaration on the Protection of All Persons from Being Subjected to Torture and Other Cruel, Inhuman or Degrading Treatment or Punishment, and the Nuremberg Code. *The international consensus against involuntary human experimentation is clear. A fortiori* the conduct charged, if it occurred, was a violation of the Constitution and laws of the United States and of the state where it occurred or where its effects were felt.[32]

The dissenters expressed astonishment that "any judicial tribunal in the world, in the last half of this dismal century, would choose to place a class of persons outside the protection against human rights violations provided by the admonitory law of intentional torts."[33]

The dissenters would have been even more astonished when, 3 years later, a federal district court judge treated the Nuremberg Code simply as a discussion document without legal force in the United States. That court also adopted one of the Nazi defenses as legitimate: In times of national emergency, research rules must take a backseat to national security. Former

Navajo uranium miners and their survivors had brought suit against the U.S. government for compensation for injuries suffered as a result of exposure to radiation during uranium mining.[34] Among the allegations was that the U.S. Public Health Service (PHS) had conducted a prospective epidemiological study of a cohort of uranium miners from 1949 to 1960 to see if they were at increased risk for cancer, lung disease, and other problems. The miners were given an annual physical exam in 1950, 1951, 1953, and every 3 years thereafter until 1960. They were told that the exam was part of a study of the health of uranium miners, but they were not warned of any suspected risks in uranium mining or told of the purpose of the study.

The study was discontinued in 1960 and replaced by the more accurate annual sputum cytology studies. In responding to the suggestion that it was a violation of the rights of the miners in this Tuskegee-like study[35] not to tell them what the real aims of the study were, the court said simply:

> The PHS epidemiological *study protocol and the conduct* of the PHS physicians participating in the study and the limits on the information given to the miners studied *were consistent with the medical ethical and legal standards of the 1940s and 1950s.* It was not until the 1964 and 1965 period that federal guidelines were established for the conduct of federally-funded research projects. This followed discussion in the legal community, the medical community, and congressional hearings after the Nuremberg trials of Nazi war criminals engaged in human experimentation in the German concentration camps. The PHS physicians here were not experimenting on human beings. They were gathering data to be used for the establishment of radiation exposure in uranium mines.[36]

In concluding that the decision not to tell the Navajo miners about the risk of uranium radiation, and why this decision was a "discretionary" one and thus not covered by the Federal Tort Claims Act (FTCA), Judge William Copple's logic is disturbing. He borrows a hypothetical example Judge Bruce Jenkins had used in *Allen v. U.S.* to illustrate the extent of the discretionary authority federal officials have under the FTCA:

> Suppose a high level decision maker says, "International pressures make open-air atomic testing highly necessary. Time is of the essence. We cannot tell our own people. We just need to do it and do it fast as we can. We know as a result of such testing some people are going to get hurt. We can't tell them they are going to get hurt. We can't even warn them what to do to minimize or prevent the hurt. *In order to preserve our way of life* some people unknown to them and unknown to us are going to give their all for the good of all."[37]

Judges Jenkins and Copple both concluded that those injured by such a government policy, in blatant disregard of human rights and human life, would have no redress because it would be as a result of a discretionary act.[38] Judge Copple went further. He concluded that the PHS decision not to inform the research subjects of the risk of continued exposure to uranium was justified "based on considerations of political and national security feasibility factors."[39]

THE DEEP DIVING EXPERIMENT

The final lower court case citing the Nuremberg Code is a civilian tort action involving a nontherapeutic experiment, a series of simulated deep-sea dives conducted at Duke University in 1981.[40] The experiment, called "Atlantis III," involved research on high-pressure nervous syndrome. The research subject, Leonard Whitlock, was an experienced diver with a degree in oceanographic technology. He had made approximately 1,500 scuba dives, 200–300 tethered air dives, 200 oxygen surface decompression dives, 50 mixed gas dives, and 6 helium-oxygen saturation dives to between 450 and 680 feet. He had also participated in an earlier experiment, Atlantis I. The Atlantis III plan was to simulate a dive to 2,250 feet, a new world record.

Prior to the experiment, Whitlock signed an informed consent form advising him of the risks of possible lung collapse, production of fluid, hearing loss, inflammation of the ear, and sinusitis. Decompression risks were described as including death, disability, and joint pain. "Unknown risks" were also possible because "the research was experimental." After the dive, Whitlock suffered permanent organic brain damage and brought suit alleging, among other things, fraudulent and negligent failure to warn of the risk of organic brain disease. The defendants moved for summary judgment, which the court granted.

On the issue of informed consent, the court cited the Nuremberg Code as authoritative in the nontherapeutic context, setting forth the entire text of principles 1, 7, and 8. The court continued:

> Two important differences to note between the Nuremberg Code and sec. 90-21.13 [North Carolina's informed consent statute] are that *the subjective consent of the subject is always required under the Nuremberg Code* whereas under sec. 90-21.13 a health care provider may escape liability if a reasonable person would have consented if the proper disclosure of information had been made; and more importantly for the purposes of this case *the Nuremberg Code requires the researcher to make known to the subject all hazards reasonably to be expected* and the possible effects upon the health and person of the subject, whereas sec. 90-21.13 only requires the health care provider to apprise the patient of the "usual and most frequent risks and hazards" of the procedure.[41]

The court thus used the Nuremberg Code as the legal standard for disclosure, properly concluding that "the degree of required disclosure of risks is higher in the nontherapeutic context." In applying this principle, however, the court found that Whitlock failed to provide any evidence that there was a foreseeable or known risk of organic brain damage associated with the Atlantis III experiment. The physician supervisor knew of no such injury that had ever been seen as a result of deep diving experiments, and none was mentioned in the literature. Therefore, it could not be concluded that organic brain disease was a "reasonably foreseeable risk" that must be disclosed.

THE U.S. SUPREME COURT AND THE NUREMBERG CODE

The U.S. Supreme Court has had occasion to mention the Nuremberg Code in only one opinion, *United States v. Stanley*, in 1987.[42] A related opinion involving access to government records of government-sponsored nontherapeutic experiments, decided 2 years earlier, helps give the *Stanley* experiments a context.

In 1953, Allen Dulles, director of the Central Intelligence Agency (CIA), issued orders for secret experiments to be conducted on the use of biological and chemical agents to alter human behavior under the code name MKULTRA. These experiments were in response to "brainwashing techniques" used on American soldiers in Korea and the desperation these techniques caused. CIA officials wanted to know how these techniques worked and if they could be countered. Almost 200 researchers at 80 institutions were eventually hired by the CIA to conduct studies, several of which involved experiments where researchers secretly administered dangerous drugs, such as LSD, to uninformed human subjects. At least two subjects died as a result of the experiments, and many others suffered serious health consequences. This type of human experimentation was finally expressly forbidden by a presidential executive order in 1982.[43]

In 1973 the CIA director ordered all records pertaining to MKULTRA destroyed. In 1977 the CIA located some 8,000 pages, mostly financial records, that had inadvertently survived the 1973 destruction. Agency Director Stansfield Turner notified the Senate Select Committee of their existence and provided the committee with a confidential list of all MKULTRA researchers and institutions. Shortly thereafter, John Sims and Sidney Wolfe filed a Freedom of Information suit to obtain this list. By the time the case reached the U.S. Supreme Court, 58 of the institutions had agreed to be identified, but the CIA continued to resist disclosing the names of the other institutions and of the individual researchers on the grounds that they were "intelligence sources" that the CIA director had a right to protect. The U.S. Supreme Court, in a decision written by Chief Justice Warren Burger, agreed with the CIA, and along the way justified almost all of the CIA's information-collecting activities as being required by the national defense and the security of the United States. All of the justices concurred in this result.[44]

Two years later, in 1987, the U.S. Supreme Court got its first chance to decide if the Nuremberg Code applied to the U.S. Army, under whose auspices the Doctors' Trial was held. Technically speaking, the Court decided only that a active duty serviceman could not sue the U.S. government for money damages for injuries sustained as a result of experimentation that violated the Nuremberg Code. On the other hand, it is fair to conclude that the Code is almost meaningless in the military context if servicemen are denied a money damages remedy for its flagrant violation. To have a right without a remedy is similar to concluding that the Nuremberg Code is an ethical code without legal standing.

The U.S. Army became interested in mind-altering drugs at about the same time the CIA did, in the early 1950s. The army's interest stemmed from intelligence information that other countries were purchasing large quantities of hallucinogenic drugs and from the worry that these might be used as an alternative to nuclear weapons to render our military forces harmless without damaging the environment or buildings. As a result, at least 13 research contracts were funded by the army, and between 1955 and 1967 the army conducted numerous in-house studies of psychedelics on military and civilian personnel.[45]

Studies were done to determine how men under the influence of LSD performed their military duties and whether LSD could be used to obtain information during interrogation. Many subjects were not informed either of the nature of the experiment or of the substance used. The problem does not appear to have been lack of guidelines, but rather lack of compliance. By 1953 the Secretary of Defense had essentially adopted the Nuremberg Code for protection of experimental volunteers in research; but the guidelines were classified "top secret" until 1974 (when new standards were adopted by the army, navy and air force), and it is unclear how seriously they were taken.[46]

James Stanley, an army serviceman, volunteered to test the effectiveness of protective clothing and equipment against chemical warfare in February 1958. Unknown to him and without his consent, LSD was administered to him pursuant to an army plan to study the effects of the drug on humans. As a result of his exposure to LSD, Stanley suffered from hallucinations and periods of incoherence and memory loss. This impaired his military performance, and on occasion he awoke in the middle of the night and "without reason violently beat his wife and children, later being unable to recall the entire incident." He was discharged from the military in 1969. One year later, his marriage ended because of the personality changes allegedly induced by LSD. In 1975 Stanley received a letter from the army soliciting his cooperation in a follow-up study of the "volunteers who participated" in the 1958 LSD studies. This was the government's first notification to Stanley that he had been given LSD in 1958. Having been denied compensation for injury by the army, Stanley filed suit under the Federal Tort Claims Act alleging negligence in the administration, supervision, and follow-up monitoring of the drug research program.

In an extraordinarily technical and abstract decision, Justice Antonin Scalia wrote the opinion for a Court split 5 to 4.[47] Without in any way characterizing the actions of the army in this case as unusual, Justice Scalia concluded that permitting Stanley to sue the army would be a judicial intrusion upon military matters that would disrupt the army itself and "would call into question military discipline and decision-making." The

Court *would* permit a suit in a civilian court "to halt or prevent the constitutional violation" of a serviceman's rights; but the Court held that such a violation provides no justification for departing from the general rule that injuries that "arise out of or are in the course of activity incident to service" shall not give rise to a cause of action for money damages. Even though this conclusion has the effect of granting military officials unqualified immunity for intentionally injuring individual serviceman, the Court refused to recognize the consequences of this effect.

Doesn't what was done to Stanley so offend not only constitutional rights, but basic human decency and civilized standards of conduct, that a remedy is required in a civilized country? The four dissenting judges thought so, and based this conclusion firmly and squarely on the Nuremberg Code. Justice Sandra Day O'Connor, writing for herself, would have found that the conduct at issue in *Stanley* could not "arise out of or in the course of activity incident to service" because the conduct "is so far beyond the bounds of human decency that as a matter of law it simply cannot be considered a part of the military mission." In her words, the *Feres* doctrine bar

> surely cannot insulate defendants from liability for deliberate and calculated exposure of otherwise healthy military personnel to medical experimentation without their consent, outside of any combat, combat training, or military exigency, and for no other reason than to gather information on the effect of lysergic acid diethylamide on human beings. *No judicially crafted rule should insulate from liability the involuntary and unknowing human experimentation alleged to have occurred in this case.*[48]

Justice O'Connor went on to quote the Nuremberg Code:

> the United States military played an instrumental role in the criminal prosecution of Nazi officials who experimented with human beings during the Second World War . . . and the standards that the Nuremberg Military Tribunals developed to judge the behavior of the defendants stated that the "voluntary consent of the human subject is absolutely essential . . . to satisfy moral, ethical and legal concepts. . . . If this principle is violated the very least society can do is to see that the victims are compensated, as best they can be, by the perpetrators. I am prepared to say that our Constitution's promise of due process of law guarantees this much.[49]

Justice Brennan wrote the other dissent, which was joined by Justices Thurgood Marshall and John Paul Stevens. Justice Brennan began by characterizing the case as one in which "the Government of the United States treated thousands of its citizens as though they were laboratory animals." He argued that if the majority is correct that our Constitution bars Stanley from recovery, then "the Court's decision, though legally necessary, would expose a tragic flaw in the document." Justice Brennan, however, argued that the majority had abdicated its responsibility to protect constitutional rights, and that the Constitution required that Stanley be provided a remedy for his injuries. Brennan framed his argument with the Nuremberg Code and cited its first principle: "The voluntary consent of the human subject is absolutely essential." After quoting the text of the last two lines of the first principle, he stated, "The United States military developed the Code, which applies to all citizens — soldiers as well as civilians."[50]

A 1959 Army Staff Study, quoted by Brennan, noted that "in intelligence, the stakes involved and the interests of national security may permit a more tolerant interpretation of moral-ethical values, but not legal limits, through necessity." It concluded, nonetheless, that legal liability for the LSD experiments could be avoided only by covering them up. A Senate report later concurred with the army's assessment. Brennan argued that "Serious violations of the constitutional rights of soldiers must be exposed and punished." He agreed with the majority that an injunction could be obtained: "An injunction, however, comes too late for those already injured; for these victims, 'it is damages or nothing.'"

Justice Brennan went on to demonstrate that the cases granting absolute immunity are relevant to the analysis, and that they demonstrate that only qualified immunity is necessary to support the public policy and military discipline objectives relied on by the majority. Moreover, as he properly noted, the people who performed the experiment on Stanley were likely civilians in any event, so that military discipline was not even implicated in this case. Brennan concluded his opinion by quoting Hans Jonas:

> The soldier's case is instructive: Subject to the most unilateral discipline, forced to risk mutilation and death, conscripted without, perhaps against, his will — he is still conscripted with his capacities to act, to hold his own or to fail in situations, to meet challenges for real stakes. Though a mere "number" to the High Command, he is not a token and not a thing. (Imagine what he would say if it turned out that the war was a game staged to sample observations on his endurance, courage, or cowardice.)[51]

Justice Brennan then continued in his own words:

> The subject of experimentation who has not volunteered is treated as an object, a sample. James Stanley will receive no compensation for this indignity. A test providing absolute immunity for intentional constitutional torts *only* when such immunity was essential to maintenance of military discipline would "take into account the special importance of defending our Nation without completely abandoning the freedoms that make it worth defending." . . . Soldiers ought not be asked to defend a Constitution indifferent to their essential human dignity.[52]

In July 1991, at a Congressional hearing on a private bill to compensate Stanley for his injuries it was alleged that some of the researchers who subjected Stanley to the LSD experiments were former Nazis brought to the U.S. under Operation Paperclip.

DESERT STORM

As a final example, in late December 1990, the FDA granted the Department of Defense (DoD) a waiver from the informed consent requirements of the Nuremberg Code and existing federal law and regulations to use unapproved drugs and vaccines on the soldiers involved in Desert Shield.[53] The basis of this waiver was military expediency. In the words of the Department of Defense: "In all peace time applications, we believe strongly in informed consent and ethical foundations . . . But military combat is different."[54] The rationale was that informed consent under combat conditions was "not feasible" because some troops might object and refuse to consent, and the military could not tolerate such refusals because of "military combat exigencies."[55] It is perhaps not remarkable that the FDA granted the request waiver and soon thereafter approved specific waivers for pyridostigmine bromide and botulinum toxoid vaccine to be administered to the troops.[56] The rule is reprinted in Appendix 5 of this volume. It did not escape everyone's attention, however, that this was the first time since World War II that any official government agency had politically sanctioned the direct violation of the Nuremberg Code (which makes no exception either for members of the military or for wartime expediencies).[57] The United States District Court for the District of Columbia refused to enjoin the regulation without even mentioning the Nuremberg Code.[58] In the court's view this was a military command decision not to be questioned by the judiciary: "The primary purpose of administering the drugs is military not scientific."[59] *The New York Times* agreed, saying that "the military is acting more like Florence Nightingale than Joseph Mengele."[60]

U.S. District Judge Stanley Harris made it clear that he had no desire to get involved with military matters. In his words, "The DoD's decision to use unapproved drugs is precisely the type of military decision that courts have repeatedly refused to second-guess." He characterized the decision as one to protect individual servicemen, and as "strategic" in nature, and thus not reviewable by a court. He went on, however, to say that if he thought he had the authority to review the decision, he would uphold it.

The Defense Authorization Act prohibits DoD from using any of its funds "for any research involving a human being as an experimental subject" unless the subject's informed consent has been obtained. This restriction was in reaction to U.S. Army experiments on servicemen using both radiation and LSD at the beginning of the cold war. Judge Harris, however, decided that "the primary purpose of administering the drugs is military, not scientific," and therefore the statutory prohibition was inapplicable.

The "not feasible" exception had previously applied only to subjects who were unable to communicate, unconscious, or incompetent. Nonetheless, Judge Harris decided the FDA could reinterpret this exception as long as its interpretation was not "arbitrary, capricious or manifestly contrary to the statute." Finally, Judge Harris rejected the claim that forced administration of unapproved drugs violates the Fifth Amendment liberty interest of servicemen. Instead he found that the military's interests in trying to prevent injury to troops, and "successfully accomplishing the military goals of Operation Desert Storm" were sufficient to justify the exception to informed consent. The Nuremberg Code was not mentioned in the decision.

At the appeals hearing, held in March, 1991, a letter was introduced from DoD to FDA saying that the military requirements for use of the two agents without informed consent had ended. DoD also informed FDA: "Central Command has recently reported that the military command in the theatre of operations decided to administer the vaccine on a voluntary basis. The pyridostigmine tablets were used without prior informed consent." On the basis of the end of the war and the DoD letter, the Justice Department argued that the case was moot and should be dismissed by the U.S. Circuit Court of Appeals.

The majority of the Court, in a 2 to 1 opinion written by Judge Ruth Ginsburg in July, disagreed.[61] The court concluded that even though DoD had withdrawn its two specific waivers, the general rule remained in effect, and therefore the use of unapproved agents was both capable of repetition and evading review. The court relied heavily on government reports concerning the proliferation of nuclear, chemical, and biological weapons systems, especially among third world nations like Iraq. On the merits, the court disagreed with the lower court that the case was beyond court review because it was military in nature. Instead the court of appeals defined the issue as a challenge to FDA's authority to issue a waiver of its consent regulations to DoD, not as an action challenging military decisions. The court of appeals did, however, agree with all the other conclusions of the lower court, and affirmed its decision in favor of the DoD. Again, no mention was made of the Nuremberg Code.

CONCLUSION

Prior to World War II, human experimentation in the United States was generally viewed by the courts as an extreme and somewhat illegitimate activity that amounted to a deviation from medical practice. Courts frequently insisted that such a deviation was itself evidence of malpractice. By World War II, experimentation that was not too extreme, and that was done with the patient's informed consent, was seen as legitimate. No nontherapeutic experiment was reviewed in U.S. courts prior to World War II.

After the war, the Nazi experiments were seldom referred to in U.S. courts. Human experimentation became a mainstream, legitimate, and valued activity. Although it continued to deviate from standard medical practice, the goal was usually to test a hypothesis. Most human experimentation, especially drug trials, was now done not to help individual patients but to find new treatment modalities. In short, human experimentation moved from the realm of quackery to the realm of science.

In this context, it is perhaps not surprising that a deep theoretical division developed between therapeutic and nontherapeutic experimentation. The former (the exclusive type reviewed by the courts before the war) was rehabilitated, with concern focusing almost exclusively on informed consent. In this regard, principle 1 of the Nuremberg Code, although rarely cited, became the primary justification for therapeutic experimentation. Much less attention was paid to the other nine principles.

On the other hand, just as therapeutic experimentation tended to be viewed as merely another type of therapy, nontherapeutic experimentation tended to be viewed as the *only* true form of experimentation and thus the only kind of research activity that the Nuremberg Code — a document fundamentally about nontherapeutic experimentation — applied to. This is reflected in the case law. The types of experiments that U.S. judges have found the Nuremberg Code useful for setting standards have involved nontherapeutic experiments often conducted without consent: psychosurgery on an involuntarily confined mental patient; secretly administering mind-altering drugs to unsuspecting soldiers and civilians; testing the effects of radiation on members of the military; and monitoring the physical effects of radiation on unsuspecting uranium miners. Many of these experiments were justified by national security considerations and the cold war. The wartime mentality expressed by the CIA and the U.S. army to justify its LSD experiments, and by the U.S. army to justify its atomic bomb exposure experiments, is almost identical to one of the major defenses presented by the Nazi physicians at Nuremberg. Remarkably, the Nuremberg Code seems to have had no effect on medical researchers even in the 1950s.

Given our belief that the Nazis were "others" and not like us, it is probably not surprising that so little attention has been paid to the Nuremberg Code in U.S. courts. However, since U.S. judges promulgated it under both natural and international law standards, it is disturbing that we have not taken it more seriously in areas where there is no question that it has direct application. The most disturbing failure to apply it for the protection of research subjects involves the U.S. military. Treating soldiers as property without basic human rights should be offensive to both us and them, and should be seen as an unacceptable and unconstitutional violation of their rights. That the U.S. Supreme Court indirectly approves of such conduct, even in the experimental context, and directly rejects the Nuremberg Code as anything more than a statement of ethics is discouraging. We are rightly horrified to hear the Nazi physician quoted in Chapter 3 tell a young doctor not to do research on herself because "We have concentration camps for that."[62] We seem content to live with U.S. army and CIA personnel who can say, "We have soldiers for that." It is very disappointing that the Court was unable to distinguish between the military mission and taking advantage of defenseless soldiers.[63]

In an age that has come to see research as necessary for progress, and progress as the new goal for humankind, it is not surprising that therapeutic research has been reinvented as simply therapy, and that many sick people actually demand it as their right.[64] It should probably not even be surprising that traditional nontherapeutic research, such as phase I cancer drug research and early research on AIDS drugs, as well as the first-of-their-kind transplants and implants, have been redefined as simply therapy, or sometimes innovative therapy.[65] What is surprising, however, is that even in those instances of nontherapeutic experimentation in which the Nuremberg Code applies directly, we have never taken it seriously ourselves and have been content to say that the rights of the individual are outweighed by national security concerns. This has been true even where those concerns are unclear or unarticulated, and where the experiments are carried out in secret and produce death and permanent disability.

The promise of the Nuremberg Code has not been fulfilled in the United States. When national security is invoked, human rights continue to take second place to the demands of state officials, and when "medical progress" is invoked, ethics continues to take a backseat to expediency.

NOTES

1. George J. Annas, Leonard H. Glantz, and Barbara F. Katz, *Informed Consent to Human Experimentation: The Subject's Dilemma* (Cambridge, Mass.: Ballinger, 1977), p. 1.

2. Ibid., p. 21.

3. See generally Arnold C. Brackman, *The Other Nuremberg: The Untold Story of the Tokyo War Crime Trials* (London: Collins, 1989), and Peter Williams and David Wallace, *Unit 731: The Japanese Army's Secret of Secrets* (London: Hodder & Stoughton, 1989).

4. This is not to say that no nontherapeutic experiments were conducted in the United States prior to the war, only that none of the participants in these experiments brought lawsuits for which we have an appellate record. The Tuskegee Syphilis study, for example, began in 1932 and continued until 1972, but no lawsuits were filed until the 1970s. See James H. Jones, *Bad Blood: The Tuskegee Syphilis Experiment* (New York: Free Press, 1981), and note 35 below.

5. *Ownes v. McClearey*, 313 Mo. 213, 281 S.W. 682, 685 (1926).

6. *Fortner v. Koch*, 272 Mich. 273, 261 N.W. 762 (1935) (emphasis added). This and other pre–World War II cases on human experimentation in the United States are discussed in more detail in Annas et al., *Informed Consent*, pp. 2–60.

7. *Stammer v. Board of Regents*, 262 App. Div. 372, 29 N.Y.S. 2d 38 (1941), *aff'd*. 287 N.Y. 359, 39 N.E.2d 913 (1942) (emphasis added).

8. *Bonner v. Moran*, 75 U.S. App. D.C. 156, 126 F.2d 121 (1941).

9. Ibid. (emphasis added)

10. David J. Rothman, "Ethics and Human Experimentation: Henry Beecher Revisited," *New England Journal of Medicine* 317 (1987): 1197.

11. See, e.g., Richard Carter, *Breakthrough: The Saga of Jonas Salk* (New York: Trident Press, 1966), pp. 123–237, and Hilary Koprowski, George A. Jervis, Thomas W. Norton, and Doris J. Nelson, "Further Studies on Oral Administration of Living Polio Virus to Human Subjects," *Proceedings, Society of Experimental Biology and Medicine* 82 (1953): 277–280.

12. T. C. Routely, "Aims and Objectives of the World Medical Association," *World Medical Association Bulletin* 1 (1949): 18–19.

13. "Organizational News," *World Medical Journal* 2 (1955): 14–15.

14. Hugh Clegg, "Human Experimentation," *World Medical Journal* 7 (1960): 77. Of course, as Grodin notes in Chapter 7 of this volume, the Hippocratic oath has nothing to say about human experimentation.

15. Quoted in W. Refshauge, "The Place for International Standards in Conducting Research for Humans," *Bulletin of the World Health Organization* 55 (supp.) (1977): 133–135 (emphasis added).

16. Ibid., 137. A 1964 physician-observer agreed:

> I think we must read the Nuremberg Code in reference to the conditions under which it was written. This is a wonderful document to say why war crimes were atrocities, but it is not a very good guide to clinical investigation which is done with high motives.

Paul B. Beeson, "Panel Discussion: Moral Issues in Clinical Research," *Yale Journal of Biology and Medicine* 36 (1964): 464.

17. CIOMS, *Protection of Human Rights in Light of Scientific and Technological Progress in Biology and Medicine* (Geneva: World Health Organization, 1974), p. 247.

18. *Strunk v. Strunk*, 445 S.W.2d 145 (Ken. Ct. App. 1969).

19. Ibid.

20. *Karp v. Cooley*, 349 F.Supp. 827 (S.D. Tex. 1972) *aff'd*. 493 F.2d 408 (5th Cir. 1974).

21. *Kaimowitz v. Michigan Dept. Mental Health*, Civil No. 73-19434-AW (Mich. Cir. Ct., Wayne Co., July 10, 1973).

22. Ibid., p. 16. For a detailed analysis of the legal regulation of psychosurgery, see Annas et al., *Informed Consent*, pp. 215–255.

23. *Aden v. Younger*, 129 Cal. Rptr. 535 (Ct. App. 4th Dist., Div. 1, 1976). See also Chester Atkins and Alison Lauriat, "Psychosurgery and the Role of Legislation," 54 *Boston University Law Review* (1974): 288–302.

24. *Pierce v. Ortho Pharmaceutical Corp.*, 417 A.2d 505 (N.J. 1980).

25. Ibid., p. 513.

26. Ibid., p. 514 (emphasis added).

27. Ibid., pp. 516–517.

28. See Chapter 9, this volume.

29. *Jaffee v. United States*, 663 F.2d 1226 (3rd Cir. 1981).

30. Ibid., p. 1240.

31. Ibid., p. 1248.

32. Ibid., p. 1249 (emphasis added).

33. Ibid., pp. 1249–1250.

34. *Begay v. United States*, 591 F.Supp. 991 (D. Ariz. 1984).

35. In the now infamous Tuskegee study, poor black men with syphilis were followed for decades so that the natural course of the disease could be studied. The men were told only that they had "bad blood," and were never informed of their diagnosis or the purpose of the study even after penicillin was discovered. The study was not discontinued until 1972. See note 4 above.

36. *Begay v. United States*, 591 F.Supp. 991, 997–998 (D. Ariz. 1984) (emphasis added).

37. Ibid., p. 1012 (emphasis added). President George Bush used similar language in justifying sending U.S. troops to Saudi Arabia in the summer of 1990 to protect "our American way of life."

38. An earlier case involving the government's act of selecting a particular strain of bacteria for use in a secret, simulated biological warfare attack on San Francisco in 1950 came to a similar conclusion. The court ruled that the family of a man who died as a result of being exposed to the bacteria had no recourse because the selection of the strain of bacteria was a discretionary function.

39. *Begay v. United States*, p. 1012. In 1986 Congressman Edward J. Markey (D. Mass.) released records detailing a series of experiments conducted by the U.S. government from 1940 to 1971 to test various aspects of radiation exposure. Many of the experiments had been published in journals. They included the injection of radium, thorium, and plutonium into patients who were believed to have a limited life span; exposure of the testicles of Oregon prisoners to test the effects of radiation on human fertility; and the intentional release of radioactive iodine in Idaho, followed in at least one case by subjects drinking milk from cows that had grazed on land contaminated with radioactivity. Only the Oregon prisoner experiments resulted in any litigation, as a result of which the U.S. Attorney in Portland, Oregon, asked state officials to cancel a program of following up released prisoners to examine their health status. For details on the radiation studies, which were conducted at some of the nation's leading educational institutions and hospitals, see "American Nuclear Guinea Pigs: Three Decades of Radiation Experiments on U.S. Citizens," A Subcommittee Staff Report for the Subcommittee on Energy and Power of the Committee on Energy and Commerce, U.S. House Representatives, October, 1986. The 1986 excuses for the experiments were predictable. Dr. J. W. Thiessen of the U.S. Department of Energy's Office of Health and Environmental Research defended the studies, saying, "You have to put yourself back in those years. They used humans because there was an urgency to find if radiation safety standards were adequate. . . . Actual exposure to those people was extremely low. We wouldn't do it now the way they did it then. But it's hard to say they were wrong even then." Larry Tye, "Radiation Tests Employed People as Guinea Pigs," *Boston Globe*, October 25, 1986, p. 3.

40. *Whitlock v. Duke University*, 637 F.Supp. 1463 (M.D.N.C. 1986).

41. Ibid., p. 1471 (emphasis added).

42. *United States v. Stanley*, 107 S. Ct. 3054 (1987).

43. *Central Intelligence Agency v. Sims*, 471 U.S. 159, 162 n. 2 (1984).

44. Ibid.

45. The issue of experimentation in the U.S. military is discussed in more detail in Annas et al., *Informed Consent*, pp. 305–311.

46. Ibid., p. 308.

47. *United States v. Stanley*, 107 S. Ct. 3054 (1987).

48. Ibid., p. 3065 (emphasis added).

49. Ibid., pp. 3065–3066.

50. Ibid., p. 3066.

51. Ibid., p. 3077, quoting from Hans Jonas, "Philosophical Reflections on Experimentation with Human Subjects," *Ethical Aspects of Experimentation with Human Subjects*, *Daedalus* 98 (Spring 1969): 219–247.

52. Ibid., p. 3077. In a mid-1991 interview, Justice Brennan described this case as "outrageous" and "incredible" and said "thank God, it hasn't shown its head again — not yet, anyway." Nat Hentoff, "The Justice Breaks His Silence," *Playboy*, July 1991, pp. 120, 154.

53. Informed Consent for Human Drugs and Biologics; Determination That Informed Consent Is Not Feasible, 55 Fed. Reg. 52,814 (1990). The regulations are reprinted in Appendix 5.

54. Ibid. at 52,815.

55. Ibid.

56. G. Kolata, *Troops May Get Unlicensed Drug*, New York Times, Jan. 4, 1991, at A10, col. 6.

57. G. J. Annas & M. A. Grodin, *Our Guinea Pigs in the Gulf*, New York Times, Jan. 8, 1991, at A21, col. 1.

58. *Doe v. Sullivan*, 756 F.Supp. 12 (D.D.C. 1991).

59. Ibid. The pyridostigmine research is reported in J. R. Keeler, C. G. Hurst, M. A. Dunn, Pyridostigmine Used as a Nerve Agent Pretreatment Under Wartime Conditions, *Journal of the American Medical Association* 266 (1991): 693–695.

60. *The Ethics of Troop Vaccination*, New York Times, Jan. 16, 1991, at A22, col. 1 (editorial). For the argument against the regulation, see G. J. Annas & M. A. Grodin, *Treating the Troops: Commentary*, Hastings Center Rep. 21 (Mar./Apr. 1991): 23–25.

61. *Doe v. Sullivan*, 938 F.2d 1370 (D.C. Cir. 1991).

62. Chapter 3, this volume.

63. And even if money damages could not be awarded, the criminal penalties provided at Nuremberg should continue to apply.

64. See Chapter 16, this volume.

65. The world's first artificial heart was described as "therapy," as was the world's first permanent artificial heart, for example. *Karp v. Cooley*, 349 F.Supp. 827. (S.D. Tex. 1972), *aff'd*. 493 F.2d 408 (5th Cir. 1974). This was also true of the world's first *permanent* artificial heart implant. G. J. Annas, "Death and the Magic Machine: Informed Consent to the Artificial Heart," *Western New England Law Review* 9 (1987): pp. 89–112.

IV

THE NUREMBERG CODE: ETHICS AND MODERN MEDICAL RESEARCH

This part presents an analysis of the importance and implications of the Nuremberg Code and its general principles for contemporary medical ethics and human experimentation. The recurrent themes in all the chapters are autonomy, subjects' rights, the balancing of benefit and harm, intentionality, responsibility, and ethical relativism. Despite the increasing sophistication and nuances of modern medical research, the Nuremberg Code and its insistence on respect for the individual serves as a foundation for all contemporary inquiry.

Chapter 12 is written by Jay Katz, a psychoanalyst and law school professor, who was one of the first scholars in the United States to formally analyze the questions surrounding the appropriate use of human subjects for experimental research. Katz has been one of the foremost advocates of the necessity of informed consent for legitimate human experimentation. Here he reexamines the centrality of informed consent in the Nuremberg Code and the influence this had on subsequent debate and contemporary practice.

In Chapter 13, bioethicist Ruth Macklin explores the problem of cultural relativism in ethics. Drawing on her examination of the claims of the Nazi doctors, and on contemporary international research projects, Macklin makes a compelling case against ethical relativism and asserts the possibility of moral progress.

In Chapter 14, bioethicist Arthur Caplan addresses the use and misuse of the Holocaust metaphor and the Nuremberg Code in modern medical ethics debates. He makes a strong claim that the complexities of contemporary clinical medicine and research are far removed from the arguments and claims of Nazi medicine. Despite the differences, however, he sees the Nuremberg Code's central focus on respect for persons as a pervasive ethos.

In Chapter 15, Marcia Angell, a physician and executive editor of the *New England Journal of Medicine*, addresses the role of journals and editors in tolerating and publishing unethical medical research. Researchers and physicians may be motivated to conduct human experiments for personal power, prestige, politics, and remuneration. Publication in peer-reviewed medical journals is a necessary step toward those goals. Thus, journal editors are in a pivotal position to judge the scientific and ethical merits of clinical investigation. Angell argues for an international standard and a consensus among journals on the ethics of research on human subjects.

In Chapter 16, attorney Wendy Mariner identifies the tension in the testing of experimental AIDS drugs between protecting the rights

of vulnerable patients and protecting their welfare. The extent to
which therapy and research have been confounded has shifted the
debate from protecting the human subject's right to refuse experimental AIDS drugs to the claim by some AIDS advocates of a right
to have access to such drugs. Mariner analyzes this debate against the
backdrop of the Nuremberg Code as a way to explore the Code's
continuing relevance.

12

The Consent Principle
of the Nuremberg Code:
Its Significance Then and Now

JAY KATZ

The Nuremberg Code is a remarkable document. Never before in the history of human experimentation, and never since, has any code or any regulation of research declared in such relentless and uncompromising a fashion that the psychological integrity of research subjects must be protected absolutely. Thus, its first principle:

> The voluntary consent of the human subject is absolutely essential. This means that the person involved should have legal capacity to give consent, should be so situated as to be able to exercise free power of choice, without the intervention of any element of force, fraud, deceit, duress, overreaching or other ulterior form of constraint or coercion; and should have sufficient knowledge and comprehension of the elements of the subject matter involved as to enable him to make an understanding and enlightened decision. . . .[1]

THE NUREMBERG CODE

The Nuremberg Code has no antecedents except, ironically, for the Regulations on New Therapy and Human Experimentation promulgated in Germany by the Reichsminister of the Interior in 1931.[2] Otherwise, the Code constitutes the first authoritative, and surely the most stringent, pronouncement on the rights of research subjects. Moreover, its unique historical significance is further highlighted by the fact that the Code's unswerving first principle was soon dethroned from its preeminent position at the 1964 Helsinki Convention of the World Medical Association.

The Nuremberg Code was relegated to history almost as soon as it was born. Yet its bold assertions about the primacy of consent could not be completely denied. The power of its appeal to respect for persons was too strong and survived, however diluted, in subsequent codifications and regulations.

While the Nuremberg Code's primary objective was to support the judgment of the Nuremberg Tribunal that the Nazi physician-scientists had been guilty of perpetrating deeds of agony, torture, degradation, and death on human beings in the name of medical science, it aspired to more than that. The Code also sought to codify "certain basic principles [that] must be observed in order to satisfy moral, ethical and legal concepts"[3] in the conduct of research.

However, the Tribunal erroneously believed that such principles, while never officially promulgated, had always been embraced by the research community in the Western world. The testimony at the Nuremberg trial of the two major American witnesses for the prosecution, Andrew C. Ivy and Leo Alexander, reinforced the judgment that the Nazi experiments were aberrational. Ivy, in particular, made much of physicians' Hippocratic commitment to protecting patients' welfare as a sufficient safeguard, even though the Hippocratic oath had nothing to say about the imperatives of science.[4] Only reluctantly did he admit on cross-examination that the American Medical Association's pronouncements on the conduct of research had been promulgated only after the extent of the Nazi concentration camp experiments had become public knowledge.

Thus, the Tribunal thought that accepted principles had been violated by the Nazi physicians, and that their violations could be attributed solely to "the ravaging inroads of Nazi pseudo-science."[5] That fatal error permitted the Tribunal to overlook that the history of human experimentation has also been a history not of ravages, but of injuries, inflicted on human beings without their voluntary consent.[6]

To be sure, nothing in the annals of medical experimentation had ever risen to conduct carried out with such massive, fiendish, thoroughgoing, and deathly intent. However, that correctly perceived difference between the Nazi experiments and those carried on in the rest of the civilized world prevented the judges from placing the Nazi experiments in their historical context. That difference also allowed physician-scientists and medical policymaking bodies to isolate the lessons to be learned from the Nuremberg Code's insistence on voluntary consent, and leave unconfronted its implications for their own past and present research practices. They did so in two contradictory ways: (1) by praising the Code as a fitting response to an unprecedented, singular aberration in the history of medical experimentation and (2) by rejecting it as an appropriate response to research practices for the rest of the Western world. It was a good code for barbarians but an unnecessary code for ordinary physician-scientists.

CONSENT TO EXPERIMENTATION

Until the Nuremberg trial, researchers at best could only heed Claude Bernard — a contemporary of Pasteur — who, at the dawn of modern medical science, had set forth the first formulation of the scientific rationale and ethical limits for human experimentation:

> It is *our duty* and *our right* to perform an experiment on man whenever it can save his life, cure him, or gain him some personal benefit. The principle of medical and surgical morality, therefore, consists in never performing on man an experiment which might be harmful to him to any extent, even though the results might be highly advantageous to science, i.e. to the health of others.[7]

Note that Bernard spoke about "our duty" and "our right"; he said nothing about research subjects' consent.

When during the late nineteenth century medicine moved into the age of science, it did so from a tradition that encouraged trying out new treatments on patients for *their* welfare, as determined by their doctors. Such interventions, being for patients' benefit, were generally performed without consent. Instead, physicians were guided in their quest to alleviate suffering, by their sacred commitment to *primum non nocere* — "first of all, to do no harm" — a principle that had served them well during the millennia when their capacity to cure was most limited. However, with the advent of the age of science, a radical break occurred in medical practice: Novel experimental interventions now served not solely — and often not at all — patients' but also future patients' or science's, interests. This decisive difference was not addressed by Bernard, Ivy, or others; instead, the distinction between patient and research subject became, and ever since has remained, blurred.

One question has not been thoroughly analyzed to this day: When may investigators, actively or by acquiescence, expose human beings to harm in order to seek benefits for them, for others, or for society as a whole? If one peruses the literature with this question in mind, one soon learns that no searching general justifications for involving any human beings as subjects for research have ever been formulated.[8] Yet, the uses of patients for multiple experimental purposes, and sometimes only for the purpose of advancing science, required such justifications. Instead, in the past and even now, it has been assumed without question that the general necessity for experimenting with human beings, while requiring regulation, is so obvious that it need not be justified. For the moment, I do not contend that it cannot be justified. I only wish to point to the pervasive silence on providing searching general justifications for this practice, and, more specifically, to the lack of separate justifications for novel interventions employed for the benefit of future patients and science, in contrast to those employed for patients' direct benefits. Even if, for argument's sake, consent can be dispensed with in therapeutic practice, it is quite a different matter to do so in research when a particular patient's best interests are not, or are only in part, at stake.

To return to Claude Bernard, his formulation did not address physicians' duties and rights in the conduct of nonclinical research. While he proscribed any experiment "which might be harmful to him *to any extent*, even though the results might be highly advantageous to science," adherence to such a formulation would have severely curtailed physician-scientists' endeavors from the late nineteenth century on, when they began to extend their research to patients irrespective of direct benefits to them. "Duty" and "right" required a careful analysis of whether experimentation in nontherapeutic settings could be justified only by asking for patient-subjects' consent. This did not occur, and what happened was inevitable.

Listen to the justification of a Swedish investigator for using young children as subjects in variola vaccine experiments:

> [P]erhaps I should have first experimented upon animals, but calves — most suitable for these purposes — were difficult to obtain because of their cost and their keep.[9]

And listen to the admonitions and consolations of a German investigator:

> [The publication of these observations] will perhaps restrain others . . . from making further experiments, often leading to the *complete wrecking of the lives* of the persons subjected to them. It would add considerably to my peace of mind in respect to the victim's fate if these experiments [were to establish the fact that the secondary stage of syphilis is contagious so that] *the suffering of a few individuals* were not too high a price to be paid by mankind for the attainment of such a truly beneficial and practical result.[10]

These and many other revelations published in the scientific literature antedating the Nazi era were unavailable to Ivy and others. Reading his testimony, one can only get the impression that he believed that such practices did not exist. Yet Ivy himself was an investigator, and he was conversant with research practices in the Western world. Thus the question: How could he have believed that the first principle of the Nuremberg Code, which he helped to formulate, comported with the ethical climate of human experimentation in the Western world?

I have already suggested that the significance of the Nuremberg Code was disregarded as soon as the Code was promulgated. Consider the Tuskegee Syphilis Study[11] begun in 1932, years prior to the concentration camp experiments, continued during the Holocaust, and not terminated until 1972, years after the promulgation of the Nuremberg Code. In this research, 400 black males suffering from syphilis were deliberately left untreated for decades in order to study the natural history of the untreated disease. The subjects had not been informed about their participation in this project. Most, if not all, did not even know that they had syphilis, and instead believed that they were receiving ordinary medical care.

Consider the Jewish Chronic Disease Hospital's experiments of 1963,[12] in which "live cancer cells" were injected into 22 chronically ill and debilitated patients without their knowledgeable consent.

Or consider the revelations of Dr. Henry K. Beecher, who concluded from an examination of 100 consecutive studies, published in 1964 in a leading medical journal, that "12 of these studies seemed unethical."[13]

These well-known revelations are only the tip of the iceberg. They speak not so much to conduct that exposed research subjects to serious physical harm (although that too) as to the disregard, if not the violation, of the first principle of the Nuremberg Code. In countless discussions with research scientists, I have learned about their tampering with the principle of voluntary consent in order to get research underway, advance science, and obtain research grants for the sake of protecting their laboratories and professional advancement. All this is done in the belief that physician-scientists can be trusted to safeguard the physical integrity of their subjects.

With respect to physical integrity, they are largely correct, yet not entirely so. However, even if they were entirely correct, their perceived role as guarantors of patients' welfare leaves unconsidered another crucial issue: voluntary consent, i.e., respect for the person as the ultimate decision maker. Unless this requirement is clearly asserted (and any exception clearly specified), the slippery slope of engineering consent stretches out before us, leading inexorably to Tuskegee, the Jewish Chronic Disease Hospital in Brooklyn, LSD experiments in Manhattan, DES experiments in Chicago.

The Nuremberg Code did not become the guiding code for the conduct of research. Instead, it was superseded by the Declaration of Helsinki and, in the United States, by the Rules and Regulations for the Protection of Human Research Subjects promulgated by the Department of Health and Human Services. Before proceeding, let me note in passing that the first principle of the Nuremberg Code, if adopted, may very well have required modification; it clearly would have required exegesis. These issues are beyond the scope of this article.

THE HELSINKI DECLARATIONS

Consider first the Declaration of Helsinki. Its latest revised version (1989)[14] sets forth 12 basic principles. They begin by stressing the importance of "medical progress"; the scientific considerations that should govern the "design and performance of the experiment"; the need to weigh "the objective [of the experiment] against the inherent risks to the subject"; and the necessity to "respect the privacy of the subject and to minimize the impact of the study on the subject's physical and mental integrity and on the personality of the subject." Clearly, the integrity of the scientific enterprise comes first, though it must be balanced against unspecified "interests of the subject."

Principle 5 is stronger: "Concern for the interest of the subject must always prevail over the interest of science and society"; yet, principle 6 speaks about "minimiz[ing] the impact of the study on the subject's integrity." What are the limits of "minimizing"? How are these two principles to be reconciled, and who decides? As suggested by principle 3, "the responsibility for the human subjects [rests] with a medically qualified person"; it does not rest with physician-investigator *and* the patient-subject.

Only later, in principle 9, is informed consent mentioned:

> In any research on human beings, each potential subject must be adequately informed of the aims, methods, anticipated benefits and potential hazards of the study and the discomfort it may entail. . . . The doctor should then obtain the subject's freely given informed consent, preferably in writing.

Contrast these statements to the Nuremberg Code, both in terms of where they are placed in the text (principle 9 rather than principle 1) and what words are used. Nothing is said in the Helsinki Code about prohibiting force, fraud, deceit, duress, overreaching, or any ulterior form of constraint or coercion. To be sure, such requirements are to some extent inherent in the legal doctrine of informed consent, but with much less stringency since it is applicable to, and has been construed for, therapeutic rather than investigative interventions. Thus, these questions: Do the admonitions promulgated by the Tribunal deserve explicit reconfirmation in any progeny of the Nuremberg Code? And if not, must any modifications be justified with relentless care?

After having set forth its basic principles, the Helsinki Code addresses the principles that should govern "Medical Research Combined with Professional Care (Clinical Research)" and "Non-therapeutic Biomedical Research Involving Human Subjects (Non-clinical Biomedical Research)." In clinical research the emphasis is not on consent but on the imperative of physicians' freedom: "[the doctor] must be free to use a new diagnostic and therapeutic measure if in his or her judgment it offers hope of saving life, reestablishing health or alleviating suffering." Questions: Whose health is considered, the health of the patients involved in research or the health of future patients? Can a new "therapeutic measure" be used with or without the patient-subject's consent?

For nonclinical biomedical research, where one should have expected some reference to disclosure and consent, they are not highlighted again. Perhaps one can argue that principle 9 is assumed to apply. But then the following statement is troublesome: "It is the duty of the doctor to remain the protector of the life and health of [the] person." Why only the protector of life and health? Why not also the protector of the dignitary interests of the person, with its implicit demand for full disclosure and consent?

The last principle concerning nonclinical biomedical research states:

> In research on man, the interest of science and society should never take precedence over considerations related to the well-being of the subject.

Had the spirit of the Nuremberg Code prevailed, that principle would have been drafted differently. Here are my modifications: "In research on man and woman, the interest of science and society should never take precedence over considerations related to the well-being of the subject *as determined by the subject, after having been fully informed by the physician-scientist, so that both can* make an understanding and enlightened decision."

Finally, a historical note: The current version of the Declaration of Helsinki, analyzed above, was preceded by a draft code (1962) and a first version, adopted by the World Health Organization in 1964. The draft code,[15] similar to the Nuremberg Code although in less encompassing language, at least opened with a statement on consent in its section on "General Principles and Definitions":

1. An experiment on a human being is an act whereby the investigator deliberately changes the internal or external environment in order to observe the effects of such a change.
2. Such change in the environment as defined should be made only if the following conditions are observed:
   (a) that the nature, the reason, and the risks of the experiment are fully explained to the subject of it, who should have complete freedom to decide whether or not to take part in the experiment.

However in the next section, "Experiments for the Benefit of the Patient," a physician is given considerable discretion to dispense with consent in clinical investigations unless he or she conducts "experiments *solely* for the acquisition of knowledge":

1. A doctor preforming an experiment for the possible benefit of his patient should not extend his experiment beyond this without the full and previous consent of the patient.
2. A doctor combining clinical research with the personal care of patients should never abuse the trust of the patient in him as a doctor by conducting experiments solely for the acquisition of knowledge, unless the full consent of the patient has been previously obtained.

As an important but only related aside, let me note that the draft code, in its section on "Experiments Conducted Solely for the Acquisition of Knowledge," proscribed the participation of specifically identified groups in experimental investigations:

(c) Prisoners of war, military or civilian, should never be used as subjects of experiment.
(d) Civilians detained in any place as a result of military invasion or occupation, or for administrative or political reasons, should never be used for human experiment.
(e) Persons retained in prisons, penitentiaries, or reformatories — being "captive groups" — should not be used as subjects of experiment; nor persons incapable of giving consent because of age, mental incapacity, or of being in a position in which they are incapable of exercising the power of free choice.

These proposed provisions were eliminated in the 1964 and 1975 versions. Considerable research done by others and by me has been unsuccessful in learning what, and at whose insistence, led to this significant alteration of the draft text.

The first official version of the Declaration of Helsinki[16] is shorter than its revised version of 1975. In the section on "Basic Principles," the requirement of consent is not even mentioned. For "Clinical Research Combined with Professional Care" the following provisions are set forth:

> 1. In the treatment of the sick person the doctor must be free to use a new therapeutic measure if in his judgment it offers hope of saving life, re-establishing health, or alleviating suffering.
>
>   *If at all possible*, consistent with patient psychology, the doctor should obtain the patient's free given consent after the patient has been given a full explanation. . . .

For "Non-therapeutic Clinical Research" the following applies:

> 2. The nature, the purpose, and the risk of clinical research must be explained to the subject by the doctor.
> 3a. Clinical research on a human being cannot be undertaken without his free consent, after he has been fully informed; . . .

Again, note the sparseness to the consent requirements in contrast to the language of the Nuremberg Code.

The Declaration of Helsinki was enacted in the shadow of the Holocaust experiments; yet, less than 20 years after the Nuremberg Code was promulgated, concerns over the advancement of science began to overshadow concerns over the integrity of the person. However, there are some hopeful signs: The 1975 revision of the Declaration of Helsinki at least reintroduced the requirement of informed consent in its ninth basic principle. Perhaps in subsequent revisions, the requirement of respect for person will become, as it was in the Nuremberg Code, more preeminent in language and in its position among the basic principles.

THE U.S. DEPARTMENT OF HEALTH AND HUMAN SERVICES' RULES AND REGULATIONS FOR THE PROTECTION OF HUMAN RESEARCH SUBJECTS

The Rules and Regulations for the Protection of Human Research Subjects promulgated by the Department of Health and Human Services[17] set forth in some detail in Section 46.116 (General Requirements for Informed Consent) the basic elements of Informed Consent:

> [T]he following information shall be provided to each subject: . . . that the study involves research, an explanation of the purposes of the research; [a] description of any reasonably foreseeable risks and discomforts . . . ; [a] disclosure of appropriate alternative procedures . . . ; [a] statement that participation is voluntary. . . .

These are commendable provisions, more consonant than the Declaration of Helsinki with the spirit of the Nuremberg Code.

They are framed by an opening statement: "[e]xcept as provided elsewhere . . . no investigator may involve a human being as a subject in research covered by these regulations unless the investigator has obtained the legally effective informed consent of the subject." yet, consider the exceptions:

> [a]n IRB [Institutional Review Board] may approve a consent procedure which does not include, or which alters, some or all of the elements of informed consent set forth above, or waive the requirement to obtain informed consent, provided . . . [t]he research could not practically be carried out without the waiver or alteration; [t]he research involves no more than minimal risks to the subjects; [t]he waiver or alteration will not adversely affect the rights and welfare of the subjects. . . .

What has happened to the Nuremberg Code? Recall its language: "The voluntary consent of the human subject is *absolutely* essential. This means [the capacity] to exercise free power of choice without the intervention of any element of force, fraud, deceit, duress, overreaching, or other ulterior form of constraint or coercion."

The Nuremberg Tribunal, by proscribing any "ulterior form of constraint," meant to convey that the claims of science cannot supersede voluntary consent; that consent is a *sine qua non*; the balancing of risks against consent is impermissible. Therefore, the Tribunal might not have countenanced the Department of Health and Human Services' requirement, in the absence of informed consent, that the "[r]isks to the subject [b]e reasonable in relation to anticipated benefits, if any, to subjects, *and* the importance of the knowledge that may reasonably be expected to result."

SUMMING UP

When I agreed to write a chapter on the significance of the Nuremberg Code then and now, I did not appreciate that my comparative reflections on "then and now" would make me conclude that the Code is a remarkable document that stands alone in its unequivocal declaration of the rights, perhaps even inalienable rights, of subjects to consent to participation in research. In its other nine principles the Code largely addresses risks to subjects — what risks can be taken and what safeguards should be provided to avoid risks. However, nowhere does it suggest that risks can be taken without prior consultation with a willing subject. Instead it admonishes investigators to consider carefully the risks prior to and during the experiment, and not to invite subjects to participate in research carelessly.

The spirit of the Nuremberg Code was not, and perhaps could not be, taken seriously. Its language was too uncompromising and too inhospitable to the advancement of science that subsequent codes reintroduced by giving physician-scientists considerable discretion in pursuing their objectives. This discretion consists of assigning to physician-investigators the responsibility for protecting research subjects' integrity and delegating to them the awesome responsibility of balancing patient-subjects' interests against the interests of the advancement of medical science.

The question "When may society, actively or by acquiescence, expose some of its members to unconsented-to harm in order to seek benefits for them, for others, or for society as a whole?" was answered differently, both implicitly and explicitly, by the draftees of the Nuremberg Code, the Helsinki Code, and U.S. regulations. The Nuremberg Tribunal saw no need to consider this question. Instead, in setting forth principles that would "satisfy moral, ethical, and legal concepts," the Tribunal wanted not only to close the door to a repetition of the violations of human decency of Dantesque proportions but also to promulgate, ironically aided and abetted by misinformation supplied by the medical experts for the prosecution, a code of research ethics that comported with its views on human decency but that until then had neither existed nor been followed. Its Code asked for both physician-scientists' unwavering allegiance to the Hippocratic ideal of *primum non nocere* and research subjects' uncompromising self-determination.

While misinformation contributed to the formulation of the Nuremberg Code, a document emerged that, if not explicitly then at least implicitly, commanded that the principle of the advancement of science bow to a higher principle: protection of individual inviolability. The rights of individuals to thoroughgoing self-determination and autonomy must come first. Scientific advances may be impeded, perhaps even become impossible at times, but this is a price worth paying.

Had the Tribunal been aware of the tensions that have always existed between the claims of science and individual inviolability, it might have made some acknowledgment of this reality. Perhaps the Tribunal would then have suggested that a balancing of these competing quests is necessary. However, in the light and darkness of the revelations at Nuremberg, it might also have concluded that the traditional balancing of the ethic of science to advance knowledge and the ethic of beneficence to benefit mankind, on the one hand, and the ethic of the sacredness of individual inviolability, on the other hand, must cease; that the former has loomed too large in physician-scientists' minds. The concentration camp experiments could have served as a telling and frightening reminder of how such a mindset can contribute to allowing Nazi physician-scientists to make common cause with the political holocaust, seizing the golden opportunity to extend the frontiers of knowledge to search for ultimate truths without constraint. The memory of these experiments could also have served as a warning that, unless rigorously controlled, even medical science can subject humans beings to abuse in the pursuit of noble goals.

Since the concentration camp experiments had been conducted with non-patients as research subjects, the Tribunal did not need to address the problem of the impact of the ideology of the medical profession on what transpired at Auschwitz. That ideology, which grants physicians great authority in the service of healing, is reflected in the Declaration of Helsinki: "In the treatment of the sick person the doctor *must be free* to use a new therapeutic measure if in *his* judgment it offers hope of saving life, re-establishing health or alleviating suffering. [Only i]f at all possible, consistent with patient psychology, the doctor should obtain the patient's freely given consent." Some of the Nazi doctors spoke to this issue at the trial by attempting to justify, for example, the typhoid vaccine studies—as an effort not only to benefit mankind but also to protect the surviving research subjects from the ravages of typhus epidemics so common in the camp.

Thus, experimenting on them was caring for them and fellow-inmates, performing *Therapia Magna Auschwitzciense*—the great therapy of and in Auschwitz. To obtain consent to participation did not occur to the Nazi doctors. To be sure, the political decision to liquidate Jews and other "inferior races" made consent unthinkable. But it must also be remembered that the investigators were physicians. Had patient consent been indelibly imprinted on their professional minds and hearts, would they have been capable of involving *Therapia Magna* as a justification? I submit that the ideology of the medical profession—which, to be sure, more in the past than now, has eschewed giving patients a more central role in deciding their medical fate—continues to contribute its share to the neglect of voluntary consent in research, particularly in situations, as is often the case, when patients serve as subjects for research.

Even if the Tribunal had been aware of these problems, I hope it would not have modified its first principle—"The voluntary consent of the human subject is *absolutely* essential." It is that assertion that constitutes the significance of the Nuremberg Code then and now. Only when that principle is firmly put into practice can one address the claims of science and the wishes of society to benefit from science. Only then can one avoid the dangers that accompany a balancing of one principle against the other that assigns equal weight to both; for only if one gives primacy to consent can one exercise the requisite caution in situations where one may wish to make an exception to this principle, but only for clear and sufficient reasons.

We must not forget that the cruel experiments conducted at Auschwitz cannot be attributed solely to the ravages of Nazi pseudoscience or to the Nazi physicians themselves. The Tribunal was mistaken in making that attribution. Auschwitz revealed, more starkly than ever, the capacity for aggression inherent in all of us. Intuitively, the Tribunal responded to this fact by formulating its first principle the way it did.

The capacity for aggression, to a considerable extent, was lost sight of again in subsequent formulations of codes and regulations for the conduct of research. As George Santayana observed: "Those who cannot remember the past are condemned to repeat it."[18] We must return to the Nuremberg Code, remember Auschwitz, reflect on the Tribunal's majestic pronouncements, and view them as not solely responsive to what transpired in the concentration camps.

In conclusion, I would like to suggest that the history of experimentation with human beings also testifies to the ubiquity of human aggression, however obscured by physician-scientists' real and caring dedication to the alleviation of mankind's pain and suffering from the ravages of disease. My colleague, the late Robert Cover, when writing about judicial sentencing, reminded us that "judges deal pain and death."[19] He went on to say that "persons [he meant judges, but he could have said it about physician-scientists as well] act within social organizations that exercise authority violently without experiencing . . . the normal degree or inhibition which regulates the behavior of those who act autonomously."[20]

The violent authority that physicians can exercise is obscured by the social organization of the caretaking institutions within which they operate, as is the violence of judges who work within the halls of justice. Many advances in medicine might have been slower in coming had physician-investigators pursued their clinical research less aggressively by not engineering consent. Would it have been a price worth paying, even though the suffering of future patients might have remained for a while longer without relief? The answer is difficult to give; but we must ponder this nagging question and not shut it out of mind.

In restudying the Nuremberg Code 30 years after I had first read it, I became aware, as I had not been before, of our indebtedness to the justices of the Nuremberg Tribunal for leaving us this legacy. We are also indebted to the victims of the medical holocaust for the Tribunal's uncompromising vision. If we wish to truly honor the victims, if we wish not to forget them — for their sake as well as ours — we must not forget the Nuremberg Code. Instead, we must study it and learn from it.

NOTES

1. *Tribunals of War Criminals before the Nuremberg Military Tribunals Under Control Council Law No. 10*, Vols. I and II (Washington D.C.: U.S. Government Printing Office, 1949), Vol. II, p. 181 (hereafter: *Trials of War Criminals*, I or II).

2. See Chapter 7, this volume.

3. *Trials of War Criminals*, II, p. 181.

4. Ibid., II, p. 86.

5. Ibid., I, p. 74.

6. See, for example, V. Veressayev, *The Memoirs of a Physician*, trans. by S. Linden (New York: Alfred A. Knopf, 1916), pp. 332–366. Reprinted in J. Katz (with the assistance of A. M. Capron and E. S. Glass), *Experimentation with Human Beings* (New York: Russell Sage Foundation, 1972), pp. 284–291 (hereafter *Experimentation with Human Beings*).

7. C. Bernard, *An Introduction to the Study of Experimental Medicine*, trans. by H. C. Greene (New York: Macmillian, 1927), pp. 101–102 (emphasis added).

8. T. L. Beauchamp and L. Walters, *Contemporary Issues in Bioethics* (Belmont, Calif.: Wadsworth, 1989), p. 416.

9. 10 *Centralblatt für Bakteriologie und Parasitenkunde* 40–44 (1892), reprinted

in *Concerning Human Vivisection — A Controversy*, (New York: American Humane Association, 1901), p. 26.

10. H. Von Hubbenet, "Observations and Experiments in Syphilis," *The Medical Military Journal* Part 77 (1860): 423 (emphasis added).

11. U.S. Department of Health, Education and Welfare, *Final Report of the Tuskegee Syphilis Study Ad Hoc Advisory Panel* (Washington, D.C., 1973).

12. Reprinted in *Experimentation with Human Beings*, pp. 9–65.

13. H. K. Beecher, "Ethics in Clinical Research," *New England Journal of Medicine* 274 (1966): 1354–1360.

14. World Medical Association: Declaration of Helsinki (revised by the 41st World Medical Assembly (Hong Kong, 1989). See Appendix 3.

15. Ethical Committee of the World Medical Association: "Draft Code of Ethics on Human Experimentation," *British Medical Journal* (2) (1962): 1119.

16. World Medical Association: "Declaration of Helsinki," *British Medical Journal* 2 (1964): 177–180.

17. Department of Health and Human Services: Rules and Regulations for the Protection of Human Research Subjects, *Code of Federal Regulations* 45 (1983): sec. 46.101–46.409.

18. G. Santayana, *The Life of Reason*, Vol. I (New York: Charles Scribner's Sons, 1905), p. 284.

19. R. Cover, "Violence and the Word," *Yale Law Journal* 95 (1986): 1609.

20. Ibid., 1615.

13

Universality of the Nuremberg Code

RUTH MACKLIN

ETHICAL RELATIVISM

A long-standing philosophical debate focuses on the question of whether ethics are relative to time and place. One side argues that there is no evident source of a universal morality, and that ethical rightness and wrongness are products of the cultural and historical milieu from which they emanate. Opponents claim that even if a universal set of ethical norms has not yet been articulated or agreed upon, ethical relativism is a pernicious doctrine that must be rejected. The first group replies that the search for universal ethical precepts is a quest for the Holy Grail. The second group responds with the telling charge: If ethics were relative to time, place, and culture, then what the Nazis did was "right" for them, and there is no basis for moral criticism by anyone outside the Nazi society.

Both sides appear to capture a kernel of truth. There is no denying that different cultures and historical eras exhibit a variety of moral beliefs and practices. The empirical facts revealed by anthropological research yield the descriptive thesis known as *cultural relativity*. But assuming that cultural relativity is an accurate descriptive thesis, whether anything follows for normative ethics is an entirely different question.

In *Patterns of Culture*, published in 1934, the anthropologist Ruth Benedict stated that "Morality differs in every society, and is a convenient term for socially approved habits."[1] In this simple statement, Benedict makes a subtle shift from a descriptive thesis to a prescriptive conclusion. Benedict's underlying assumption is the view that whatever members of a society approve of is right, and whatever they disapprove of is wrong. But that view is easily rebutted. If *morality* were simply a convenient term that described socially approved habits, the accepted medieval practice of torturing criminals, the government-sanctioned institution of slavery, and the subjugation of women historically and in various parts of the world today would all have to stand as morally acceptable because of societal approval at those times and places.

The philosopher Bernard Williams calls relativism "possibly the most absurd view to have been advanced even in moral philosophy."[2] Williams characterizes the "vulgar" form of relativism as consisting of three propositions:

> that "right" means (can only be coherently understood as meaning) "right for a given society"; that "right for a given society" is to be understood in a functionalist sense; and that (therefore) it is wrong for people in one society to condemn, interfere with, etc., the values of another society.[3]

Williams argues that the thesis of ethical relativism, characterized by these three propositions, is logically inconsistent. This is because "it makes a claim in its third proposition, about what is right and wrong in one's dealings with other societies, which uses a *nonrelative* sense of 'right' not allowed for in the first proposition."[4] This results in a "logically unhappy attachment of a nonrelative morality of toleration or noninterference to a view of morality as relative."[5]

If ethical relativism were a logically coherent position, it would not only follow that members of one culture or historical era could never criticize on moral grounds the socially approved practices of another time or place. In addition, there could be no such thing as moral progress. Abolition of slavery could not be seen as a moral victory, but only as political change. The Eighth Amendment to the U.S. Constitution, prohibiting cruel and unusual punishment, could be viewed only as a product of the beliefs of the framers of the Bill of Rights. Granting social and economic equality to women and to blacks, thereby overturning centuries of injustice, could only be viewed as peculiarities of mid-twentieth-century political movements.

If moral beliefs and practices of other cultures and earlier eras cannot be criticized or compared from an ethical point of view, the notion of moral progress is conceptually incoherent. But it does make sense to be able to say that the practices of one time or place are more or less ethically acceptable than those of another. If this is a good reason for rejecting ethical relativism, on what basis can cross-cultural or transhistorical ethical judgments be made?

One answer is offered by the philosopher Walter T. Stace. In order to render cross-cultural judgments about higher or lower degrees of moral progress meaningful, we must appeal to some sort of absolutist ethical theory.[6] This suggestion has the unfortunate consequence of abandoning the frying pan of ethical relativism for the fire of ethical absolutism.

Stace characterizes ethical relativity as "any ethical position which denies that there is a single moral standard which is equally applicable to all men at all times."[7] He contends further than any form of ethical relativity can be shown to be equivalent to radical subjectivism, which reduces ultimately to the position that there is nowhere "to be found a moral standard binding upon anybody against his will. . . . Even judgments to the effect that one man is morally better than another become meaningless. All moral valuation thus vanishes."[8] Stace's absolutist, on the contrary, "believes in moral commands, obedience to which is obligatory on all men, whether they know it or not, whatever they feel, and whatever their customs may be."[9]

Something is amiss if ethical theory allows only these two alternatives: an ethical relativism that reduces to radical subjectivism, an "anything goes" morality; or an ethical absolutism that posits the existence of moral commands obligatory for everyone, but neither universally acknowledged nor clearly articulated. I think there is an alternative to these two unacceptable philosophical positions. One way of spelling out that alternative lies in an analysis of the concept of moral progress. This concept is explicated as resting on two basic normative principles, which can serve as criteria for judging whether moral progress has occurred.[10] However, adherence to the principles does not require a prior acceptance of some particular absolutist ethical theory in order to make cross-cultural or transhistorical judgments about comparative degrees of moral progress.

THE CONCEPT OF MORAL PROGRESS

The first of these two principles can be termed the principle of *humaneness*: One culture, society, or historical era exhibits a higher degree of moral progress than another if the first shows more sensitivity to (less tolerance of) the pain and suffering of human beings than does the second, as expressed in the laws, customs, institutions, and practices of the respective societies or eras.[11]

The second principle I call the principle of *humanity*: One culture, society, or historical era exhibits a higher degree of moral progress than another if the first shows more recognition of the inherent dignity, the basic autonomy, or the intrinsic worth of human beings than does the second, as expressed in the laws, customs, institutions, and practices of the respective societies or eras.[12]

The key terms in these two principles are admittedly somewhat vague. They denote properties that are hard to measure, such as "sensitivity to" or "tolerance of pain and suffering," and "recognition of the dignity, autonomy, or intrinsic worth of human beings." Despite this vagueness, the application of the principles is based on clear, observable evidence drawn from laws, customs, and allowable practices in particular societies or historical eras. For example, the prohibition of cruel and unusual punishment is a sign of moral progress over earlier eras when the hands of thieves were cut off for stealing and when criminal offenders were tortured on racks or pilloried in public. A further indicator of moral progress is found in the sorts of arguments given to justify changes in laws and allowable practices.

It is also clear when one culture or historical era exhibits greater respect for the inherent dignity, the basic autonomy, or the intrinsic worth of human beings. An example is the Bill of Rights, which guarantees people the preservation of their dignity and autonomy in the form of certain freedoms. Any attempt to change laws or social institutions in order to enhance human dignity or promote justice and equality is intended to achieve moral progress. Fair employment legislation, child labor laws, equal rights amendments, and judicial decisions aimed at rectifying discriminatory practices all exemplify conscious efforts to ensure the preservation of the autonomy and dignity of all citizens. To the degree that laws, practices, and ethical beliefs change in the direction of greater recognition of these human attributes, to that extent moral progress has taken place.

The growing acknowledgment of human rights throughout the world provides evidence that certain fundamental ethical principles are now recognized as universally valid. As we know too well, there remain in power some individuals, along with their military forces, and perhaps a few cultures as a whole, that violate ethical prohibitions against torture, maiming, degradation, and exploitation. But these instances are not counterexamples to the universality of fundamental ethical principles. Instead, they represent malevolent, corrupt, inhumane, or insensitive behavior, conduct that violates fundamental ethical precepts rather than being ethically valid alternatives.

A judgment that moral progress has occurred does not entail the proposition that human nature has changed. Nor does it mean that there have been no lapses or regressions by individuals in power or even by entire societies. The Nazi era in general, and the behavior of Nazi doctors in particular,[13] serve to show that despite a general historical progression toward greater humaneness and humanity, egregious regressions and moral backsliding have occurred.

ULTIMATE PRINCIPLES VERSUS SPECIFIC STANDARDS

There have been other notable attempts to resolve the question of what cultural relativism as a descriptive thesis implies for ethical relativism as a normative view. One philosopher has sought to distinguish between ultimate moral principles and specific moral standards or rules. Paul Taylor notes that both can be called *norms*, and the descriptive relativist often overlooks this distinction. The key to rebutting ethical relativism lies in understanding that an ultimate moral principle can "be consistent with a variety of specific standards and rules as found in the moral codes of different societies."[14]

Taylor gives examples of specific moral standards, such as personal courage or trustworthiness, and specific rules of conduct, such as "Do not tell lies for one's own advantage," which prescribe how people ought or ought not to act. He contrasts these to ultimate moral principles, which are universal propositions about the conditions under which a standard or rule is to be used to judge *any* person or action. Taylor offers utility as one example of an ultimate moral principle: Right actions or practices are those that result in an increase in everyone's happiness or a decrease in everyone's unhappiness.

Applying this general principle of utility to different societies, we find that a specific standard or rule that increases people's happiness in one culture will not increase but rather decrease people's happiness in another. Taylor uses the well-known example of letting elderly people die when they can no longer contribute to economic production. When that practice is necessary for the survival of everyone else, it accords with the principle of utility. In a society of abundance, however, old people can easily be supported when they are no longer productive.

> Thus the principle of utility would require that in the first society the rule "Do not keep a person alive when he can no longer produce" be part of its moral code, and in the second society it would require a contrary rule. In this case the very same kind of action that is wrong in one society will be right in another. Yet there is a single principle that makes an action of that kind wrong (in one set of circumstances) and another action of that kind right (in a different set of circumstances).[15]

Taylor's analysis is useful for distinguishing between ultimate moral principles and specific rules of conduct. But that analysis stops short of another foundational problem in ethics: how to determine which of several *ultimate* moral principles to accept in cases where they conflict. The principle of utility, which Taylor uses to illustrate the consistency of having a single ultimate principle while allowing for different specific rules of conduct, is not the only ultimate ethical principle. Another leading candidate is the Kantian categorical imperative: "People are to be treated as ends, never merely as means to the ends of others." What happens when these two fundamental principles clash?

APPLYING ULTIMATE PRINCIPLES TO HUMAN SUBJECTS RESEARCH

Consider how the principle of utility operates in the context of research involving human subjects. If utility were the only fundamental ethical principle, there would be no need to obtain informed consent from research subjects when the research is likely to yield great benefits to future patients while posing little risk of harm to the subjects themselves. A favorable risk-benefit ratio is a specific ethical standard governing research design, a requirement justified by the general principle of utility. In the research context, it is referred to as *beneficence*. The obligation of researchers, according to the principle of beneficence, is to "maximize possible benefits and minimize possible harms."[16]

This specific standard is ethically necessary but not sufficient for addressing the ethical concerns of human subjects research. A second and crucial requirement is the need to obtain voluntary, informed consent from research subjects. Indeed, this second ethical requirement is the foremost precept of the Nuremberg Code. The Code begins by stating that "the voluntary consent of the human subject is absolutely essential. This means that the person involved . . . should be so situated as to be able to exercise free power of choice without the intervention of any element of force, fraud, deceit, duress, overreaching, or other ulterior form of constraint or coercion and should have sufficient knowledge and comprehension of the elements of the subject matter involved as to enable him to make an understanding and enlightened decision."

This requirement constitutes a different specific ethical standard from that of beneficence and is justified by a quite different ultimate moral principle from that of utility. Drawn from the Kantian tradition in moral philosophy, this principle is commonly referred to as *respect for persons*. As formulated by the National Commission for the Protection of Human Subjects of Biomedical and Behavioral Research: "Respect for persons incorporates at least two ethical convictions: first, that individuals should be treated as autonomous agents, and second, that persons with diminished autonomy are entitled to protection."[17]

The propositions spelled out in the Nuremberg Code state a set of moral precepts that serve as criteria for evaluating the conduct of biomedical research. Actual research practices, both before and after the Nuremberg Code was enunciated, can be judged against the moral standards articulated in the Code.

The Nuremberg Code contains ethical principles that ought to have applied to biomedical research, whether or not Nazi physicians acknowledged or recognized them. An example is principle 4: "The experiment should be so conducted as to avoid all unnecessary physical and mental suffering and injury." This principle reflects a fundamental moral belief about how human beings should treat one another, namely, that it is wrong to cause unnecessary pain or suffering. It is not a principle peculiar to the ethics of research involving human subjects. Nor is it a moral principle that first emerged in the mid-twentieth century. It is a variant of the utilitarian principle that enjoins moral agents to minimize pain or unhappiness and to maximize pleasure or happiness.

Some ethical defenses of the form "We didn't have these rules back then" can be valid. For example, a rule requiring ethical review by an independent committee, such as an Institutional Review Board, stipulates a mechanism for trying to ensure that research involving human subjects is ethically sound. This is a procedural rather than a substantive ethical requirement. There may be other ways of accomplishing this or other procedural requirements. Generally speaking, in ethical contexts, procedural rules fall under Taylor's category of "specific rules of conduct." Although some specific rules of conduct have substantive ethical content, others are merely procedural.

NAZI VIOLATION OF ULTIMATE MORAL PRINCIPLES

The Nazi doctors violated fundamental moral principles governing the conduct of human beings toward one another, specifically, that it is wrong to inflict unnecessary pain or suffering. In addition to this general moral principle, Nazi doctors *as physicians* belonged to a professional tradition going back to ancient Greek medicine that embodied maxims such as "Do no harm."

Nazi doctors conducted experiments on hypothermia in order to develop survival techniques for German pilots shot down over the North Sea. To simulate these conditions, hundreds of Dachau inmates were immersed in vats of freezing water until their body temperatures fell to 79.7°F. Many died of exposure.[18]

Another series of experiments related to the Nazi war effort involved high-altitude studies in decompression chambers. One

> was a continuous experiment on a 37-year-old Jew in good general condition.
> . . . Breathing continued up to 30 minutes. After 4 minutes, the experimental
> subject began to perspire and wiggle his head, after 5 minutes cramps occurred,
> between 6 and 10 minutes breathing increased in speed and the experimental
> subject became unconscious; from 11 to 30 minutes breathing slowed down to
> three breaths per minute, finally stopping altogether.[19]

The doctrine of ethical relativism was invoked explicitly at various points in the Nuremberg trial. For example, under direct examination, Dr. Andrew C. Ivy, an expert witness for the prosecution, was asked about ethical standards and practices in the United States. An objection was raised by Dr. Sauter, defense counsel for the defendants Ruff and Romberg:

> The question asked here is always what the opinion of the medical profession in
> America is. For us in this trial, in the evaluation of German defendants, that is
> not decisive. In my opinion the decisive question is for example, in 1942, when the
> altitude experiments were undertaken at Dachau, what the attitude of the medical
> profession in Germany was. . . . [W]e are not interested in finding out what the
> ethical attitude of the medical profession in the United States was. In my opinion
> a German physician who in Germany performed experiments on Germans cannot
> be judged exclusively according to an American medical opinion, which moreover
> dates from the year 1945 and was coded in the years 1945 and 1946 for future use;
> it can also have no retroactive force.[20]

This objection implicitly defends both claims of the relativist thesis: that ethics is relative to place and to time. As invoked in this example, the point that ethical standards vary according to time is truly bizarre. A gap of 3 or 4 years is presumed to justify a variation in ethical standards. If genuine ethical standards could change so radically in so short a time, how could anyone be expected to keep up?

To accept Dr. Sauter's contention that standards developed later can have no retroactive force would mean that practices in earlier times could never be subjected to subsequent ethical judgments. We could not morally condemn slavery, cruel and unusual punishment, or other practices in the array of inhumane activities to which history bears witness. The human experiments carried out by the Nazis were not the sort of behavior that might ethically be defended by pointing out that rules for conducting biomedical research were developed later. Nazi experiments violated fundamental moral principles known to the Germans and applicable throughout the Western world for centuries.

It is surely true that some research on human subjects conducted in earlier eras did violate fundamental moral principles, but probably not in the systematic, egregious manner of the Nazi experiments. Historically, many experiments failed to accord with more recently established ethical standards, such as the requirement to obtain informed consent. Nazi doctors violated all previously existing ethical precepts of medical practice in carrying out their experiments, not just a failure to obtain the subjects' informed consent. The fact that doctors in earlier eras experimented on human subjects without their knowledge or consent, and that such behavior was widely practiced and approved, cannot ethically justify such conduct. Yet those common practices of earlier times were used by the defense in the Nuremberg trials. One argument for the defense asserted that

> evidence has now proved that in recent decades and even earlier, numerous experiments were carried out on human beings, . . . of the nature and degree of danger of which they could not have been aware and to which they would never have agreed voluntarily. The only conclusion that can be drawn from these facts is that during recent decades views on this question have changed. . . . [21]

In this passage and elsewhere in the transcript of the trials, the defense emphasized the widespread practice of conducting experiments on human beings without their voluntary consent. The fact that a practice is widespread at any time or place does not mean that it is ethically sound, but only that it is accepted or tolerated. The ethical relativist's claim is that the acceptability of an action or practice at any given time or place is the *only* criterion for its ethical rightness. Arguments for the defense in the Nuremberg trial repeatedly invoked this contention of the relativist. As one example:

> Experiments that time and again have been described in international literature without meeting any opposition do not constitute a crime from the medical point of view. . . . In view of the complete lack of *written* legal norms, the physician, who generally knows only little about the law, has to rely on and refer to the admissibility of what is generally recognized to be admissible all over the world. [22]

The Nazi experiments not only violated specific procedural rules of conduct, they also violated specific substantive moral precepts embodied in widely accepted, ultimate moral principles. Although the specific rules governing human experiments were not promulgated until the Nuremberg Code was enunciated, after the Nazi experiments had been carried out, Nazi doctors could not justify their actions by saying "We didn't have those rules back then."

THE CHARGE OF "ETHICAL IMPERIALISM"

It cannot be denied that the leading precepts of biomedical ethics articulated over the past several decades have a bias that reveals their origins in Western philosophical thought. With roots in both the Kantian moral tradition and British liberal philosophy, the bias appears in injunctions that mandate truth telling, self-determination, and respect for privacy and confidentiality. These values are integral to the political philosophy of liberal individualism and are rarely as prominent, if they exist at all, in non-Western societies.

This fact was pointed out by some participants from developing countries at a conference sponsored by the World Health Organization (WHO) in December 1980. At the conference, WHO's "Proposed International Ethical Guidelines for Human Experimentation" were first presented. One conference participant from the United States described the guidelines as "essentially based on American standards of ethical review as well as on the international codes"—the Nuremberg Code, the Declaration of Helsinki, and the Tokyo Amendment.[23]

Put more precisely, the guidelines embody not peculiarly American ethical *standards*, but rather American *procedures* for review of research. Ethical standards and procedures for implementing them should be clearly distinguished. The ethical standards of the WHO guidelines are embodied in the international codes. Procedures such as the use of Institutional Review Boards, like those in the United States, may vary from one country to another without violating the ethical standards spelled out in the codes.

The critics from developing countries at the WHO conference objected to what they called "ethical imperialism." "How far, they wondered, can Western countries impose a certain concept of human rights? In countries where the common law heritage of individuality, freedom of choice, and human rights does not exist, the . . . guidelines may seem entirely inappropriate."[24] The reply given at the conference did not exactly meet this objection. "Several delegates pointed out that when first introduced in the United States, ethical review and IRBs were also considered to be idealistic and an imposition on the rights of researchers."[25]

This reply addresses the fact that medical researchers in the United States were now required to adhere to a set of constraints and procedures that had not existed in the past. But the reply overlooks the fact that the values embodied in these new ethical requirements have long endured in Western culture. Such values as self-determination, the right to be informed, and the right to confidentiality have been widely acknowledged and embraced outside the realm of medical research. They are all associated with individualism, which is more characteristic of Western societies than of African or Asian cultures. What the participants from developing countries were really objecting to was not the constraints imposed on researchers, but rather the imposition of Western individualistic values that were alien to their own societies.

A slightly revised version of the Proposed International Guidelines was endorsed in October 1981 by the 23rd Session of the WHO Advisory Committee on Medical Research. The Proposed Guidelines go beyond the 10 basic principles stated in the Nuremberg Code, both in detail and in scope. For example, one ethical concept not even mentioned in the Nuremberg Code, but discussed explicitly in the Guidelines, is confidentiality.

Confidentiality is not mentioned in the Declaration of Helsinki either, but it is broadly implied. Principle 6 of the Declaration states: "The right of the research subject to safeguard his or her integrity must always be respected. Every precaution should be taken to respect the privacy of the subject and to minimize the impact of the study on the subject's physical and mental integrity and on the personality of the subject."[26]

The section on confidentiality in the Proposed International Guidelines is close to the federal regulations governing National Institutes of Health (NIH)-sponsored research in the United States. The WHO statement says:

> Research may involve the collection and storage of data relating to individuals, which, if disclosed to third parties, might cause harm or distress. Consequently, arrangements should be made by investigators to protect the confidentiality of such data, as for example by omitting information which might lead to the identification of individual subjects, by limiting access to the data, or other appropriate means.[27]

Is this ethical imperialism? Privacy and confidentiality are largely contemporary Western concepts. Almost 20 years ago, Victor Sidel, a physician widely known for his national and international work in public health, visited China for the first time. When he encountered common public health practices that required people to reveal highly personal information, Sidel asked: "Don't people object to this? Don't they consider it an invasion of their privacy?" His Chinese interpreter replied that the concept of privacy did not have a Chinese equivalent. The interpreter could not translate the question.

Public posting in medical clinics of highly personal information about individuals' health status, inoculations, women's menstrual cycles, and other data is commonly practiced in some developing nations. If, like China, these societies do not even have a concept of privacy or confidentiality, can such practices be ethically wrong? Would it be an imposition of alien ethical concepts to insist that privacy and confidentiality be respected in the research setting? If people do not perceive an act or practice as harmful, can they nonetheless be harmed by it? These questions are not easily answered.

One approach to this issue is to hold that privacy is a derivative moral concept, not a fundamental one. It derives from a philosophy of individualism, as does the "respect for persons" principle discussed earlier in connection with informed consent. But the principle demanding respect for persons is fundamental. The wrongness of acts or practices such as enslavement, exploitation, torture, and degradation is a moral judgment not culturally limited to the perspective of Western individualism. These acts are violations of a moral prohibition that ought to be universally acknowledged.

In contrast, invasion of privacy in Western societies is one of numerous ways of failing to respect a person. In Japan or China, a different specific act might constitute a violation. More needs to be said to support my contention that privacy is a derivative rather than a fundamental moral concept. I propose it as a suggestion that needs fleshing out by supplying an underlying theory capable of explicating the distinction between fundamental and derivative ethical concepts.

When research involving human subjects is carried out on an international scale, in the form of collaborative research or under the auspices of an international organization, then the most well-developed ethical standards should apply. This is necessary to prevent researchers from countries in which research is highly regulated from taking their operations elsewhere. It can also serve to introduce ethical standards in settings where they do not yet exist. The introduction of these standards should not be construed as ethical imperialism, but rather, as an instance of moral progress.

ILLUSTRATION: WHO-SPONSORED RESEARCH

This is essentially the approach taken by WHO in the international research it sponsors. I currently serve on a standing committee that conducts ongoing scientific, technical, and ethical reviews of WHO-sponsored research on human reproduction.[28] Most of the research on fertility regulation, male contraceptives, and natural family planning methods is carried out in developing countries. The ethical standards used by WHO in guidelines issued to investigators are those embodied in the latest revision of the Declaration of Helsinki.

In my work with the review group, I anticipated some problems of confidentiality and informed consent arising out of a set of research proposals studying infertility. A few of these studies seek to enroll both husbands and wives as participants. The studies typically investigate infertility in women as secondary to previously contracted sexually transmitted diseases. Studies are carried out at or in conjunction with local clinics where the woman (or couple) normally receives health services. When I encountered the first of these protocols, to be carried out in a country in which women are still the virtual property of their husbands, I asked whether information supplied by a woman would be kept confidential from her husband, especially in cases where both partners were enrolled in the study. No one on the committee knew the answer, but all became concerned about the possibility. Committee members knowledgeable about the prevailing customs confirmed my supposition about the relationship between husbands and wives in this culture.

My question and the ensuing discussion by committee members led to the formulation of a new statement on confidentiality of research subjects, which was subsequently added to the WHO Program's Guidelines for preparation of applications. The statement reads as follows:

> HRP guidelines require the consent form to state that all records are confidential. However, if absolute confidentiality cannot be guaranteed, subjects should be told whether anyone might have access to records of the study. In cases where both members of a married couple are study participants, each partner should be informed of the extent to which confidentiality will be maintained. In cultures in which husbands normally exercise considerable control over their wives, women must be advised in advance of becoming a study participant whether information they disclose might be revealed to their spouses.

Including this statement about confidentiality in the guidelines does not, of course, guarantee that a physician conducting research will not disclose information to a demanding husband when both men — researcher and subject — are from a culture in which husbands own their wives. It does, however, show that despite its Western origins, the precept of confidentiality should now be considered sufficiently universal to be mandated in WHO-sponsored research. Given the sensitive nature of information about a woman's history of sexually transmitted disease, which might be disclosed to her husband, to adhere to the culturally approved practice of not respecting a wife's confidentiality could cause her harm. Imposing a requirement of confidentiality is thus justified by the more general moral principle embodied in the Nuremberg Code's principle 4: "The experiment should be so conducted as to avoid all unnecessary physical and mental suffering and injury."

ETHICAL STANDARDS AND RELIGIOUS DICTATES

A different problem of ethical relativism arises when the moral rules of a culture are dictated by a single dominant religion. In several Islamic countries, religious dictates may preclude acceptance of some of the leading precepts of biomedical ethics. Consider what one health care professional, who is chief psychologist at the psychiatric hospital of Kuwait, has to say about Islamic values in bioethics:

> . . . the patient's right to know the truth about his medical condition is highly promoted in Western medical practice. The Islamic interpretation of this right has a different emphasis: The physician is responsible for ensuring the calm and peaceful life of the patient. If, in his judgment, knowledge about terminal, non-contagious disease would be counterproductive, withholding the truth from the patient, even if the patient wished to be fully informed, would not be sinful.[29]

This position serves as a reminder that medical paternalism is still very much alive in some parts of the world. *Even if the patient wished to be fully informed*, the Islamic ethic permits the doctor to withhold the truth about his medical condition. Setting aside the standard therapeutic context, what are the implications for the research setting? I am ignorant of the extent to which medical research is carried out in Kuwait, but it is clear that withholding information from terminally ill patients is inconsistent with informed consent to a research maneuver. If experimental drugs for cancer are available in Kuwait, a patient with advanced metastatic cancer could not be enrolled in a clinical trial without first being informed of the purpose of the research. Revealing that, along with the potential risks and anticipated benefits, would entail informing the patient about the nature and prognosis of the disease.

Failure to disclose this information to the patient in the research context would violate principle 1 of the Nuremberg Code. Specifically: "the person involved should have . . . sufficient knowledge and comprehension of the elements of the subject matter involved as to enable him to make an understanding and enlightened decision. This latter element requires that before the acceptance of an affirmative decision by the experimental subject there should be made known to him the nature, duration, and purpose of the experiment . . . and the effects upon his health or person which may possibly come from his participation in the experiment." It follows from principle 1 of the Nuremberg Code that a cancer researcher in Kuwait must disclose the truth about a terminal condition to a patient, even if the researcher judges that such knowledge "would be counterproductive."

Is it unacceptable to impose this Western-derived precept of informed consent on an Islamic society? Ethical debate may continue to swirl around the purely therapeutic context. But for research, the universality of the Nuremberg principle should prevail. A physician could always take the option of deciding not to enroll as research subjects any patients to whom disclosure of terminal illness would be counterproductive in ensuring a calm and peaceful life. If it is objected that this would deny such patients the potential benefits of the experimental drug, one reply is that the Nuremberg Code is silent on the ethical issue of justice in equitably distributing the benefits and burdens of research.

The psychologist from Kuwait made a second point:

> The management of suffering and death produces tensions for the Islamic practitioner. For a Muslim patient long-term suffering presents an opportunity to show courage and faith in the God who tests his patience. And the Islamic position on euthanasia is very clear: Life cannot be terminated either actively or passively because that interferes with God's will. Continued aggressive therapy is always demanded.[30]

This point also poses a problem in the research setting. Suppose that the research involved implantation of an artificial heart. Suppose, further, that the heart was powered by an external source to which the patient had to remain tethered, as were Barney Clark and the others who received the Jarvik artificial heart. The Islamic position on withdrawing treatment is very clear: "Life cannot be terminated either actively or passively because that interferes with God's will. Continued aggressive therapy is always demanded."

However, principle 9 of the Nuremberg Code states: "During the course of the experiment the human subject should be at liberty to bring the experiment to an end if he has reached the physical or mental state where continuation of the experiment seems to him to be impossible." The solution proposed in connection with the example of cancer research could be used here as well: Such research might have to be forgone altogether in an Islamic state. In the case of the Jarvik heart, that might well have been a benefit rather than a loss to the potential subjects. But in the case of other experimental drugs that prolong life, such as new therapies for AIDS, the inability of patients to withdraw would violate their rights as research subjects.

COLLABORATIVE RESEARCH: WHOSE ETHICAL STANDARDS?

Are ethics relative to time and geography? Although there is no single "yes" or "no" answer to this question, I have tried to show that a careful ethical analysis tends to support a "no" rather than a "yes" answer. I conclude with a brief account of a 1989 meeting in which I participated at the U.S. Centers for Disease Control (CDC) in Atlanta.

A group was invited to discuss a number of ethical issues that arose in a proposed collaborative study between the CDC and medical researchers in the People's Republic of China. The study was to be placebo-controlled and randomized. The Chinese collaborator was resisting the CDC-imposed requirement of informed consent. Some CDC officials thought that the Chinese researcher's objections were valid, given the differences in biomedical research and practice between the United States and China. Our standards of informed consent to treatment seem rarely to apply in China, and there have apparently been very few clinical trials similar to those common in the United States and Europe.

The Chinese physician was opposed to the informed consent requirement on two grounds. First, consent is an alien notion in Chinese medical practice, so informed consent in a research context would be totally unfamiliar to Chinese participants. Second, if subjects were told that half would get a placebo, no one would enroll because the concept of a placebo (or, at least, a placebo-controlled study) is unheard of in China.

Lengthy discussion ensued on whether it was ethical imperialism to impose on China research requirements drawn from U.S. regulations. Several of us managed to convince the larger group that it was not specific U.S. government regulations that were being imposed, but rather worldwide principles articulated in the Declaration of Helsinki, an international statement adopted by the World Medical Association at four separate congresses, most recently in 1989.

After much discussion, the group also agreed that the use of placebos in research is unethical when subjects are *not* informed that they will receive either active medication or placebo. The discussion was complicated by the literal translation offered by the Chinese researcher. He proposed a Chinese translation of the phrase "makes people comfortable." The group insisted that he should use different Chinese words that would convey the true meaning of *placebo* in the research context.

Near the end of the meeting, one or two people who knew Chinese asked the physician to write the Chinese characters that would be used on a consent form. When he wrote the ideograph for *informed consent*, one American was puzzled. Hesitantly, she asked that the ideograph be interpreted. The Chinese physician explained the ideograph, which turned out to mean "*informal* consent." That had been his understanding all along of what is conveyed by our English words *informed consent*.

One moral of this story is that biomedical researchers themselves need to be fully educated about the ethical principles embodied in the Nuremberg Code and the Declaration of Helsinki before these principles can be implemented in regions where such ethical requirements for research do not exist. Nazi doctors could not make a valid defense that they did not know their hideous experiments violated ultimate moral principles. Nor can medical scientists anywhere today circumvent the need to comply with the basic principles of research ethics endorsed throughout the world.

A second moral of the story pertains to moral progress. The consensus reached at the CDC meeting was that research ethics are universal, and that imposing the requirement of informed consent on biomedical research carried out in China would serve to raise the standards of physicians and the expectations of patients. In conforming to the "respect for persons" principle, attaining these new standards would be an instance of moral progress.

The week that followed the CDC meeting saw the march of events at Tienanmen Square, in which Chinese soldiers fired on civilian demonstrators, political prisoners were taken, and government repression squelched the democracy movement. The Chinese government was condemned by nations throughout the world for the many violations of human rights that occurred during the ensuing weeks and months. An ethical relativist would have no basis for that moral condemnation. The conclusion is compelling that when it is a matter of fundamental human rights, ethics are not relative to time and geography.

CONCLUSION

It would be a moral understatement to conclude that the Nazi experiments were wrong because voluntary, informed consent was not obtained from the subjects. The moral evil of these experiments lay in the torture and killing of human beings for the ostensible purpose of obtaining useful information for the German war effort. Two fundamental ethical principles were simultaneously violated: the prohibition against inflicting suffering on human beings and the Kantian categorical imperative prohibiting the use of persons as mere means to the ends of others.

In reaction to the Nazi experiments, specific ethical rules for conducting research on human subjects were fashioned and embodied in the principles of the Nuremberg Code. In addition to principle 1, stating that "the voluntary consent of the human subject is absolutely essential," other key principles are as follows:

4. The experiment should be so conducted as to avoid all unnecessary physical and mental suffering and injury.
5. No experiment should be conducted where there is an *a priori* reason to believe that death or disabling injury will occur.
7. Proper preparations should be made and adequate facilities provided to protect the experimental subject against even remote possibilities of injury, disability, or death.
10. During the course of the experiment the scientist in charge must be prepared to terminate the experiment at any stage, if he has probable cause to believe, in the exercise of the good faith, superior skill, and careful judgment required of him, that a continuation of the experiment is likely to result in injury, disability, or death to the experimental subject.

These principles embody an ethical ideal, one that is universally applicable. Conduct that comports with this ideal is possible to achieve in the day-to-day practice of biomedical research. Medical experiments conducted before the articulation of the Nuremberg Code can still be judged by the extent to which they approximate the ideal. All present and future research involving human subjects should comply with this ideal, now internationally recognized as embodying ethical standards that must be applied in actual practice.

The closing brief for defendant Ruff in the Nuremberg trial called for just such an international agreement:

one has to strive toward obtaining an international basis to represent the present international opinion on human experiments, one which for decades, if not for centuries, will form the criterion for the permissibility of human experiments. We, as jurists, can only render a service to the development of medical science and therewith to humanity if we endeavor to establish an incontrovertibly clear view of today's international opinion on human experiments. . . .[31]

The international basis representing international opinion was eventually established in the Declaration of Helsinki, for which the Nuremberg Code served as the cornerstone.[32] It is the ongoing obligation of biomedical researchers, sponsors of the research, and members of ethical review committees to exercise constant vigilance to ensure that the principles stated in the Nuremberg Code are universally applied.

NOTES

1. Ruth Benedict, *Patterns of Culture* (New York: Mentor Books, 1934).

2. Bernard Williams, *Morality: An Introduction to Ethics* (New York: Harper & Row, 1972), p. 20.

3. Ibid.

4. Ibid., p. 21.

5. Ibid.

6. Walter T. Stace, "Ethical Relativity," in Paul W. Taylor, ed., *Problems of Moral Philosophy* (Encino, Calif.: Dickenson, 1972), pp. 51–65.

7. Ibid., p. 51.

8. Ibid., p. 61.

9. Ibid., p. 57.

10. See, generally, Ruth Macklin, "Moral Progress," *Ethics* 87 (1977): 370–382.

11. Ibid., pp. 371–372.

12. Ibid., p. 372.

13. See, for example, Robert J. Lifton, *The Nazi Doctors: Medical Killing and the Psychology of Genocide* (New York: Basic Books, 1986); and Robert N. Proctor, *Racial Hygiene: Medicine Under the Nazis* (Cambridge, Mass.: Harvard University Press, 1988).

14. Paul W. Taylor, *Principles of Ethics: An Introduction* (Encino, Calif.: Dickenson, 1975), p. 17.

15. Ibid.

16. National Commission for the Protection of Human Subjects of Biomedical and Behavioral Research, *The Belmont Report: Ethical Principles and Guidelines for the Protection of Human Subjects of Research* (Washington, D.C.: U.S. Government Printing Office, 1979), p. 4.

17. Ibid.

18. Beryl Byman, "Bitter Fruit: The Legacy of Nazi Medical Experiments," *Minnesota Medicine*, 62 (1989): 582–586.

19. Quotation cited in ibid., p. 581.

20. Extracts from the Testimony of Prosecution Expert Witness Dr. Andrew C. Ivy, *Trials of War Criminals Before the Nuremberg Military Tribunals Under Control Law 10* (Washington, D.C.: Superintendent of Documents, U.S. Government Printing Office), *Military Tribunal I*, case 1, *United States v. Karl Brandt et al.*, October 1948–April 1949, Vol. II, p. 85.

21. Selection from the Argumentation of the Defense, Extract from the Final Plea for Defendant Gebhardt, *Military Tribunal I*, Vol. II, p. 72.

22. Extract from the Closing Brief for Defendant Ruff, *Military Tribunal I*, Vol. II, p. 92.

23. Emily Miller, "International Trends in Ethical Review of Medical Research," *IRB: A Review of Human Subjects Research* 3(8) (1981): 9.

24. Ibid., 10.

25. Ibid.

26. Version adopted by the 18th World Medical Assembly, Helsinki, Finland, 1964, and revised by the 29th World Medical Assembly, Tokyo, Japan, 1975.

27. Proposed International Ethical Guidelines for Human Experimentation (Geneva: CIOMS, 1982), p. 34.

28. The committee, called the "Scientific and Ethical Review Group," is convened under the auspices of the Special Programme of Research, Development and Research Training in Human Reproduction (abbreviated HRP) of the World Health Organization.

29. Marwan Al-Mutawa, "Health Care Ethics in Kuwait," *Hastings Center Report* 19, Special Supplement (1989): 11.

30. Ibid.

31. Extract from the Closing Brief for Defendant Ruff, *Military Tribunal I*, Vol. II, p. 93.

32. See Chapter 7, this volume.

14

The Doctors' Trial and Analogies to the Holocaust in Contemporary Bioethical Debates

ARTHUR L. CAPLAN

What is the relevance of the Holocaust for contemporary bioethics? It defies credibility that those in bioethics have spent so little time trying to answer this question. This is not simply because crimes on a staggering scale were committed in the name of public health by doctors and nurses. The tone and tenor of current debates concerning moral choices in biomedicine give this question particular urgency. References and analogies to the Holocaust, to Nazi Germany, and to the crimes of German medicine abound in contemporary discussions of bioethical subjects. Yet many who are quick either to invoke the Holocaust or to deny its relevance to contemporary events do so with an inadequate understanding of what Nazi doctors and scientists actually did and why.

It is only during the past 5 years that serious scholarship aimed at understanding biomedicine's role in the Holocaust has emerged. This work shows that medicine, public health, and the biological and social sciences all played key roles in the rise to power of the Nazis and in the implementation of the "Final Solution."[1] Even though serious analyses of how those in biomedical sciences justified their embrace of Nazism are still rare,[2] the Holocaust and the crimes of Nazi medicine and biomedical science command wide attention in contemporary bioethical discussions and debates.

One reason for the relative silence of bioethicists concerning the rationales and justifications given by German scientists and physicians during the Nazi era is that it is troubling for those concerned with bioethical issues to contemplate the possibility that those who supported the Nazi regime, who helped supply key elements of the epistemological and ideological foundations of Nazism, and who implemented or quietly endorsed the genocidal policies of the Third Reich did so from firm moral convictions. It is hard to accept the idea that those who committed terrible crimes against helpless persons were, when placed on trial for these actions, willing to present serious moral arguments in their defense. It is easier and less disturbing to simply dismiss the crimes of biomedicine under Nazism as the vicious acts of a small group of lunatics, deviants, and second-rate minds. It is easier, but it is also false.

Once the extensive role of mainstream doctors, nurses, public health officials, and other biomedical scientists in the rise and reign of Nazism is acknowledged, it becomes impossible to avoid an examination of the ethical views and rationale that fueled biomedicine's embrace of Nazism. One of the obvious, if too long ignored, places to turn to begin the examination is the Nuremberg trials. The first set of defendants placed on trial after the War Crimes Trial were 26 physicians and public health officials in what has come to be known as the "Doctors' Trial." The Doctors' Trial focused primarily on the actions of the defendants with respect to medical experiments conducted in concentration camps. Many of the charges concerned abuse carried out in research on human beings. In the area of human experimentation, the Doctors' Trial has become paradigmatic of the extremes of abuse that can occur.

The doctors who stood trial at Nuremberg were also, however, charged with a broad assortment of crimes that had nothing to do with research or human experimentation. They were charged with crimes against humanity, including genocide and murder. They were accused of carrying out forced sterilization. They were charged with complicity in the selection of persons for slave labor or extermination. These crimes have received far less attention, partly because the Nuremberg Code, which was promulgated at the conclusion of the trial, focused exclusively on the legal and ethical obligations and rights of those involved in human experimentation.

The emphasis on human experimentation was partly a response to the fact that it was easier for the prosecution to make those charges stick. While the legal foundation of the indictments concerning the abuse of human subjects was somewhat shaky,[3] it was far more solid than the legal foundations for the indictments pertaining to crimes against humanity, forced sterilization, and genocide.[4] These were crimes of such a horrid nature that few governments had bothered to write laws prohibiting them. Moreover, it was easier to prove that the defendants had taken direct roles in carrying out abuses against specific human subjects, some of whom had survived and could give evidence, than it was to prove that a particular defendant had directly caused the death of a particular person in a concentration camp by means of poison gas.

Research, more than the ethics of public health or of therapy, dominated the Doctors' Trial and the Nuremberg Code that resulted from it. Nonetheless, the ethics of research and the ethics of medical practice with respect to therapy and the promotion of public health were all inextricably intertwined in the Doctors' Trial. While it is true that the Nuremberg Code is explicitly aimed at regulating research involving human subjects, the trial proceedings provide clear insight into the moral rationales that motivated the defendants, as well as the many others who were not on trial but who supported the Nazi Reich. The moral rationales given for the conduct of cruel and sometimes lethal experiments were also those cited in defense of participation in infanticide, genocide, murder, sterilization, and torture.

The moral arguments of those in biomedicine who supported and carried out the policies of the Nazi regime must be taken seriously, if for no other reason than to understand how it was that doctors and public health officials came to play such a central role in the Holocaust. The moral arguments and rationales offered at Nuremberg are also important for the light they shed on one of the most important arguments invoked in contemporary bioethical debates — the Nazi analogy.

Nowhere has the Nazi analogy been more in evidence than in the controversy over the propriety of withdrawing life-extending care from Nancy Cruzan and in the dispute over efforts to use fetal tissue obtained from elective abortions in clinical research aimed at helping those with Parkinson's disease and diabetes. Given the gravity of the charge, whenever the Nazi analogy is invoked, the appropriateness and validity of analogies to the Holocaust and Nazism regarding biomedicine must be carefully evaluated and assessed. The only way to analyze the similarities and differences between what happened in Germany and what is going on now in the United States, Germany, or any other nation is to strive to understand what the Nazis did and why they did it. The Doctors' Trial and the specific moral rationales presented by the biomedical defendants at that trial provides an invaluable source of evidence for the assessment of analogies to the Holocaust with respect to both contemporary research and contemporary therapeutic practices.

THE CRUZAN CASE AND THE NAZI ANALOGY

Those who argue against withdrawing food and fluids from Nancy Cruzan, and from others in the same state of permanent unconsciousness, are sometimes quick to draw analogies between stopping her medical care and the actions of Nazi physicians and nurses who engaged in active euthanasia in mental hospitals, nursing homes, and concentration camps.[5] Are these comparisons appropriate? Do those making the analogies know what they are talking about when they suggest that the attempt by Cruzan's parents to have her feeding tube withdrawn is analogous to the actions of doctors and nurses who killed handicapped infants, the mentally ill, and the demented elderly as part of Nazi Germany's euthanasia programs? Are they accurate in drawing comparisons between the Cruzan case and attempts to conduct research on euthanasia techniques in concentration camps using methods such as gasoline injections, pistols, and phosgene gas? In drawing analogies between this case and the Nazi euthanasia experience, are the events of the Holocaust being treated with caution, care, and respect?

In June 1990, the U.S. Supreme Court issued a ruling in *Cruzan*.[6] At the time of the ruling, Nancy Cruzan had been in a permanent coma for almost 7 years. Her parents had made repeated requests to physicians and administrators at the Missouri Rehabilitation Hospital to withdraw all her lifesaving medical interventions, including food and water. They said that they did not believe Nancy would want to exist in a state of permanent unconsciousness. The State of Missouri decided to oppose their requests to stop life-extending medical care on the grounds that the state's interest in preserving life overrode the Cruzan family's desire to not have her life prolonged by medical technology. Neither the State of Missouri nor Nancy's doctors denied the fact that she had no hope of recovering from her comatose state. The state did not attempt to discredit the beneficent intent of Nancy's parents in requesting that treatment be stopped. Nor did the state deny that Nancy had made oral statements indicating that she would not have wanted to be maintained in a permanently comatose state by artificial means.

The Missouri Supreme Court had previously ruled that the state could decide that life had to take precedence over the expression of the parents' wishes to terminate medical care for their daughter in situations where the specific wishes of Nancy Cruzan could not be documented. The court thus denied the request of the Cruzan family to have the nursing home stop the provision of food and fluids. The U.S. Supreme Court affirmed this ruling, stating that while competent persons have the right to control all aspects of their medical care, it is not unconstitutional for a state to require "clear and convincing" evidence of a patient's wishes before life-extending treatment can be stopped for an incompetent person.[7]

Subsequent to the Supreme Court's decision, new witnesses came forward who stated that they had had extensive conversations with Nancy before her accident in which she had clearly stated that she would not want to be maintained in a vegetative state by artificial means. A new trial was convened based on this evidence. The State of Missouri chose not to contest the new evidence. The treating physicians and the independent guardian assigned to Nancy agreed that stopping her food and fluids was in her best interest. In December 1990 Judge Charles Teel, Jr., ordered that Nancy Cruzan be disconnected from her feeding tube. She died on December 26, 1990.

Some of those who supported the original position of the State of Missouri against allowing the cessation of medical treatment for an incompetent person in a state of permanent unconsciousness frequently made analogies to the practice of euthanasia and the mass murder of the disabled in Nazi Germany.[8] They argued, and have argued with reference to similar cases in other states, that permitting the withdrawal of life-extending medical treatments for those in a state of permanent unconsciousness is the first step on a road that leads inevitably to the death camps of Dachau and Auschwitz.[9] By allowing Cruzan to die, our society enters on to a slippery slope to mass murder from which there is no turning back and no return.[10]

Some critics of withdrawing care also maintain that discussions of the "quality of life" or the "burden of treatment," which often characterize disputes about what treatment to provide to persons in Nancy Cruzan's condition, parallel the language used by Nazi physicians and ideologists to justify the elimination of the demented elderly, disabled children, the congenitally retarded, Jews, and Gypsies. To talk of "quality of life" or "burdens" with reference to an incompetent patient is to talk the language of Nazism.[11] Others maintain that the same attitudes that allowed doctors to torture and kill millions in the concentration camps are evident in the indifference of physicians to the suffering that those in Nancy Cruzan's circumstances will endure if allowed to starve to death.

The comparisons and analogies invoked between Cruzan and those who were murdered by the Nazis are wrong. Indeed, they are odiously wrong. Put aside the question of whether the U.S. Supreme Court, the Missouri Supreme Court, her guardian, or her parents decided wisely about the fate of Nancy Cruzan. Ignore the issue of whether the provision of food and fluids constitute medical treatment or something else. Put aside the fact that the provision of food and fluid is ordinary, routine therapy, and not experimental or innovative in any way. Analogies to the crimes of the Nazis still have no place in discussions of Nancy Cruzan's death or the public policies that ought to govern the fates of others in the same situation in the United States today. To invoke them is to allege a theory of moral equivalence between Nazi Germany and the United States that is false, pernicious, and an insult to those murdered by the Nazi regime.

The assessment of the endless comparisons between Nazi euthanasia policies and the struggles within American society to reach a consensus about the application and withdrawal of medical technologies — both those intended for therapy and those clearly recognized as experimental interventions, for those who are terminally ill, suffering intractable pain, or permanently comatose — require an understanding of exactly what the Nazis did during the Holocaust. The analogies stand or fall on the similarities that exist between what Nazi physicians said in settings such as the Doctors' Trial about their conduct and what courts, parents, friends, guardians, and health care professionals say today about those from whom life-supporting technology is withdrawn.

No such understanding is in evidence in the inflammatory analogies that have been made by those opposed to the withdrawal of care from Nancy Cruzan. Nor is it at all evident in the comparisons drawn between the Nazi era in Germany and the moral climate that prevails in the United States with respect to the use of sophisticated medical technologies.[12] Before examining why analogies to the Holocaust are wrong, offensive, and abhorrent in the context of discussions of *Cruzan* and other cases like it, consider another hotly contested topic where analogies to Nazism and the Holocaust abound—the use of fetal tissue from elective abortions for medical research, including innovative forms of transplantation.

THE USE OF FETAL TISSUE FROM ABORTIONS FOR TRANSPLANT: THE NAZI ANALOGY

There are many conditions for which fetal tissue transplants have been attempted, including Parkinson's disease, diabetes, severe immunodeficiency disease, and hereditary storage disorders such as Gaucher's, Hurler's, and DiGeorge's syndromes.[13] All but one form of fetal tissue transplants is highly experimental. Unlike the *Cruzan* case, which involves ending treatment, fetal tissue transplantation has evoked a host of analogies to barbarous Nazi experimentation on human subjects. Many persons who believe that elective abortions are immoral fear that the use of fetal remains might weaken the case for making abortions illegal, since such use will legitimate abortion.[14] Others believe that the use of tissue from a practice, elective abortion, which they see as morally abhorrent, makes those who use fetal tissue complicit in the evil of abortion. To make the case against the use of fetal tissue for transplants, some draw analogies between the arguments of those who support the use of fetal tissue for transplantation and the arguments used by Nazi scientists and physicians to justify conducting research on the inmates of concentration camps.[15]

They argue that in both situations, Dachau in Nazi Germany circa 1942 and the University of Colorado or the University of Lund circa 1990, researchers claimed that they were not responsible for the occurrence of evil but, instead, were only taking advantage of sad or tragic circumstances to create something of value. Moreover, some critics of fetal tissue transplantation contend that, just as the Nazi researchers could not evade moral responsibility for experimenting on prisoners in camps by arguing that they were only taking advantage of the availability of those condemned to death, transplant surgeons and tissue procurement agents cannot avoid complicity in the evil of abortion by arguing that they bear no responsibility for the decision to abort if they knowingly utilize tissues that result.[16]

Others claim to see a moral equivalence in the attitudes toward the fetus among those who conduct research with fetal tissue and those who froze or shot concentration camp inmates to study hypothermia and exsanguination. Those who use fetal remains for research or therapy must, according to some critics of these practices, view the fetus as worthless, nonhuman, and of no inherent moral value, just as the Nazi held that the lives of Jews and the mentally disabled were worthless.[17] Not all who draw analogies to the conduct of Nazis in arguing against the use of fetal tissue from elective abortions bother with an argument to support the comparison. Some merely label anyone who would use tissues from an abortion as a Nazi and let it go at that.

WHAT WOULD JUSTIFY THE NAZI ANALOGY?

What would justify an analogy between the millions of murders committed by the Nazis and the decision to honor the requests of parents to stop life-extending medical treatment for their daughter? Is it legitimate to equate those who would attempt to use fetal tissue from elective abortions for transplants with Mengele, Rascher, Brandt, Rose, and others who conducted or approved of barbarous experiments at Dachau and Auschwitz? The dimensions of the moral horror that was the Holocaust demand the highest standards of evidence and argument on the part of those who wish to make the claim of moral equivalence between then and now.

More than similarities in overt conduct are required. Disconnecting a respirator or stopping dialysis may or may not be the moral equivalent of giving a patient a lethal injection of potassium. The moral assessment of these acts depends not only on the death of the patient but on the reason the action was taken and the motives of those involved. Merely noting similarities in conduct, rhetoric, or context does not prove that two actions are the same. Two actions can appear to be substantively the same, but unless some insight is available about motives, intentions, capacities, and goals, it is impossible to tell whether they are morally equivalent. If I go to the store, buy rat poison, and pour it into my wife's coffee in the hope of inheriting her fortune, this is a very different course of conduct from a situation in which my wife dies as a result of drinking rat poison that I inadvertently put in her cup thinking it to be sugar. The former is murder; the latter is at most negligence, and probably nothing more than a tragic mistake.

Similarities in the outcome of behavior are not sufficient to ground an analogy between events in contemporary medicine and in medicine during the Nazi era. The death of Nancy Cruzan from starvation and dehydration when her feeding tube was removed is not, despite the inflamed rhetoric of some commentators, obviously morally equivalent to a German physician gassing a physically handicapped person on the grounds that doctors have a duty to eliminate threats to the well-being and health of the Reich. Transplanting tissues obtained from an elective abortion into the brain of someone with Parkinson's disease in an effort to learn how to palliate the patient's symptoms is not patently the moral equivalent of transplanting bones between two female inmates at the Buchenwald concentration camp without benefit of anesthesia or antiseptics in order to test a hypothesis about repairing gunshot wounds. In order to ascertain the propriety of drawing analogies between the conduct of Nazis and current or proposed biomedical practices, and the propriety of the claim of moral equivalence, it is essential to understand the rationales behind the Nazi euthanasia program, research on camp inmates, and ultimately, medicine's role in the Holocaust itself. The fact that Nazi doctors, politicians, and public health officials used terms such as *euthanasia* or *quality of life* and contemporary physicians, judges, bioethicists, parents, or legislators use these same terms does not in and of itself mean that any contemporary exponent of these words is a Nazi.

The requisite foundation for drawing parallels and analogies between the conduct of the Nazi doctors and the conduct of American doctors, a foundation that is inexcusably absent in nearly all comparisons that have been drawn to date, is an examination of what German doctors and public health officials who engaged either directly or indirectly in torture, murder, the abuse of subjects in human experimentation, sterilization, genocide, and other crimes against humanity said about their actions. What were the motives and intentions of those in medicine, nursing, and public health who participated in or provided the ideological underpinnings for the Holocaust? One obvious, if underutilized, way to answer these questions and, in turn, to be in a position to assess the appropriateness of analogies to the conduct of the Nazi biomedical community in discussing contemporary issues in American medicine is to examine what was said by the defendants in the Doctors' Trial. Only by examining the rationales and justifications offered by Nazi doctors for their acts can any judgment be made as to the utility and propriety of comparisons between the abuses of that time and the alleged abuses of our time.

THE DOCTORS' TRIAL

The focus of the charges brought by the Allied prosecution team at the Doctors' Trial was the exploitation, torture, and killing that occurred, primarily in the name of medical experimentation, in various concentration camps.[18] This is a bit puzzling, since those who were on trial had also participated in, or were aware of and did nothing to protest, the mass murder of millions of innocent persons in these same camps. While the medical experiments conducted on prisoners were exceedingly cruel and gruesome, they involved, at most, only a few thousand people.[19] Why didn't genocide and mass murder form the heart of the prosecution's charges against those placed on trial? The answer lies in the vulnerability of the prosecution's case with respect to mass murder and genocide.[20] It was the concreteness of the crimes committed in the context of human experimentation that moved medical experimentation to center stage at Nuremberg.

Incredibly, it was easier to find evidence of experimental abuse against particular persons who were on trial than it was to assign specific responsibility to particular persons for the murder of millions.[21] Moreover, as the defense team noted time and time again throughout the trials, the charges of genocide and crimes against humanity rested on very shaky legal ground. It was easier for the prosecution to win convictions by prosecuting specific instances where the accused were directly involved in the abuse of human subjects than to try to prove their complicity in crimes such as genocide or mass murder, which had not been formally recognized as crimes in the legal systems of the Allied nations.

Astonishingly, and rarely noted by those who do not hesitate to invoke the Nazi analogy to argue for the moral equivalence between biomedical conduct today and an action carried out during the Nazi era, none of those on trial begged forgiveness from the judges. Nor did they show any signs of remorse for what they had done. In fact, almost no one accused of a crime actually denied that he had done what the prosecution alleged. Rather, those on trial attempted to recast what they had done in different terms. They tried vigorously to explain and justify their actions to the judges on ethical grounds.

Their arguments are crucial for understanding the relevance of what they did in evaluating the propriety of analogies to what doctors, nurses, and scientists now do or might do in the future. Similarities between events that took place during the Third Reich and those that took place in a state nursing home for the severely disabled in Missouri more than 40 years later must be more than superficial to be meaningful. They must also be more than superficial in order to be adequately respectful of the nature of the crimes and abuses that millions were forced to endure compared to the agony of parents trying to do what they thought was best for their daughter. If the charge of Nazism is to stick, if there is to be any force to claims of the slippery slope, it is imperative to be clear about exactly what is the same and what is different in the rationales for action then and now.

EXCUSING THE INEXCUSABLE

Those who stood trial at Nuremberg advanced a variety of moral arguments in defense of their conduct.[22] Six of these arguments are of special interest in light of contemporary efforts to impugn physicians and biomedical scientists with the Nazi analogy. One of the key rationales of those put on trial was that only people who were doomed to die were used in medical research. Time and again, the doctors who froze screaming subjects to death, watched their brains explode as a result of rapid decompression, or examined the most efficacious agents for euthanasia stated that only prisoners condemned to death were used. When the prosecutors asked why animals or human volunteers were not used, those on trial responded that they did not have the time to design careful, nonlethal experiments. The desire to obtain answers, especially in research sponsored by the military or with military applications that could supply answers that might save the lives of German soldiers, obligated them to get results in the fastest possible manner. If that meant conducting potentially lethal experiments on prisoners condemned to die, so be it. Since there were large numbers of subjects available who were going to die anyway, it was morally justifiable to use them in research that could benefit others.

Another rationale given for their behavior toward camp inmates was that participation in research offered expiation to the subjects. By being injected, frozen, or transplanted, subjects could cleanse themselves of their crimes. One of the defendants argued vociferously that participation in medical experimentation gave prisoners an opportunity to make up for their crimes, whatever they might have been. Presumably, he knew he was referring to crimes such as being a Gypsy, a homosexual, a political dissident, a Jehovah's Witness, a prisoner of war, or a Jew.

Some defendants provided a third rationale for their conduct. They claimed that no wrong had been done because those who had been subjects had volunteered. Prisoners might be freed, some defendants noted, if they survived the experiments. Indeed, the defense team noted that medical experiments had been conducted by one of the prosecution's expert witnesses, Dr. Andrew Ivy, in the Statesville, Illinois, prison, using prisoners who were told that they might receive early parole or reductions in their sentences if they participated. The prospects of release and pardon were mentioned frequently during the trial, since they were the basis for the claim that people participated voluntarily in the experiments. Inmates were told that if they survived, they might be freed. This incentive, the defendants claimed, induced some to volunteer.

A fourth rationale offered during the trial, one that is especially astounding even by the standards of self-delusion in evidence throughout the proceedings, was a lack of moral expertise and, thus, of moral responsibility. Some of the defendants invoked what is in essence a philosophical doctrine, logical positivism, in their defense. While they did not actually use these words, they maintained that scientists and doctors are not responsible for and have no knowledge of values. They are only responsible for discovering and explaining empirical facts. Thus, they felt no moral responsibility for what they had done or what had occurred in the camps because they did not have any expertise concerning moral matters. Consequently, they had left decisions about these matters to others. All actions—euthanasia, genocide, and experimentation—were done with appropriate orders from a higher authority.

A fifth justification for what had happened was that the defendants had acted for the defense and security of their country. All actions—genocide, euthanasia, experimentation, sterilization—were done to preserve the Reich during a time of total war. Total war, war in which the survival of the nation hangs in the balance, justifies exceptions to ordinary morality, the defendants maintained. Allied prosecutors had much to ponder in thinking about this defense in light of the fire bombing of Dresden and Tokyo, and the dropping of atomic bombs on Hiroshima and Nagasaki.

The line of moral justification of most interest from the point of view of assessing the validity of the Nazi analogy was that it was reasonable to sacrifice the interests of the few, even to cause their deaths, in order to benefit the majority. The most distinguished of the scientists placed on trial, Gerhard Rose, the head of the Koch Institute of Tropical Medicine in Berlin, said that while he initially opposed performing lethal experiments on camp inmates, he came to believe that it made no sense not to involve 100 or 200 people in research, even lethal research, in pursuit of a vaccine for typhus when the Reich was losing 1,000 men a day to this disease on the Eastern front. What, he asked, were the deaths of 100 men compared to the possible benefit of developing a prophylactic vaccine capable of saving tens of thousands? Other versions of utilitarian arguments were made during the trial, but Rose, because he admitted that he had anguished about his own moral duty when asked by the Wehrmacht to perform the typhus experiments in a concentration camp, was the most convincing proponent of the position. Ethical arguments based on utilitarian justifications seem to have played a key role in the stress placed on informed consent in the Nuremberg Code, since consent ensures that the rights of the individual will not be sacrificed to the needs or interests of the majority.

In closely reviewing the statements that accompany the six major moral rationales for murder, torture, and mutilation conducted in the camps — only the condemned were used, expiation was a possible benefit, freedom was a possible benefit, a lack of moral expertise, the need to preserve the state in conditions of total war, and the morality of sacrificing a few to benefit many — it becomes clear that the conduct of those who worked in the concentration camps was guided by a biomedical paradigm of the mortal danger facing their nation. Time and again, the physicians and public health officials at the trial referred to the threat posed by "inferior races" and "useless eaters" to the welfare of the Reich. This paradigm of the state facing a physical threat to its overall well-being that could be alleviated only by medical interventions is reflected in the medical literature and training of health care professionals both before and during the war.[23]

Physicians justified their actions, whether direct involvement with euthanasia and lethal experiments or merely support for Hitler and the Reich, on the grounds that the Jew, the homosexual, the congenitally handicapped, and the Slav posed a biological threat to the existence and welfare of the Reich. The appropriate response to such a threat was to eliminate it, just as a physician must eliminate a burst appendix using surgery or a dangerous bacterium using penicillin. Viewing specific ethnic groups and populations as threatening the health of the German state permitted, and in the view of those on trial demanded, the involvement of medicine in mass genocide. The overarching biomedical paradigm provided the theoretical basis for allowing those sworn to the Hippocratic principle of nonmaleficence to kill in the name of the state and was the backdrop against which the various moral defenses of the crimes committed in the camps unfolded.

THE RESPONSE: THE NUREMBERG CODE

The Doctors' Trial did not conclude with the condemnation of the barbarities performed by those on trial and the pronouncement of punishments. It ended with the promulgation of what we now call the Nuremberg Code. The judges understood that the ethical arguments of those they had tried had to be addressed, and the Code was their attempt to articulate standards for the conduct of medical experimentation in the future. The Code places extraordinary emphasis on informed, voluntary consent. Its first and strongest injunction is that "The voluntary consent of the human subject is absolutely essential." Those who created the Code realized that they had to find a powerful moral foundation for rejecting the crass utilitarianism so much in evidence in the arguments used by those on trial to justify their actions. The Nuremberg Code explicitly rejects the moral argument that the creation of benefits for many justifies the sacrifice of the few. Every experiment, no matter how important or valuable, requires the express voluntary consent of the individual. The right of individuals to control their bodies trumps the interest of others in obtaining knowledge or benefits from them.[24]

Dr. Gerhard Rose was, according to the Code, simply wrong. It is immoral to kill 100 people over the span of a few weeks to save 1,000 who will die every day with predictable certainty from disease on the battlefront. The individual must retain autonomy over the use of his or her body for biomedical purposes. Consent, according to the Code, is not negotiable.

The Code also emphasizes the obligation researchers have to assess the risks associated with their studies in order to decide whether to allow anyone to participate. Research that is likely to be fatal should not be done. Even if a particular experiment is deemed reasonably safe by researchers, subjects must still be given sufficient information to make informed choices about whether or not to participate. The requirements that researchers not engage in dangerous research and try to convey adequate information about hazards and risks appear to have been motivated by the desire of the Nuremberg Tribunal to counter the justification of those who claimed they did no harm since only those condemned to die were made the subjects of experimentation. Even prisoners under the sentence of death, the Code maintains, should not be subjected to dangerous research. Being a prisoner does not obviate the person's right to full information in order to decide whether or not to participate in research.

The Code does not address the other key ethical rationales that the Nazi doctors and health officials proffered. It says nothing about the standards that should guide those concerned with the protection or advancement of public health or about the duties of those engaged in medical therapy. This is unfortunate, since the crimes for which the defendants were tried and the key rationales they offered in defense of their conduct ranged far beyond abuses of human subjects.

For example, the Code remains silent about the logical positivism defense, the contention that doctors lack expertise in morality and thus cannot be held accountable for actions such as genocide or sterilization undertaken at the behest of legitimate government authorities who are, presumably, in possession of the requisite moral expertise. Nor is anything said about whether or not the circumstances of total war permit the state to institute extreme measures in order to protect itself, including the waiving of the Code with respect to human experimentation. While one might read the Code between the lines to imply that there are no circumstances under which its provision may be waived, it does not explicitly state that this is so. The Code makes no mention of the underlying paradigm that supported the specific moral arguments offered by the defense: that medicine must respond and doctors must do whatever is needed when called upon to protect the health and welfare of the state.

The major moral message of the Code is that voluntary consent, if taken seriously, can provide an adequate prophylactic against rampant utilitarianism. In the decades since the promulgation of the Nuremberg Code, consent has come to occupy center stage in all bioethical and legal discussion in both research and therapy. For example, most committees today charged with monitoring the welfare of human research subjects spend the bulk of their time mulling over and refining consent documents.

ANALOGIES, DISANALOGIES, AND MISLEADING COMPARISONS

What is the relevance of the Holocaust in general and the crimes of Nazi medicine and biomedical science in particular for contemporary arguments about the moral permissibility of withdrawing feeding tubes or using fetal tissue from abortions for transplants? Is there any similarity between what Nazi doctors and biomedical scientists thought they were doing and honoring the request of parents to have a feeding tube removed from their comatose daughter?

The answer is that there is little similarity between then and now. It distorts the monstrosity of the crimes conducted during the Holocaust to draw direct analogies between the Nazi involvement with euthanasia and the Cruzan case or Nazi research on camp inmates and the use of fetal tissue for experimental transplants. This is not to say that no convincing moral arguments can be made against discontinuing life support for Nancy Cruzan and other incompetent patients or against the use of fetal tissue in research. It is to say that the invocation of analogies to the conduct of the Nazis requires an understanding and caution that are notably absent in many of those who glibly make the claim of moral equivalence in drawing the Nazi analogy.[25]

The Cruzan case lacks similarity to Nazi euthanasia when seen in the light of what the Nazis did in the camps and the ethical arguments presented to defend what was done at the Doctors' Trial. First and foremost, nearly all of those targeted for death under German public health laws as threats to the welfare of the state were competent persons. Nancy Cruzan was never competent throughout the course of her medical care. Nor had she been sentenced or convicted of any crime. Therefore, moral arguments focusing on what health care professionals can do in caring for the condemned do not apply.

Time and again during the Doctors' Trial, Karl Brandt and his co-defendants noted that they had become involved in genocide from a sense of duty to protect the state against the threat posed by groups such as Jews. Can anyone not blind to the facts of the Holocaust and to the facts of the Cruzan case seriously believe that Nancy Cruzan's parents, her former friends, her independent guardian, her doctor, or the judge who issued the order allowing her tube to be removed wanted her to die because they viewed her as a biological or genetic threat to the well-being of the United States or the State of Missouri? Whatever else is true of the Holocaust, it was rooted in racism. The Cruzan case had nothing to do with race. There is no link between the request by parents to have a feeding tube removed on the grounds that it is what their daughter would have wanted and the murder of the mentally ill or genetically "inferior" because a physician believes that the racial composition of the German nation must be kept pure.

There is no parallel, no similarity, and no commonality between the outlook that motivated those on trial at Nuremberg and the beliefs that drove the Cruzan family's requests concerning the fate of their daughter. Again, those who argue for the cessation of Nancy's care, including her own parents, may be wrong, but if they are wrong, the reasons have nothing to do with the motives and goals of those who planned, supported, or implemented the Nazi euthanasia program.

It might be argued that there is still a similarity in that Cruzan's family or others who favor allowing medical treatment for the incompetent to be stopped do so on grounds concerning the quality of life or burden to the patient. These are concepts analogous to those used by those who administered the Nazi euthanasia program. But this is simply nonsense.

In 1917, patients in psychiatric hospitals in Germany were given low priority for food under government wartime rationing schemes.[26] The government decided that the mentally ill should be excluded from scarce rations, since they were not making a productive contribution to the well-being of the nation. Is this notion of burden at all akin to what motivated the Cruzans' request to stop their daughter's life support? Is it not an affront to those who secretly starved to death as a result of a government fiat in the psychiatric hospitals of Germany to suggest otherwise?

Many books and articles were written in the years between the two world wars in Germany about the burdensome nature—moral, economic, and emotional—to the state of certain groups: the mentally ill, the demented elderly, the congenitally handicapped, and interracial children. These groups were alleged to pose not only a threat to the economic solvency of Germany but also to the moral fiber of the nation, since interbreeding with "inferiors" would lead inevitably to moral degeneracy.[27] The arguments gained special favor among the members of the emerging Nazi party and were eventually put into public policy in the late 1930s.

Restrictions on marriage and intercourse between people of different racial and ethnic backgrounds were enacted to protect the genetic health of the Reich. Children who were the product of interracial sexual relationships were sterilized. The killing of the mentally ill through neglect, dating back to World War I, was next, motivated by a desire to protect the German *Volk* from the burden of racial inferiority. Finally, the euthanasia program was created and extended to the incurably ill, the demented elderly, and children born with birth defects. The "burdens" that made life worth living or not were assessed on genetic and economic grounds, not for the individual but for the state. This is not analogous to the moral reasons advanced for allowing treatment to be withheld or removed from incompetent persons on the grounds of a substituted judgment standard.

Euthanasia under Nazism refers to the active killing, usually surreptitiously and always without the consent of the person killed or the next of kin, for racial and economic reasons. These motivations have nothing to do with the current debate about whether or not life-extending care and treatment should be withdrawn at the request of parents such as the Cruzans, who are universally believed to love and cherish a daughter who was no longer in a position to make decisions about her own medical care.

The thesis of moral equivalence is also grievously flawed when drawn between Nazi experiments on camp inmates and the use of fetal tissue from aborted fetuses for experiments. Once the moral rationales for the use of Jews, Gypsies, political prisoners, and prisoners of war in barbaric experiments are made clear, the thesis of moral equivalence inherent in the Nazi analogy is not only wrong, it is outrageously wrong. Those who object to the use of fetal tissue in experimentation do so on the grounds that it violates the rights of the fetus if the tissue must be obtained from elective abortions.[28] No one who proposes to use fetal tissue from aborted human fetuses for transplantation does so because he believes that the fetus is condemned to die. The fetus, whether rightly or wrongly, is already dead. It is plausible to consider the morality of complicity in the act of abortion in arguing against the use of fetal tissue for transplants.[29] It is also plausible, even if it is likely false, to claim an analogy between the moral rationales that allowed a scientist to use a concentration camp inmate in a potentially lethal typhus vaccine trial and those that permit a surgeon to recruit a person with Parkinson's disease to participate in a clinical trial of fetal tissue transplantation. It is not plausible, and it is especially demeaning, to equate the moral rationale that allows a biomedical scientist to feel justified in performing experiments using the remains of a dead fetus after an elective abortion and performing lethal and painful experiments on a live Jew, political dissident, or Soviet prisoner of war.

No one believes that the fetus will achieve expiation by serving as a source of tissue. And no one has argued that it is moral to recruit subjects to accept tissue in the form of experimental transplants because they will somehow feel less guilt or responsibility for their condition. Some worry that mothers may feel expiation from any possible guilt they may have about choosing an abortion, but it is an inexcusable confusion to equate the supposed expiation offered a living subject with the expiation that some fear may be indirectly obtained by a mother who chooses to abort her fetus.

No one who seeks to use fetal tissue for research believes that the fetus stands to benefit in any way from such use. The German doctors who did some of the experiments may have believed that their subjects would obtain early release from the camps, although in fact, insofar as available records and testimony indicate, no one ever did. No one can possibly believe that researchers seek to use fetal tissue from the motive of national security or as a result of the demands of total war on the state.

No one who proposes to use tissue from aborted human fetuses chooses to do so because they believe that the sacrifice of a few fetuses can be justified by the potential benefits to the transplant recipients. Since they are seeking the opportunity to transplant tissues from fetuses that are already dead, the notion of sacrifice has no bearing on the assessment of their argument. No one who proposes to justify the use of fetal tissue does so based on the view that scientists and doctors have no moral expertise or moral responsibilities.

In short, none of the arguments invoked by the Germans who conducted experiments in the camps has any parallel to the arguments against complicity or legitimation cited by those who would outlaw or forbid the practice of fetal tissue transplant experiments in the United States or other nations. The concern of those who object is not for the experimental subjects who have tissue implanted, but for the fetuses who die because of elective abortions.[30] But the Nazi scientists and doctors who performed horrible experiments in the camps did not believe that their conduct required any defense against complicity in an evil practice on a par with the supposed evil of abortion, since they did not see the systematic exploitation and extermination of Jews, Gypsies, and other enemies of the state as evil.

The most troubling error in the claim of moral equivalence between the use of prisoners in concentration camps and the use of fetal remains from elective abortions in research is the equation of causing harm to living adults with manipulating the remains of fetuses. There is a great moral difference between causing a young man to freeze to death slowly and using tissue from the brain of a dead fetus to transplant cells to another person. Both may be unethical, but they are not unethical for the same reason, and to equate them is to insult the memory of those who suffered and died solely as a result of who they were and what they believed.

Once superficial similarities are cleared away, there is no basis for the claim of moral equivalence between the conduct of Nazis and the conduct of the Cruzans or of researchers doing fetal tissue experiments. The questions of whether it is right to allow parents to remove a feeding tube from their daughter on the grounds of substituted judgment, or for scientists to find fetal brain tissue amid the remains of an abortus and transplant it to someone with parkinsonism, are open to moral debate. The appropriateness of analogies and claims of moral equivalence between the actions, policies, and deeds of Nazi medicine with respect to these activities is not. Those who wish to use the Nazi analogy can certainly do so, but they must do so with greater care and caution than has been in evidence in discussions of the Cruzan case and fetal tissue research.

Analogies to the Holocaust must be carefully constructed and justified. The Doctors' Trial and the Nuremberg Code have taught us that while themes recur, history does not repeat itself. The enormity of the violations of human dignity perpetuated by Nazi physicians in the name of science is a lesson for all mankind. The significance for bioethics discourse is far-reaching, but analogies must be used with caution lest we lose their ethical significance.

NOTES

1. B. Muller-Hill, *Murderous Science* (Oxford: Oxford University Press, 1988); R. Proctor, *Racial Hygiene* (Cambridge, Mass.: Harvard University Press, 1988); M. Kater, *Doctors Under Hitler* (Chapel Hill: University of North Carolina Press, 1989).

2. P. Steinfels. "Biomedical Ethics and the Shadow of Nazism," *Hastings Center Report*, special Supplement (1976); N. Hentoff, "The Nazi Analogy in Bioethics," *Hastings Center Report* 18 (1988): 29–30.

3. See Chapter 7, this volume.

4. Caplan, oral presentation at conference entitled "The Meaning of the Holocaust for Bioethics," May 17, 1989, Minneapolis, Minnesota.

5. D. Andrusko, ed., *A Passion for Justice* (Washington, D.C.: National Right to Life, 1988); G. Crum, "Nazi Bioethics and a Doctor's Defense," *Human Life Review* 8 (1982): 55–69; N. Hentoff, "Nazi Bioethics and a Doctor's Defense," *Hastings Center Report* 18 (1976) 29–30 (1988); E. Skoglund, *Life on the Line* (Minneapolis: World Wide Publications, 1989); E. Spannaus, K. Kronberg, and E. Everett, eds., *How to Stop the Resurgence of Nazi Euthanasia Today* (Washington, D.C.: EIR, 1988).

6. *Cruzan v. Director, Missouri Department of Health*, 110 S. Ct. 2841 (1990).

7. G. J. Annas, "Nancy Cruzan and the Right to Die," *New England Journal of Medicine* 323 (1990): 670–673.

8. Andrusko, *A Passion for Justice*; Hentoff, "The Nazi Analogy in Bioethics"; Skoglund, *Life on the Line*; Spannaus et al., *Resurgence of Nazi Euthanasia*; F. Wertham, *The German Euthanasia Program* (Cincinnati: Hayes, 1988).

9. F. Wertham, *A Sign for Cain* (New York: Warner, 1973); Hentoff, "The Nazi Analogy in Bioethics."

10. Andrusko, *A Passion for Justice*.

11. Hentoff, "The Nazi Analogy in Bioethics"; Spannaus et al., *Resurgence of Nazi Euthanasia*; Wertham, *A Sign for Cain*; Wertham, *The German Euthanasia Program*.

12. Wertham, *A Sign for Cain*; Wertham, *The German Euthanasia Program*.

13. D. Vawter, W. Kearney, K. Gervais, et. al., *The Use of Human Fetal Tissue* (Minneapolis: Center for Biomedical Ethics, 1990).

14. J. Burtchaell, "Case Study: University Policy on Experimental Use of Aborted Fetal Tissue," *IRB* 10 (1988): 7–11; J. Burtchaell, *The Giving and Taking of Life* (Notre Dame: University of Notre Dame Press, 1989); J. Burtchaell and J. Bopp, "Statement of Dissent," Human Fetal Tissue Transplantation Research Panel (Bethesda, Md.: NIH, 1988), pp. 1–31.

15. Ibid.

16. J. Burtchaell, "Case Study"; L. Bond, "NRL News Special Report: Fetal Tissue Transplants," *NRL News* (January 22, 1989), pp. 1–14.

17. Bond. "NRL News Special Report."

18. T. Taylor, "Opening Statement of the Prosecution," *Trials of War Criminals*

Before Nuremberg Military Tribunals Under Control Law No. 10, The Medical Case (Washington, D.C.: U.S. Government Printing Office, 1946), Vol. I, pp. 27–75.

19. Caplan, Supra note 4.

20. Ibid.

21. Ibid.

22. See Chapter 7, this volume.

23. R. J. Lifton, *The Nazi Doctors* (New York: Basic Books, 1986); Proctor, *Racial Hygiene*; Kater, *Doctors Under Hitler*.

24. See Chapter 12, this volume.

25. J. Goodall, *Through a Window* (Boston: Houghton Mifflin, 1990); Hentoff, "The Nazi Analogy in Bioethics."

26. Muller-Hill, *Murderous Science*; Proctor, *Racial Hygiene*.

27. Ibid.

28. Vawter et al., *The Use of Human Fetal Tissue*.

29. Ibid.

30. G. Annas and S. Elias, "The Politics of Transplantation of Human Fetal Tissue," *New England Journal of Medicine* 320 (1989): 1079–1082.

15

Editorial Responsibility: Protecting Human Rights by Restricting Publication of Unethical Research

MARCIA ANGELL

The Third Reich was so abhorrent in so many ways that we tend to use it as an example for anything we wish to condemn. Thus, heads of state whom we do not like are referred to as "Hitlers," and those who counsel conciliation are termed "Chamberlains." Similarly, unethical research readily evokes comparisons with the Nazis. We may be too inclined, however, to draw parallels between the Nazi medical experiments conducted on prisoners in the death camps and the unethical research that is done today. In a sense, the Nazi experiments were incidental — sadistic sidelights in a uniquely evil society dedicated to eradicating entire populations because of their race, religion, or nationality. It is difficult to believe that such systematic torture and killing of helpless people by the state in the name of medical research could occur again. Indeed, the Doctors' Trial was conducted for the primary purpose of preventing the recurrence of this barbarism, and adherence to the Nuremberg Code would preclude any recurrence.

Nevertheless, there are real concerns about the use of human subjects in clinical research. In therapeutic research, for example, there is an inherent tension between the ethical imperative to do what is best for each patient and the scientific requirement to gather information that will be useful to others. Doing one's best (or what one *believes* to be best) for each patient is, of course, highly individualistic. Scientific requirements, on the other hand, necessitate viewing subjects to some extent as members of a group and making decisions statistically. There is no way to eliminate this tension altogether. For example, in most clinical trials comparing two treatments, the study is continued until a statistically significant difference in effectiveness or toxicity between the treatments is found. But the difference becomes apparent to the clinician even before it is deemed statistically significant by the conventional scientific standard. According to the statistical standard, a difference is not significant unless there is a less than 5 percent possibility that it can be explained by chance. The trial must go on for some time after the difference becomes apparent to reach this degree of certainty. What of patients who enter a trial when a difference has become apparent, but there is, say, a 7 percent possibility that it arose by chance? This is not statistically significant by scientific conventions, but it is certainly close enough that most of us would bet on the treatment that looked better at this point. Is it ethical for patient-subjects to receive the treatment that is *probably* inferior?[1] This is the sort of problem that inheres in even the most ethical research using human subjects who have the disease that the intervention under study is designed to help.

In addition to such arguable problems, I believe that there are more clear-cut violations of the interests of human subjects, in enlightened societies committed to human rights, and in work that is not dedicated to torture and killing, but rather to alleviating suffering and extending life. The current breaches of research ethics are clearly less monstrous than those of Nazi Germany, but that, of course, is weak justification for them. They cover a broad spectrum of offenses, some of which are obvious and some of which are arguable. I will set forth three principles of ethical research, and then describe a few of these offenses and some of the pressures and misconceptions that lead to unethical research. Finally, I will discuss the appropriate response of the scientific community to unethical research, especially the response of journal editors.

SOME PRINCIPLES

Three principles underlie my point of view. The first is the familiar moral precept that the ends do not justify the means. In clinical research, this means that human subjects cannot be seen merely as tools. On the contrary, concern for the individual subject's welfare and autonomy must take precedence over the interests of science and society. All enlightened codes and regulations, beginning with the Nuremberg Code and including the Helsinki Declarations and the U.S. federal regulations, appeal to and buttress this principle.[2] In a therapeutic trial, particularly one in which subjects stand to gain greatly, they may be willing to take proportionately great risks, and this may be ethically permitted. In a nontherapeutic trial, however, where no benefit is expected for the subjects themselves, the risks should be vanishingly small, or "minimal," in the words of the federal regulations. Trials expected to yield intermediate benefits to the subjects may permissibly entail intermediate risks. The Nazi experiments, which were nontherapeutic, obviously grossly violated this proportionality between risks and benefits.

The second principle that underlies my view is that informed consent by human subjects is necessary but not sufficient. It does not absolve researchers of the responsibility to ensure that benefits and risks are commensurate. There is usually an asymmetry in the relationship between researcher and subject that makes consent almost inevitably less than free. The researcher is, for example, more knowledgeable about the issues. The asymmetry is particularly great when the researcher is also a physician and the subject is a patient who may feel dependent on the physician's good will. Nontherapeutic research is especially problematic in this situation. No matter what the physician says, the subject may be reluctant to believe that what the researcher is proposing is not therapeutic. Furthermore, some patients may agree to participate in research studies because they wish to please their physicians. Thus, informed consent cannot transform an inherently unethical experiment into an ethical one. Having stated this, however, I am not so ready to dismiss or disparage the importance of informed consent as are many others who emphasize the asymmetry between researcher and subject. Most of the critics of informed consent are actually objecting to the way it is obtained in practice, not to the principle. They are correct in believing that obtaining informed consent is often a legalistic ritual, designed more to obfuscate than to clarify. If the effort to inform the patient is genuine, however, the concept is unarguable, and it is perhaps the strongest barrier against unethical research.[3] This principle, so unequivocally stated in the Nuremberg Code, has unfortunately been diluted and deemphasized in later codes and in the U.S. federal regulations.[4]

The third principle is that whether research results are important is immaterial in judging the ethics of the research. It is tempting to adjust our evaluation of the ethics of a study on the basis of its scientific rigor and the social impact of the results. If, for example, human subjects are exposed to moderate risks without a chance of benefit, but the research yields an effective treatment for a disorder that afflicts many other people, it is tempting to overlook the ethical lapse. But to do so would be to regard the subjects as means to an end, albeit a worthy end, and judgments about the implications of research results would come to replace judgments about the ethics of the study. Thus, as stated in the Massachusetts General Hospital's Guiding Principles for Human Studies of 1981, "a study is ethical or not at its inception. It does not become ethical because it succeeds in producing valuable data."[5]

UNETHICAL RESEARCH

The end of Nazi Germany did not mean the end of unethical research. Henry Beecher, in a widely publicized 1966 article in the *New England Journal of Medicine*,[6] described violations of the rights of human subjects, as spelled out in the Nuremberg Code, that occurred in the United States after World War II. One example was the Willowbrook, New York, hepatitis study, in which hepatitis was studied by deliberately infecting institutionalized retarded children with the virus. This was done, incidentally, with the permission of the parents of the children. A second example, not mentioned by Beecher, was the Tuskegee Syphilis Study, in which treatment was withheld from men with syphilis, without their consent, to observe the natural course of the disease. This study lasted from 1932 to 1969, long after penicillin had become available and long after the Nuremberg Code was formulated.

Since the publication of Beecher's paper, ethical violations have become less frequent and certainly less egregious. Some of this change reflects the increasing emphasis on informed consent generally, which in turn reflects the importance of informed consent in malpractice litigation.[7] Over the past 20 years, we have come to grips more explicitly with the issue of unethical research by defining it and taking steps to prevent it. In addition to the international and federal codes and regulations, many institutions have developed their own codes. Institutional Review Boards (IRBs) have also been established to evaluate the ethical aspects of proposed research. Nevertheless, some unethical research continues. Usually, I believe, it stems from the desire to obtain unambiguous answers to scientific questions as rapidly as possible in a highly competitive research environment.

It is important to understand the atmosphere that can give rise to ethical violations in human studies. In biomedical research, the competition for funding is growing increasingly intense. An important criterion for funding is evidence of past productivity. To receive a grant from the National Institutes of Health, the source of most funding, a researcher must submit a proposal that includes an account of past work, with a list of prior publications. Thus, there is a strong incentive to complete and publish as many studies as possible. In addition, status and promotion at the researcher's institution depend on a strong record of past work, in particular on a long list of publications—the tangible measures of past work.[8]

In this atmosphere, there is an understandable desire to do studies that are both scientifically rigorous and capable of being completed quickly. Unfortunately, it is often easier and more efficient to get answers to scientific questions if the rights of human subjects are violated. An example is the Willowbrook study. What better way to study hepatitis than to infect human subjects with the virus? Any other method is necessarily slower and less certain. Similarly, if a researcher wanted to study the natural history of AIDS, one efficient way would be to infect human subjects deliberately. One could learn a great deal by doing so. Obviously, we cannot do that. What we have had to do instead is to study people who have contacted AIDS from blood transfusions, go back to try to identify when the contaminated transfusion occurred, and then try to reconstruct what happened. Alternatively, we must rely on prospective studies of very large numbers of people at high risk for AIDS in order to piece together slowly, and sometimes incorrectly, the natural course of the disease.

Although it is clear to anyone living in the 1990s that it is unethical to produce disease in human subjects simply to study it, there are other, more subtle, ethical violations that are fairly frequent.[9] One is including subjects in an experiment without making certain that they understand how the study will be carried out. The notion of randomization in a therapeutic clinical trial is often dismaying to patients, who prefer to think that their doctors know what the best treatment for them is and will provide it.[10] Rather than take the time to explain the necessity of randomization to patients, with the attendant risk to the researcher that they will decide not to participate, researchers may be tempted to gloss over this aspect of the experiment. They may also devise stratagems for avoiding the dilemma.[11] This is because researchers usually want to include as many subjects in their trials as quickly and efficiently as possible, in part for good scientific reasons. Thus, patients may be denied the full information necessary for voluntary consent.

Another frequent ethical violation is the inappropriate use in therapeutic clinical trials of placebo groups or groups receiving a treatment known to be inferior to the experimental treatment. An ethical condition for doing clinical trials is that the researchers have no reason to believe that one group of subjects in the trial will fare any better than the other group or groups. In other words, researchers must be genuinely in doubt about which treatment is better, considering both risks and benefits, or whether a treatment is better than a placebo. If there is not genuine doubt, the researchers would be *knowingly* giving patients inferior treatment, and this is unethical. Many researchers, however, make compromises with this ethical requirement. Sometimes these compromises involve self-delusion in that researchers convince themselves that they do not know what they really do know. Sometimes the compromises involve ingenious methods of denying themselves access to information that would make the trial ethically impossible to continue. And, as previously mentioned, at some point in a trial, clinically one treatment may look much better than another, but not with scientifically acceptable statistical reliability. How should subsequent patients asked to enter such a trial be dealt with? Thus, the spectrum of unethical research extends from the clearly barbaric through the thoughtless to more subtle and even arguable violations.

THE PUBLICATION OF RESEARCH RESULTS

Most researchers intend to publish their work. Publication is, after all, the tangible result of their efforts and the accepted way of communicating their findings (and priorities) to the scientific community. It is also the primary yardstick for measuring success and doling out rewards in the biomedical research community. So important is the length of the bibliography in evaluating biomedical researchers that it is an incentive to cut corners, both scientific and ethical, to produce a publishable manuscript. Given this emphasis on publication, what should editors of biomedical journals and their peer reviewers do when faced with work that they believe may be, or is, unethical?

The responsibility of editors in responding to work they consider unethical has been intensely debated among editors and within editors' organizations. The Declaration of Helsinki of 1975 is quite clear on this point; its eighth principle states: "Reports on experimentation not in accordance with the principles laid down in this Declaration should not be accepted for publication." Nevertheless, editors have tended not to invoke this principle, and it is likely that most are unaware of it. The reluctance of editors to reject work that they believe to be unethical, so long as the violations were not egregious, probably stems from several considerations. First, editors are reluctant to accept responsibility for evaluating the ethics of a study; there is a tacit assumption that this is the job of the institution where the research was done. Particularly after 1983, when IRBs were first required for federal funding, editors could view the question of unethical research as out of their purview. Furthermore, the growing importance of publication to the success of a researcher increased the reluctance of editors to deny it on so "soft" a ground as questionable ethics. Moreover, with the completed manuscript in hand, editors are influenced by the importance of the results. If the study is of great practical significance — that is, if it might save lives — it is difficult to deny publication. Thus, research ethics have received relatively little attention from editors until quite recently.

Nonetheless, over the past decade, a consensus has been emerging among some groups of editors that clearly unethical research should not be published. In part, the lack of an earlier stance on research ethics by editors reflected the fact that there were no cohesive editors' organizations to formulate policies on this or any other issue. Journals were largely private, although they published the results of publicly funded research, and each editor was on his own, answerable only to the owners of the journal.

In 1979 a group of editors of general medical journals formed the International Committee of Medical Journal Editors (ICMJE), also known as the "Vancouver Group." This organization has grown increasingly influential in developing common policies for many journals. At first, it addressed only strictly editorial matters, such as the proper form for references in manuscripts. Later, it began to address much broader concerns, including allegations of fraud, redundant publication, and editorial independence. Although the ICMJE is a small group, its Uniform Requirements are now accepted by several hundred journals. On the subject of ethics in clinical research, the ICMJE has stated: "When reporting experiments on human subjects, indicate whether the procedures followed were in accordance with the ethical standards of the responsible committee on human experimentation (institutional or regional) or with the Helsinki Declaration of 1975, as revised in 1983."[12] Unfortunately, this statement emphasizes process rather than substance and avoids the issue of what editors should do when they believe a study unethical, despite IRB approval and informed consent. Nevertheless, it requires attention from editors to the ethics of the work they publish.

The Council of Biology Editors is an older and larger group but has perhaps had less impact on editors of biomedical journals, in part because of its heterogeneous membership. Concerns of biomedical editors are not necessarily central to the organization as a whole. Nevertheless, its Editorial Policy Committee has developed a position on the role of editors in responding to unethical research on human subjects as a part of its book, *Ethics and Policy in Scientific Publication*.[13] It contains a stronger statement on ethics that concludes: "Editors can and should play their part in upholding ethical standards by refusing to publish reports of work that violates human rights, even if the work seems scientifically valid and important."

The policy of rejecting for publication reports of unethical research has three justifications. First, it is likely to deter unethical work. Because publication is central in the reward system in scientific research, very few researchers would knowingly jeopardize their chances for publication. On the other hand, any other policy would lead to more unethical work, because cutting ethical corners would often enable researchers to get clearer answers faster and thus give them a competitive edge. Second, refusing to publish reports of unethical work protects from erosion the principle of the primacy of the research subject. This is true even when the violations are small. Small lapses, if permitted, invite bigger ones. Third, refusal to publish unethical work serves notice to society at large that even scientists do not consider scientific knowledge the ultimate good in society.

The primary kinds of unethical research that occur today seem to result from a failure of attention to relatively subtle matters of ethics, from a failure of analysis, and from counterincentives, rather than from lack of compassion or deliberate callousness. Unfortunately, in the past, editors and reviewers contributed to this situation by being more willing to forgive ethical lapses than to forgive scientific lapses. There are, however, signs that this disparity is changing.

UNCERTAINTY ABOUT ETHICS

Denying publication may be appropriate in the case of clearly unethical research, but what about work in which the ethics are merely doubtful? I believe editors have an obligation to evaluate work for its ethical content as well as for its scientific content, and that they should seek answers when ethical questions arise, just as they do when scientific questions arise. They should ask authors for clarification. For example, it may be helpful to see the informed consent document. In making an ethical evaluation, editors must be willing to override the judgment of local IRBs, although they should not do this without careful deliberation. All those involved in the research enterprise at each step in the process—investigators, IRBs, funding agencies, reviewers, and editors—have an obligation to evaluate the ethical content of a work just as they evaluate the scientific content, for analogous reasons.

Those who believe that the determination of the IRB should be decisive need to remind themselves that these committees are often not unanimous, nor do they necessarily agree with one another when they are presented with the same type of problem. Unless violations are major, there are often disagreements as to what constitutes an ethical study and what does not. Furthermore, IRBs are subject to local pressures. In particular, they often reflect ethical relativism; a study that would be disapproved in one society would be approved with little trouble in another.[14] Editors are one more link in a chain guarding against unethical research. They should override the judgment of IRBs only reluctantly, after careful deliberation, but they should not publish work that they consider to be unethical, just as they would not publish work that they considered scientifically invalid. When the issue is arguable, other journal editors, who reach a different conclusion, may be willing to publish the work.

AN EXAMPLE

Many of the points I have made about unethical research and the role of editors in dealing with it can be illustrated by a paper *The New England Journal of Medicine* received for consideration. This paper did not come from the United States. It reported a study of virus X (I cannot give more specific details about a paper not published), a virus carried asymptomatically by much of the normal adult population. Before describing the study, it is necessary to give some brief background. For about 10 years it has been known that virus X, although harmless in normal adults, can be lethal or cause devastating disease in premature newborns. Since the infection can be transmitted by blood transfusions, it is recommended in the United States that premature newborns who need blood transfusions for whatever reason receive blood donations only from people who are free of virus X. Whether the donor is free of the virus (seronegative) or infected (seropositive) can be determined by a blood test.

The paper we received concerned the study of a new method to make seropositive blood safe by removing the virus. The authors did a randomized clinical trial in premature newborns who required blood transfusions. All infants received blood from untested donors, but in half of the cases the blood was treated by the new method. As expected, some of the patients in the control group received infected blood, and became sick or died. The new method worked; there were no cases of virus X in the experimental group. The study had been approved by the IRB, and the parents had given informed consent. The *New England Journal of Medicine* refused to publish this report on the grounds that the researchers had knowingly exposed some of their subjects to unacceptable risks.

The researchers believed this decision was unfair for several reasons. First, they pointed out that most blood banks in their country did not routinely use seronegative blood for premature infants; therefore, they were not exposing half of their study subjects to harm, but rather offering protection to the other half. Second, they said that it was their intention to demonstrate as dramatically and clearly as possible the necessity of changing the routine practice in their country, and that they had done so. Demonstrating the efficacy of their method in other ways — for example, by comparing it with historical controls — would not have had the same impact, nor would it have been as scientifically compelling.

Some of their arguments were cogent, particularly the argument that denying publication would mean that premature infants in their country would continue to receive untested blood and thus run the same risk for infection as their control group had. They were outweighed, I believe, by three considerations. First, as emphasized by all the relevant codes, laudable goals do not justify unethical means. They had knowingly allowed harm to come to subjects in their care. Second, clinical trials are justifiable only when researchers are genuinely uncertain as to which group will fare better. In this case, they knew very well which group was likely to fare better. And third, the world is too small for this type of ethical relativism. Instead of demonstrating locally what they already knew, these researchers should have worked to educate their colleagues about the world literature, which showed clearly that giving untested blood to premature infants is dangerous. A review article on this subject in a local journal would probably have been more effective, as well as more ethical, than collecting more data for an international journal.

CONCLUSION

Our sensitivity to ethical issues is still growing and evolving. As it does, the line between unethical and ethical research will be increasingly finely drawn, and not everyone will agree where it should be drawn. It is important that all of us participate in the process of drawing it, and that once drawn, we make absolutely certain that it is observed. In this regard, the Nuremberg Code serves as a beginning, not an end, to the analysis.

NOTES

1. M. Angell, "Patients' Preferences in Randomized Clinical Trials," *New England Journal of Medicine* 310 (1984): 1385–1387.

2. T. L. Beauchamp and J. F. Childress, eds., *Principles of Biomedical Ethics*, 2nd ed. (Oxford: Oxford University Press, 1983), pp. 338–343; OPRR Reports, *Protection of Human Subjects*, 45 CFR 46 (Washington, D.C.: Department of Health and Human Services, 1983).

3. See Chapter 12, this volume.

4. See Chapter 8, this volume.

5. *Guiding Principles for Human Studies* (Boston: Massachusetts General Hospital, 1981).

6. H. K. Beecher, "Ethics and Clinical Research," *New England Journal of Medicine* 274 (1966): 1354–1360.

7. C. B. Chapman, *Physicians, Law, and Ethics* (New York: New York University Press, 1984), p. 125.

8. R. Petersdorf, "The Pathogenesis of Fraud in Medical Science," *Annals of Internal Medicine* 104 (1986): 252–254.

9. M. Angell, "The Nazi Hypothermia Experiments and Unethical Research Today," *New England Journal of Medicine* 322 (1990): 1462–1464.

10. K. Taylor, R. G. Margolese, and C. L. Soskolne, "Physicians' Reasons for Not Entering Eligible Patients in a Randomized Clinical Trial of Adjuvant Surgery for Breast Cancer," *New England Journal of Medicine* 310 (1984): 1363–1367; D. Marquis, "Leaving Therapy to Chance," *Hastings Center Report* 13 (1983): 40–47.

11. For example, M. Zelen, "A New Design for Randomized Clinical Trials," *New England Journal of Medicine* 300 (1979): 1242–1245; and S. S. Ellenberg, "Randomization Designs in Comparative Clinical Trials," *New England Journal of Medicine* 310 (1984): 1404–1408.

12. International Committee of Medical Journal Editors, "Uniform Requirements for Manuscripts submitted to Biomedical Journals," *New England Journal of Medicine* 324 (1991): 424–428.

13. Editorial Policy Committee, Council of Biology Editors, *Ethics and Policy in Scientific Publication* (Bethesda, Md.: Council of Biology Editors, 1990).

14. M. Angell, "Ethical Imperialism? Ethics in International Collaborative Clinical Research," *New England Journal of Medicine* 319 (1988): 1081–1083; Chapter 7, this volume.

16

AIDS Research and the Nuremberg Code

WENDY K. MARINER

The Nuremberg Code has served as the formal basis for virtually all subsequent ethical codes concerning experimentation with human beings. Yet the ways in which the Code's principles have been restated and embellished in the ensuing years have created different visions of ethically defensible objectives and methods of research involving human subjects. Chapter 8 describes how the Declaration of Helsinki and the World Health Organization/Council for International Organizations of Medical Sciences Proposed Guidelines shifted the primary focus of research ethics from (a) ensuring that a subject voluntarily consents to participate in research to (b) independent review of the risks and benefits of proposed research.[1] At least some of this shift in emphasis appears to derive from expanding opportunities for therapeutic medical research — research with people who are ill or disabled that is intended to find or develop ways to help them — research that is conducted, for the most part, by physicians.

The Doctors' Trial was concerned with experimentation by physicians. Nonetheless, the Nuremberg Code does not refer to therapeutic research. The judges at the Doctors' Trial were confronted with obviously *nontherapeutic* research — experiments intended to collect information of no use or benefit whatsoever to the subjects themselves. Although the defense argued that the Nazi doctors' cruel experiments were research, there was no pretense that they were intended to be therapeutic. Thus, it is not surprising that the concept of therapeutic research is absent from the Code that emerged from the judges' decision.[2]

After Nuremberg, codes of ethics that relied on the Nuremberg Code have generally distinguished between therapeutic and nontherapeutic research.[3] The Declaration of Helsinki contains a brief statement distinguishing between therapeutic medical research, "in which the aim is essentially diagnostic or therapeutic for a patient," and nontherapeutic medical research, "the essential object of which is purely scientific and without direct diagnostic or therapeutic value to the person subjected to the research."[4]

The more recent codes' attention to research involving patients as subjects seems to have arisen out of the rapid growth of medical knowledge and resources in the last half-century. Therapeutic research is the largest area of experimentation today. Because it may sometimes help the people who serve as research subjects, its research identity is sometimes submerged beneath its ostensibly beneficent purpose.

While the broad goal of research has always been to discover new or generalizable knowledge, research projects focus on specific substantive questions and specific people. It is these more specific elements of the research project that create quandaries in judging the ethical merit of research. The fact that new information might be gained by an experiment does not, by itself, make the experiment ethically desirable or even justifiable. The Doctors' Trial at Nuremberg made abundantly clear, if it was not already obvious, that experiments can hurt people. That is why we control research—to protect people from needless harm.

The Nuremberg Code embodies this basic concern for protecting human subjects of research in lasting general principles. How are we, as its heirs, to use this rich legacy? How, if at all, does it apply to therapeutic research? We know that the Code does not contain specific rules for all new research circumstances, so that it cannot be applied verbatim to answer specific questions about every new situation. For example, is it fair to exclude some people from participation in a research study they believe will save their lives? Is it appropriate to use pregnant women in an experiment that might endanger their fetuses? What research can be done on embryos? In essence, these questions ask, what are the scope and limits of ethical research? This is also the Code's question. Although it is being asked in new circumstances, and partly answered in new codes, the fundamental question remains the one asked at Nuremberg.

To illustrate how this question haunts contemporary research, this chapter considers an example of therapeutic research—new drugs for AIDS—that has generated controversy among the research community and the general public and has challenged our concepts of research and human subjects.

THE RISE OF THERAPEUTIC DRUG RESEARCH

Studies of experimental pharmaceuticals (drugs) may be the most visible example of new biomedical research activity. Indeed, modern pharmacology and the development of synthetic drugs to treat disease are distinctly postwar phenomena.[5] The organic chemical industry grew to considerable size after the First World War but apparently engaged in little fundamental research.[6] Until the 1930s, most drugs produced were plant derivatives,[7] such as opium, quinine, digitalis, and salicylates. And apart from insulin,

penicillin, and the sulfonamides, little was added to the world pharmaco-
poeia before the 1940s.

Rapid change in the development of new synthetic chemical drugs began
after the Food, Drug and Cosmetic Act of 1938[8] was enacted. The most
dramatic growth in the scientific knowledge of chemical entities and their
effects on disease and illness came in the 1950s and 1960s. Such advances as
cortisone, chloroquine, polio vaccine, tranquilizers, anticholinergics, anti-
hypertensives, and diuretics were introduced. In 1963, sociologist Richard
Titmuss wrote, "In most Western countries some 80 to 90 percent of the
prescriptions are written today for drugs not on the market ten to fifteen
years ago."[9] This explosion of therapeutics inspired new faith in the powers
of medicine to alleviate and even cure diseases that theretofore were assumed
to be untreatable. But unlike the snake oils of an earlier era, these new drugs
were not automatically accepted as ordinary consumer products, dispensed
with a simple *caveat emptor*. In Europe and North America, public opinion
favored regulating potentially harmful chemicals in order to forestall the
exploitation of a public with little knowledge of new drugs.[10]

THE APPEAL OF DRUG RESEARCH WITH HUMAN SUBJECTS

Controlled testing of experimental drugs in human beings is also largely a
postwar phenomenon. Gaddum noted that "when the first edition of [his]
textbook *Pharmacology* appeared in 1940, properly controlled clinical trials
were almost unknown, and the section dealing with them was theoretical."[11]
Lasagna found examples of experiments using controls as far back as Neb-
uchadnezzar's time described in the Book of Daniel. But he noted that "the
widespread use of control groups" in therapeutic research began only in the
1940s.[12] Undoubtedly, the cruel experiments with Nazi prisoners sensitized
the world to the dangers of uncontrolled experimentation. The need to
understand the effects of new chemical substances in human beings, and
especially whether they worked well enough to be publicly distributed, fos-
tered new methods of testing experimental drugs in scientifically controlled
trials. Subjects received the experimental drug and their responses were
compared with those of controls, subjects who received placebo or nothing
at all.

Perhaps as much was learned about *how* to study drugs as about the drugs
themselves. In the 1960s, controlled clinical trials became widely accepted.[13]
They also became more sophisticated, with subjects distributed randomly
(by chance) into treatment and control groups. The randomized clinical trial
became the gold standard in drug research because it was the best-known
method of isolating and demonstrating the effects of an experimental substance as distinguished from the results achieved without the drug. The
method most often thought necessary for accuracy in research is the double-
blind, randomized clinical trial, in which neither the subject nor the researcher knows which of the drugs being compared a given subject has re-

ceived in order to avoid researcher and subject bias in looking for specific results.[14]

As new drugs and methods of testing them became more sophisticated, the distinction between experimental and approved drugs crystallized. Experimental drugs were used in increasingly structured research formats. Federal law now forbade interstate distribution and marketing of new drugs unless they were approved as safe and effective by the federal Food and Drug Administration.[15] A clear division emerged: Drugs that were approved and licensed by the federal government were accepted therapies; those that were not formally approved were experimental.

At the same time, the beneficent aura of experimental drugs grew. New drugs are intended to treat or prevent illness. Testing new drugs in human beings can be seen as a necessary step to identify ways to help people by preventing, alleviating, or even curing disease. While it is generally appreciated that experimental substances may cause unforeseeable serious adverse reactions or side effects, it is also understood that, ultimately, the only way to find out whether a drug is safe and effective for people is to test it on human beings. Thus, testing experimental drugs in human beings is now ordinarily welcomed as desirable experimentation. It seems far removed from the types of experiments conducted on Nazi prisoners. Subjects are not placed in life-threatening conditions just to observe their survival time. They are not deliberately infected with a disease they did not have to see if they can be cured. They are not mutilated to monitor the effects. Instead, in therapeutic experiments, subjects are given a chemical or biological substance to see if it is safely tolerated and whether it works to cure disease. Moreover, the results of this research have been generally positive. The array of drugs that have been developed to alleviate pain and suffering is impressive.

By the time the National Commission for the Protection of Human Subjects in Biomedical and Behavioral Research issued the *Belmont Report*, to identify the ethical precepts underlying human experimentation as a basis for regulating research in 1979, the need for ethical principles explicitly governing therapeutic research was widely recognized. The differences in the history and nature of therapeutic drug research from those of the Nazi doctors' obviously nontherapeutic experiments tend to distance the Nuremberg Code from current tests of experimental drugs. The Declaration of Helsinki reflects a more benign modern attitude toward biomedical research: "Medical progress is based on research which ultimately must rest in part on experimentation involving human subjects."[16] Introducing the Helsinki principles, the World Medical Association stated that it prepared its recommendations "because it is essential that the results of laboratory experiments be applied to human beings to further scientific knowledge and to help suffering humanity."[17] The Helsinki Declaration was written by physicians for physicians. It embodies a general faith in the methods and achievements of medical science and an acceptance of the premise that scientific success depends upon testing new substances in human subjects.

As pointed out in Chapter 8, the Nuremberg Code's first and strongest principle—that the voluntary consent of the human subject is absolutely essential—is relegated to the ninth of twelve basic principles in Helsinki. Helsinki's first basic principle requires compliance with "generally accepted scientific principles."[18] This is intended to ensure that any experiment involving human subjects is justified by scientific knowledge and design, as stated in the third principle of Nuremberg. Yet it can be seen as deeming "generally accepted scientific principles," rather than the subject's consent, the *sine qua non* of proceeding with an experiment. It seems most at home in the field of therapeutic research. It should come as no surprise, then, that when the Food and Drug Administration issued regulations specifying the ethical principles that should govern experimental drug research, it adopted the Declaration of Helsinki, not the Nuremberg Code, as part of its regulations.[19] Helsinki fit best with an enterprise whose purpose is generally therapeutic.

The success of drug development has buttressed the idea that research with experimental drugs is not only necessary but highly desirable. The corollary is that testing experimental drugs in human subjects is similarly desirable. It is understood to produce beneficial products, sometimes "magic bullets." Even though very few of the drugs that are initially developed make it to market, the successes tend to drive the system.[20] Both the public and practicing physicians are made aware of new drugs that can treat disease more effectively and are eager to have them. Thus, where ethical principles do not specifically prohibit the use of human subjects to test new drugs, there is desire and pressure to do so. The operant question for contemporary researchers, and for most of the public, is not whether the use of human subjects in any proposed experiment can be justified, but how to get the experiment done.

THE DEMAND FOR EXPERIMENTAL DRUGS

The public appeal of most drug research may help explain the willingness, indeed the eagerness, of many patients to become research subjects. This attitude is most evident among persons with diseases or conditions for which no generally accepted cure or treatment exists. Patients with cancer have a relatively lengthy history of participating in clinical trials of experimental cancer drugs.[21] In the absence of any demonstrably effective treatment for many types of cancer, patients who want to "do something" have to submit to some experiment, be it with drugs, radiation, or surgery. Experimental drugs, or chemotherapy, have become the treatment of choice for many cancer patients.

Traditionally, experimental drugs have been distributed to patients as part of a controlled clinical trial. In the United States, the Food, Drug and Cosmetic Act prohibits the distribution of drugs outside of clinical trials until they are approved (licensed) for marketing.[22] This means that as a

general rule, patients who wish to take an experimental drug must participate in the trial as subjects.[23] Experimental drugs are occasionally given by
physicians to patients who have not responded to any accepted treatment.[24]
The purpose of using them is largely therapeutic, to benefit the patient
directly. Still, this "compassionate use" of experimental drugs is nonetheless
an experiment, with information on the patient-subject's response collected
and added to the research data to evaluate the drug. However, from the
patient's point of view, the experimental drug may have the same purpose as
an approved drug—to help him recover. The fact that his use of the drug
becomes part of research may be ignored. For such patients, the distinction
between treatment and experimentation has become blurred. Thus, experimental drugs sometimes metamorphose into therapy because patients use
experimental drugs the same way as approved drugs. Similarly, the distinction between being a patient and being a research subject may become lost if
access to the experimental drug, which is thought of as therapy, is contingent on joining an experiment.

Patients who want to become research subjects in this sense are not limited to those with cancer. People who are dying understandably seek a cure.
The most visible recent example concerns people with acquired immunodeficiency syndrome (AIDS) or human immunodeficiency virus (HIV) infection. Here again, there is no real cure for a fatal disease, although zidovudine has extended the lives of many patients.[25] The best hope for treating
either HIV infection or many of the opportunistic infections that take the
lives of so many patients lies in the future, in experimental drugs now being
developed and tested. It should not be surprising, therefore, that persons
with AIDS have insistently sought access to experimental AIDS drugs.[26]

But AIDS activists pose a new challenge to therapeutic drug research.
They have organized forceful objections to the design of AIDS drug trials,
questioning the need for randomization, controls, dosage requirements, limits on eligibility to participate, and rigid adherence to academic scientific
standards for evaluating results.[27] Not only have they demanded access to
drugs in clinical trials, they have challenged the distinction between research
and therapy as unnecessary, as a manifestation of elitist control over science
and patient care, and as contrary to a deep sense of individual autonomy. In
this view, the subject is respected best not by protection against research
risks but by ensuring freedom of choice and participation in research.

AIDS patients appear to make one or both of two types of demands. One
is to participate in clinical trials in order to obtain a drug that is being tested.
The other is to obtain experimental or other drugs outside of clinical trials.
In both cases, the demand is based on the desire for the drug itself. However,
in the first case, individuals seek to become subjects in order to obtain the
drug in a clinical trial,[28] while in the second case, they effectively dismiss the
concept of subjects of research.

The desire to participate in a clinical trial of experimental anti-HIV drugs
is similar to that of many other seriously ill patients seeking a cure. These
individuals have little hope for their condition as patients unless they can

also become research subjects. The second demand makes a much stronger claim. Those who make this demand claim personal entitlement to all experimental and unapproved drugs as a matter of principle. Further, it is the patient, not the physician or the investigator, who claims the right to choose what drugs to use. Finally, the patient claims the right to the drugs whether or not they are in clinical trials. In other words, this demand is not a claim to become the subject of an experiment, but to obtain a drug for personal use and possible benefit, free of any external regulation or control.

Both demands spring from the hope that a particular drug will help one's condition or save one's life. But AIDS activists have built a revolutionary conception of access to drugs on this premise. In this view, if there is no approved cure, all options are experimental. If no one knows what will work, then all options are equally promising and equally risky. Because it is the patient who suffers the illness, it is argued, the patient should be the one to choose what risks he or she takes to overcome the illness.[29]

AIDS CHALLENGES TO ETHICAL PRINCIPLES OF HUMAN EXPERIMENTATION

Students of research ethics have always been more concerned about protecting subjects involved in nontherapeutic research than those involved in therapeutic research. The opportunities for harm and exploitation are most obvious in nontherapeutic experiments. Conventional wisdom holds that there is less likelihood of harm in therapeutic research because the investigator's ultimate goal is to help the subject. But subjects in therapeutic experiments can misunderstand or be misled into believing that they are receiving an accepted treatment, not helping to answer a question. For this reason, in discussing therapeutic research, ethical principles have stressed the distinction between research and therapy.

The demand for experimental AIDS drugs challenges traditional assumptions underlying human experimentation and raises difficult questions. Is there any meaningful difference between research and therapy or between patients and research subjects? Who should decide what constitutes an experiment and by what criteria? Are there any limits on the risk of harm to which a person may be subjected or voluntarily submit?

It is possible to think of the demand to participate in anti-HIV drug trials as a demand for what has come to be called *innovative* or *nonvalidated* therapy. An innovative therapy is an experimental drug or procedure offered to a patient, generally as a last resort, in the hope that it might save the patient's life or improve a serious illness.[30] Not only experimental drugs, but also such surgical procedures as heart transplants, were called innovative therapies when the physician sought to use them to save a patient's life before their effectiveness was known.[31] Such experimental efforts tend to deny the difference between formal therapeutic research and accepted medical therapy because they are at the same time experimental and ostensibly for the sole benefit of an individual.[32]

If, during the course of therapy, all accepted medical techniques fail and a physician tries an experiment with one patient, is this research or therapy? Should it matter whether the physician is trying to benefit the patient or is testing the new drug or procedure to see if it could work? Should research be characterized by *what* is done or *why* it is done?

A practical definition of research is an experiment or study conducted for the purpose of obtaining generalizable knowledge.[33] The Declaration of Helsinki also describes biomedical research in terms of its purpose: "to improve diagnostic, therapeutic and prophylactic procedures and the understanding of the aetiology and pathogenesis of disease."[34] Yet this cannot mean that giving new, untested substances to human beings is research only when the physician decides that it is.

Although the Nuremberg Code does not define research, its very existence presupposes that research differs significantly from ordinary human activities, including, presumably, medical care. Why else lay down principles defining ethically acceptable conduct? The prosecutors at the Doctors' Trial argued that those who conducted the experiments were "for the most part, on trial for murder."[35] Neither the prosecution nor the defense, however, argued the cases in terms of the crime of murder alone. Both saw the critical conduct performed in the context of research. The Nazi doctors tried to defend themselves on this ground. But the prosecution and the judges rightly saw their actions as all the more heinous because camouflaged as medical experimentation. Introducing the 10 principles of the Code, the judgment emphasized that medical experiments must conform to certain basic principles. Acts committed in the guise of research were subject to more, not fewer, norms than the crimes of murder and torture alone. The judges undoubtedly were concerned about the increased vulnerability of people who might think that their lives and health were under the watchful care of physicians who pursued science rather than mayhem. Murder and torture could be prohibited. But the researcher could accomplish both more subtly where the harm was disguised by a scientific purpose.[36]

All ethical principles of research appear to be solidly built on the premise that experimentation differs from other voluntary human conduct. Research subjects also assume that people who participate in research as subjects have a status in addition to that of an ordinary civilian. They perform a unique function that demands that they be protected from unnecessary, as well as unconsented to, harm. Codes of ethics governing experimentation with human subjects were developed to protect human beings against unwarranted experimentation and harm. What are we to do when potential subjects reject such protection?

Carole Levine has noted that while Nuremberg began with the premise that "people have the right *not* to be research subjects," the current claim is that people have the right to *be* research subjects.[37] The experimental drug can be seen as part of personal medical care. For some, there is no difference between experimental and nonexperimental drugs. There are only drugs that may or may not save their lives. This conception, however, leaves experiments to be defined without reference to the experimental substance being used. Alternatively, it leaves the definition of experimentation to the individual subject (or nonsubject). Research would be in the eye of the beholder, a wholly subjective concept. If experimentation cannot be objectively defined, how can the intended beneficiaries of the Nuremberg Code be protected?

People who demand access to experimental drugs they believe may save their lives present an especially compelling case for making an exception to the basic assumptions about medical research. Yet it is unclear how such an exception could be defined without undermining the noncontroversial general principles of ethical research. It would be difficult to argue that the exception should lie in excusing the physician from the remaining ethical obligations, such as avoiding unnecessary suffering and using care to protect the subject during the experiment. If the distinction between research and therapy were eliminated, what would a physician's responsibilities be? Could there be any objective measure of reasonable care for a patient? The reason physicians are charged with the duty to use accepted medical practices is that such practices have been demonstrated to be effective. A physician who departs from accepted practices does so at his peril.[38] He is constrained to do so only when he has a very good reason to believe that his patient will be better off than with accepted therapy. If there is no way to differentiate the departure from the norm, should physicians be accountable for all harm that befalls a patient, or for none?

The appeal of much of modern drug research, coupled with the desperate need of so many who are ill, poses a fundamental challenge to the vitality of ethical principles of medical research. There is obvious tension between the need to distribute potentially beneficial drugs fairly to those who are ill and the need to protect human subjects against unwarranted harm in medical experimentation. General ethical research principles offer no obvious accommodation of any public demand for experimental drugs. This is why it has proved so difficult for even the World Health Organization to recommend specific guidelines for experimental AIDS drugs. To scrap all of our codes of ethics merely to satisfy such demands would return us to the days before Nuremberg. It is not at all clear that the need for explicit ethical principles is past. Examples of the misuse and ill treatment of human beings for the sake of research, such as the Tuskegee and Willowbrook experiments,[39] are all too contemporary, and are evidence of the need for reminders of the basic ethical obligations of all those who use human beings in the search for knowledge. The codes embody principles of respect for persons that should apply whether or not the definition of research is altered. No one has suggested that such basic prerequisites as consent to participation be eliminated in order to liberalize access to investigational drugs. Yet the demands for such access will not go away. Whether and how they can be accommodated represents a major challenge to the legacy of the Nuremberg Code.

Can the demand for experimental drugs be satisfied without sacrificing an essential respect for persons? We can begin to answer this question by asking again the basic question addressed by the Nuremberg Code: What are the scope and limits of justifiable research with human subjects? Even if there are hard cases that challenge the limits of research, it is too late to pretend that there is no difference between research and therapy. We should recall the warning implicit in the judgment at the Doctors' Trial. Human beings may be most vulnerable to misuse when they are asked to submit to experiments in the name of science. Therapeutic research, while ordinarily more beneficent than nontherapeutic research, may have greater potential to mislead people because of its implicit promise of personal benefit. Indeed, the recent tendency to forget that an experiment is involved when research is labeled "medical" argues for a stronger emphasis on the research aspect.

To be meaningful, research must be defined in objective, not subjective, terms. This means that the purpose and content of research should be discernible to independent observers, regardless of the personal objectives of the participating investigators and subjects. In other words, the applicability of ethical principles should not depend on the participants' willingness to have them apply in any particular case. To protect people from unjustified harm, then, there must be an objective basis on which to judge justifiable risks. This cannot depend on the subject's willingness to take particular risks any more than a person's agreement to be a slave justifies slavery. At the same time, the nature of justifiable risks can be flexible enough to permit knowledgeable subjects to expose themselves voluntarily to risks when there is a reasonable expectation of greater benefit.

This emphasis on the difference between research and therapy seems to make it more difficult to obtain experimental drugs. After all, there is no right to be a research subject. But one can make a more credible moral claim to accepted therapies. Thus, a better argument from the principle of justice seems available if experimental drugs are treated as accepted therapies.

The arguments against entitlement to experimental drugs are both practical and normative. The most salient practical argument is that if experimental drugs are universally available, controlled research will no longer be feasible and it will be impossible to determine which drugs do and do not work. Although some individuals may be better off for serendipitously having used the right drug, others, and society as a whole, will be worse off. Some people will use drugs that either cannot help them or turn out to harm them. And there will be no way for people to identify drugs that can help them. The counterargument is similarly empirical: The use of experimental drugs is not likely to be so widespread as to jeopardize the conduct of valid research. Although only the future can reveal which position will prove true, there seems to be general agreement that research will not be expedited by the universal availability of experimental drugs. If so, society and most seriously ill people will wait longer than necessary to identify drugs with real benefit.

The normative argument against entitlement to experimental drugs is that people are entitled to protection from avoidable risks. Most people are not in a position to evaluate the risks and benefits of an experimental substance, especially when science is uncertain about them. Thus, society has an obligation to identify therapeutic measures and to prevent exploitation of and harm to its members. The counterargument is that as long as there is uncertainty, it should be up to the person who takes the risk—the subject—to decide whether or not to use the drug. Thus, society has no right to preclude access to freely chosen goods. Yet this leaves us with no basis for judging any risk unacceptable. The same principle that rejects limits on drug availability as paternalistic also rejects safety standards for automobiles and other consumer products, and, most relevantly, prohibitions against illicit drugs such as heroin and cocaine. If it is conceded that some risks should not be permitted, even if a subject is willing, then the principle of line drawing has been embraced. The only question is where to draw the line.

One can agree that a line should be drawn between justifiable and unjustifiable risks and still argue that the current line is inappropriate, at least in some cases;[40] or that more efficient research methods could accurately identify safe and effective drugs more quickly.[41] This does not undermine the need to make the identification or to protect individuals from risks still deemed unwarranted.

CONCLUSION

Many AIDS activists define what research is justifiable by the desire for the knowledge sought and by the consent of the human subject rather than scientific benefit-risk analysis and design. In this view, there are no limitations on experimentation by researchers, and consent is the only limitation on participation by human subjects. It permits experimentation wherever there is a subjective desire for knowledge. Since consent merely identifies the people who are willing to undergo the experiment, it cannot define the scope of permissible research.[42]

The Nuremberg Code was premised on the fact that some experiments cannot be justified by reference to a single principle. Neither scientific interest nor subject consent is sufficient by itself to warrant abusing people. If the narrow conception of consent were applied to research with embryos and fetuses, it would preclude all such research, for embryos and fetuses have no capacity to consent or decline to participate in research. If, on the other hand, fetal or embryo research were justified solely on the basis of the need for knowledge, there would be no limits to the use of fetuses and embryos in research.[43]

The legacy of the Doctors' Trial at Nuremberg is that knowledge is not the supreme value. If it were, on what ground could the Nazi doctors' experiments be condemned? The doctors argued that they were seeking information about human survival and expanding general knowledge. Yet objectively, what they did was to torture and murder people. Thus, the investigator's subjective statement cannot be dispositive of the value of information or any particular experiment. The Nazi doctors tried to bolster their defense by arguing that a national emergency or war justified the nature of their experiments. The idea that desperate times call for desperate acts is a familiar one. But without some clear concept of how desperate one must be and how desperate the acts can be, it invites abuse.

The Nuremberg Code recognized that any calculus justifying research with human beings embodies several principles that are not self-evident in the concept of a search for knowledge. Not just any information, but knowledge that is useful for the benefit of humankind, justifies the effort. This requires a valid scientific basis. Moreover, the way in which information is obtained matters. For this reason, the principles include requirements for the qualifications of researchers and the design of the experiment. Most important, perhaps, is the insistence that risks to human beings be minimized and that these risks be acceptable in light of the reasonably foreseeable benefits. Such principles have endured. Perhaps the fact that they have required elaboration in more complex circumstances is an affirmation of the Code's original insight: that no single principle is sufficient to justify an experiment.

Although the Code insisted on the voluntary, informed consent of subjects, it appreciated that people are not always in a position to give valid consent. Their autonomy can be compromised in many ways. Under such circumstances, these vulnerable people are entitled to protection against harm. Reasonable people may disagree on what constitutes a vulnerable population or harm. Pregnant women, for example, argue that they are not as vulnerable as others have thought.[44] The Nuremberg Code does not define vulnerability. But it recognizes that even people who agree to participate in experiments may be vulnerable in ways that they themselves may not appreciate. Therapeutic research, including new drug trials and promises of experimental cures outside of organized trials, have the potential to mislead people into forgetting that experiments can hurt as well as help.

Therapeutic biomedical research—in particular, new drugs for AIDS—has challenged the legacy of the Nuremberg Code. The Code, and virtually all later statements of ethical principles, insist that researchers cannot decide what is and what is not a justifiable experiment solely on the basis of the need for knowledge. Neither can people who may become research subjects. There must be a distinction between justifiable and unjustifiable research. Neither the Nuremberg Code nor any of its progeny tells us precisely where the line should be drawn in each case. It is up to us, the evolving society, to make distinctions as science gathers more evidence on what is and is not beneficial. We may disagree on where to draw the line in a particular case. But that does not mean that no line can be drawn today, any more than it meant that no line could be drawn at Nuremberg.

NOTES

1. See Chapter 8, this volume.

2. The Code's second principle states that an experiment "should be such as to yield fruitful results *for the good of society*" [emphasis added], suggesting that using an experimental drug or other treatment in the hope of helping a patient is not contemplated. Physicians are not referred to in their capacity of ministering to the sick, but only as scientists in charge of the experiment, or as potential subjects themselves in experiments in which death or disabling injury is expected: "The individual who initiates, directs or engages in the experiment" (principle 1); "scientifically qualified persons" (principle 8); and "the scientist" (principle 10). Moreover, the Code never refers to subjects of research as patients.

3. The National Commission for the Protection of Human Subjects of Biomedical and Behavioral Research differentiated research from the practice of accepted therapy: "For the most part, the term 'practice' refers to interventions that are designed solely to enhance the well-being of an individual patient or client and that have a reasonable expectation of success. The purpose of medical or behavioral practice is to provide diagnosis, preventive treatment or therapy to particular individuals. By contrast, the term 'research' designates an activity designed to test a hypothesis, permit conclusions to be drawn, and thereby to develop or contribute to generalizable knowledge (expressed, for example, in theories, principles, and statements of relationships)." National Commission for the Protection of Human Subjects of Biomedical and Behavioral Research, *The Belmont Report: Ethical Principles and Guidelines for the Protection of Human Subjects of Research* (Washington, D.C.: Department of Health, Education and Welfare, 1979), pp. 2–3.

4. Declaration of Helsinki, Introduction, para. 6. The former is called "medical research combined with professional care (clinical research)" and is made the subject of 6 principles (Part II), in addition to the basic 12 of the Declaration. The latter is called "non-therapeutic biomedical research involving human subjects (non-clinical biomedical research)" and is subject to four additional principles (Part III). Read literally, these definitions state not a distinction between therapeutic and nontherapeutic research, but the difference between research and therapy, as described in the *Belmont Report*. The therapeutic research definition focuses on a single patient, not on patients with a particular condition. It contains no reference to scientific knowledge being sought. This is reserved for the definition of nontherapeutic research, which also excludes any direct value to the subject. Indeed, the definition of nontherapeutic research sounds more like that contemplated in the Nuremberg Code. It should not be surprising, then, that those who rely on the Helsinki definitions tend to confuse therapeutic research with therapy or ordinary treatment. Even so, the Helsinki Declaration intends to describe research alone. Its definition of therapeutic research, however, seems pertinent only to studies intended to establish whether an intervention should be *accepted* by the medical community as useful for a patient. At the same time, the two definitions are not mutually exclusive. The tendency of some researchers to confuse therapeutic research with accepted therapy (medical care of a patient) may be rooted in the peculiar language in the Helsinki definitions.

5. Austin Smith, president of the Pharmaceutical Manufacturers Association in 1960, was reported to have said that "only with World War II did the American pharmaceutical industry come of age." J. H. Young, "Social History of American Drug Legislation," in P. Talalay, ed., *Drugs in Our Society* (Baltimore: Johns Hopkins University Press, 1964), p. 227, citing F.D.C. Reports, Dec. 19, 1960.

6. J. Stieglitz, ed., *Chemistry in Medicine* (New York: The Chemical Foundation,

Inc., 1928), p. 720; J. P. Swann, *Academic Scientists and the Pharmaceutical Industry* (Baltimore: Johns Hopkins University Press, 1988), p. 30.

7. E. B. Chain, "Academic and Industrial Contribution to Drug Research," *Nature* 200 (1963): 441–453.

8. 21 U.S.C. 301 *et seq.*

9. R. Titmuss, "Sociological and Ethnic Aspects of Therapeutics," in Talalay, *Drugs in Our Society*, p. 243.

10. P. Starr, *The Social Transformation of American Medicine* (New York: Basic Books, 1982), pp. 127–134.

11. J. H. Gaddum, "A Perspective on Pharmacology," in Talalay, *Drugs in Our Society*, pp. 21–22.

12. L. Lasagna, "On Evaluating Drug Therapy: The Nature of the Evidence," in Talalay, *Drugs in Our Society*, p. 92.

13. Ibid.

14. The term *double-blind* is thought to have been coined by Dr. Harvey Gold and colleagues in 1959. H. Gold, in D. R. Laurence, ed., *Quantitative Methods in Human Pharmacology and Therapeutics* (London: Oxford University Press, 1959).

15. 21 U.S.C. §355.

16. Declaration of Helsinki, Introduction, para. 5.

17. Ibid., para. 8.

18. Ibid., I, 1.

19. 21 C.F.R. §312.20–.29 (1988).

20. For every drug that the FDA approves for marketing in the United States, many more are abandoned as unsafe or ineffective on the basis of laboratory tests, animal studies, or clinical trials with human beings. Little is publicly known about new drugs that are not pursued beyond initial laboratory or animal tests. The negative results of some clinical trials may be published in the scientific or medical literature. But it is the drugs that are demonstrated to be safe and effective that receive the most attention. Studies of their efficacy should appear in prominent medical journals. Investigators who report original research demonstrating an effective new therapy may expect the rewards of increased prestige and academic honor. Pharmaceutical companies may be quick to advertise a drug soon after FDA approval. Print and broadcast media may carry stories about a new drug and how it may help people, especially if it is intended to treat a disease for which no alternative therapy is available or if it represents a significant advance over existing treatments. Physicians may recommend the drug with enthusiasm, sometimes even for uses that differ from its approved use. For a critical account of drug development and marketing, see M. Silverman and P. R. Lee, *Pills, Profits, and Politics* (Berkeley: University of California Press, 1974). For a more sympathetic analysis, see H. Edgar and D. J. Rothman, "New Rules for New Drugs: The Challenge of AIDS to the Regulatory Process," *The Milbank Quarterly* 68, Supp. 1 (1990): 111–142.

21. R. J. Levine, *Ethics and the Regulation of Clinical Research*, 2nd ed. (Baltimore: Urban and Schwarzenberg, 1986).

22. Ordinarily, new drugs are tested in a series of experiments and clinical trials to gather data sufficient to demonstrate their safety and effectiveness in order to gain FDA approval. Typically, a new drug is tested first in the laboratory and then in animal studies. If the drug is promising, the sponsor will want to proceed with testing it in human subjects. In order to ship the drug to clinical trial investigators, sponsors must obtain an exemption from the prohibition against distributing unapproved drugs in interstate commerce by submitting to the FDA a Notice of Claimed Investi-

gational Exemption for a New Drug, known as an IND. (21 C.F.R. §312). Clinical trials generally are conducted in three phases. Phase 1 trials observe the pharmacological effects and the disposition of the drug in a small group of subjects, usually between 20 and 80 healthy volunteers. A phase 1 study also collects data on human tolerance of different doses, as well as adverse reactions and drug toxicity. Phase 2 trials also study drug safety issues and gather preliminary information on the drug's effectiveness, usually in several hundred subjects. Phase 3 trials collect sufficient evidence of the drug's effectiveness and safety to permit FDA approval. They typically involve larger numbers of subjects and attempt to identify the specific use of the drug, as well as more common side effects. After a drug is approved, phase 4 studies may be conducted to refine knowledge about the drug.

23. This general rule has been altered by the FDA in recent years to permit the use of experimental drugs for treatment purposes in certain circumstances. See W. K. Mariner, "New FDA Drug Approval Policies and HIV Vaccine Development," *American Journal of Public Health* 80 (1990): 336–341; W. K. Mariner, "Equitable Access to Biomedical Advances: Getting Beyond the Rights Impasse," *Connecticut Law Review* 21 (1989): 571–603. The most recent initiative is the parallel track, or expanded access, used to distribute experimental drugs to treat HIV infection. See note 24.

24. Although the general rule has been that investigational drugs may not be distributed for use outside clinical trials that are subject to an FDA-approved IND, the FDA has permitted exceptions. Many of these have been loosely called the "compassionate use" of investigational drugs. Since the 1960s, physicians familiar with the drug development process have occasionally obtained FDA approval to use an investigational drug to treat a patient outside a clinical trial, when there was no alternative effective treatment. Technically, this required the physician to become an investigator, whether or not attached to an existing clinical trial, or to submit his or her own independent IND application. P. B. Hutt, "A Brief History of FDA Policy on Investigational Drugs for Treatment Purposes," presented at the Institute of Medicine Round Table on Expanding Access to Investigational Therapies, March 12, 1990.

Sometimes drugs have been made available to patients by keeping the drugs on investigational status. This excused the sponsor from submitting a formal application for new drug approval (NDA) when it might not have been granted. For example, there might be too few subjects with whom to test a new drug for a rare disease (orphan drug), or the clinical trial results might be insufficient to permit FDA approval (Group C drugs for cancers), but no other therapy for the disease existed. In some cases, the FDA has permitted subjects who seem to benefit from an investigational drug to continue to take it after the clinical trial has ended. This "open-label" IND allows subjects to remain on a drug while it is being reviewed for approval and before it is marketed.

None of these informal policies were incorporated in either the Food, Drug and Cosmetic Act or FDA regulations. While they were used for humanitarian reasons, they were difficult to reconcile with the governing statute. Until the late 1980s, the only regulatory exception to the statutory structure was emergency use, which permits a physician to use an investigational drug in an emergency with a single patient without conducting research. In 1987 the FDA adopted regulations providing for a treatment IND, which combined research objectives with the compassionate use of investigational drugs. 21 C.F.R. §312.34 (1988). Investigational drugs "intended to treat a serious or immediately life-threatening disease" for which no alternative therapy exists may be used to treat patients while clinical trials with human subjects are ongoing. More recently, the Public Health Service has proposed a new policy to distribute investigational drugs to persons with HIV infection or AIDS who are unable to participate as subjects in clinical trials of the drugs. Public Health Service, "Expanded Availability of Investigational New Drugs Through a Parallel Track Mechanism for People with AIDS and HIV-Related Disease," *Federal Register* 55 (May 21, 1990): 20856–20860. Known as *parallel track* or *expanded access*, this procedure would permit HIV-infected persons to obtain investigational drugs for personal use as soon as they were available for use in phase 2 clinical trials. A similar approach was used to distribute dideoxyinosine to patients at the beginning of phase 2 clinical trials.

25. M. A. Fischl, D. D. Richman, M. H. Grieco, et al., "The Efficacy of Azidothymidine (AZT) in the Treatment of Patients with AIDS and AIDS-Related Complex: A Double-Blind, Placebo-Controlled Trial," *New England Journal of Medicine* 317 (1987): 185–191; M. A. Fischl, C. B. Parker, C. Pettinelli, et al., "A Randomized Controlled Trial of a Reduced Daily Dose of Zidovudine in Patients with the Acquired Immunodeficiency Syndrome," *New England Journal of Medicine* 323 (1990): 1009–1014.

26. G. J. Annas, "Faith (Healing), Hope and Charity at the FDA: The Politics of AIDS Drug Trials," *Villanova Law Review* 34 (1989): 771–797; W. K. Mariner, "Equitable Access to Biomedical Advances: Getting Beyond the Rights Impasse," *Connecticut Law Review* 21 (1989): 571–603.

27. R. Bayer, "Beyond the Burdens of Protection: AIDS and the Ethics of Research," *Evaluation Review* 14 (1990): 443–446.

28. For many, an additional reason to seek participation in a clinical trial is to obtain access to health care services that are otherwise unavailable to them, either for lack of health insurance or financial resources or because of inability to locate a physician willing to care for them. See J. D. Arras, "Noncompliance in AIDS Research," *Hastings Center Report* 20 (1990): 24–32. Where medical examinations and treatment for medical conditions are provided in tandem with research, people understandably see drug trials as their only realistic chance to enter the health care system. This has prompted several groups to call for the provision of adequate health care services for people with AIDS. See National Commission on AIDS, *Report Number One: Failure of U.S. Health Care System to Deal with HIV Epidemic*, Dec. 5, 1989; National Institutes of Health, Acquired Immunodeficiency Syndrome Program Advisory Committee, "Recommendation to the Secretary of Health and Human Services," November 20, 1990. Because such circumstances, however deplorable, do not implicate the need for research or drugs, they are not considered here.

29. M. Delaney, "The Case for Patient Access to Experimental Therapy," *Journal of Infectious Disease* 159 (1989): 416–419.

30. S. E. Lind, "Innovative Medical Therapies: Between Practice and Research," *Clinical Research* 36 (1988): 546–551; B. Freeman et al., "Nonvalidated Therapies and HIV Disease," *Hastings Center Report* 19 (1989): 3.

31. G. J. Annas, "Consent to the Artificial Heart: The Lion and the Crocodiles," in *Judging Medicine* (Clifton, N.J.: Humana Press, 1988), pp. 391–396.

32. Annas has argued, however, that some physicians may have pursued an experiment in order to test the procedure itself rather than with any reasonable expectation of benefiting the person. G. J. Annas, "Baby Fae: The 'Anything Goes' School of Human Experimentation," in *Judging Medicine*, pp. 384–390.

33. The *Oxford English Dictionary*'s definition of research is "A search or investigation directed to the discovery of some fact by careful consideration or study of a

subject; a course of critical or scientific inquiry." (Oxford: Oxford University Press, 1971), Vol. II, p. 2505.

34. Introduction, para. 3.

35. Chapter 7, this volume.

36. Justice Brandeis expressed this concern aptly in his dissent in *Olmstead v. United States*, 277 U.S. 438 (1928): "Experience should teach us to be most on our guard to protect liberty when the government's purposes are beneficent. Men born to freedom are naturally alert to repel invasion of their liberty by evil-minded rulers. The greatest dangers to liberty lurk in insidious encroachment by men of zeal well-meaning but without understanding."

37. C. Levine, "Has AIDS Changed the Ethics of Human Subjects Research?" *Law, Medicine and Health Care* 16 (1988): 167–173.

38. J. H. King, Jr., *The Law of Medical Malpractice*, 2nd ed. (St. Paul, Minn.: West Publishing, 1986); A. R. Holder, *Medical Malpractice Law*, 2nd ed. (New York: Wiley, 1978).

39. See J. Katz, *Experimentation with Human Beings* (New York: Russell Sage Foundation, 1972).

40. For example, it is possible to argue that AIDS drug trials with human subjects may begin with fewer or different indications of safety or effectiveness than are expected for other drugs on the grounds that laboratory and animal studies have not always proved to be reliable models for predicting AIDS drug activity in human beings. This approach raises the threshold of risk but does not remove it. The FDA has proposed to accelerate its review and approval of new drugs for AIDS (and other "life-threatening and severely-debilitating illnesses") by combining phase 2 and 3 trials. Food and Drug Administration, "Investigational New Drug, Antibiotic, and Biological Drug Product Regulations: Procedures for Drugs Intended to Treat Life-threatening and Severely Debilitating Illnesses," *Federal Register* 53 (October 21, 1988): 41516–41524. The procedure is intended to encourage expeditious clinical trials of sufficiently high quality to demonstrate safety and effectiveness, and therefore permit FDA approval as promptly as possible.

41. New approaches to designing clinical trials are being discussed. See, e.g., D. P. Byar, D. A. Schoenfeld, S. B. Green, et al., "Design Considerations for AIDS Trials," *New England Journal of Medicine* 323 (1990): 1343–1348; S. B. Green, S. S. Ellenberg, D. Finkelstein, et. al., "Issues in the Design of Drug Trials for AIDS," *Controlled Clinical Trials* 11 (1990): 80–87. See, generally, L. Lasagna, "Clinical Trials in the Natural Environment," in C. Steichele, U. Abshagen and J. Koch-Weser, eds., *Drugs Between Research and Regulation* (Darmstadt: Steinkopff Verlag, 1985). In addition, the AIDS activist and medical communities have developed community research initiatives to conduct trials without rigid adherence to traditional academic standards of scientific rigor. See V. Merton, "Community-based AIDS Research," *Evaluation Review* 14 (1990): 502–537.

42. Consent may operate to influence the scope of research undertaken by investigators in practice, however. If researchers believe that there is no need to weigh risks and benefits in order to justify a particular experiment, they may believe that anything is permissible, and that subjects can decide whether or not to take the risks. The risk-benefit analysis is shifted to the prospective subjects, who must decide for themselves whether the risks are worth the benefits. Although such an analysis should be part of all subjects' deliberations about entering research, used this way it is transformed from a personal analysis to a substitute for determining whether *anyone* should be invited to participate.

43. Fetuses and embryos can be used both as subjects of research and as research material. They are research subjects when they are manipulated in an experiment intended to alter a genetic or congenital abnormality they have. Fetal tissue can be used as research material, as when tissue from dead fetuses is transplanted to an adult human subject in an attempt to alleviate that person's medical condition. Embryos can be research material when used in *in vitro* fertilization experiments. Public attitudes on such uses are hardly unanimous. Several national commissions have recommended that embryo research should be limited to a short period after fertilization, usually 14 days, the time at which the primitive streak normally develops or the embryo is individually differentiated. Ethics Advisory Board, Department of Health, Education and Welfare, *HEW Support of Research Involving Human In Vitro Fertilization and Embryo Transfer* (Washington, D.C.: U.S. Government Printing Office, 1979); *Report of the Committee of Inquiry into Human Fertilization and Embryology* (Chairman, Dame Mary Warnock), Cmnd 9314 (London: Her Majesty's Stationery Office, 1984); Committee to Consider the Social, Ethical, and Legal Issues Arising from In Vitro Fertilization (Chairman, Louis Waller), *Report on the Disposition of Embryos Produced by In Vitro Fertilization* (Melbourne: Government of Victoria, 1984); Ontario Law Reform Commission, *Report on Human Reproduction and Related Matters*, Vol. II (Ontario: Ministry of the Attorney General, 1985). They generally agree that the embryo ought to be treated with respect, although they are less specific on what this respect entails.

The United States has restricted the type of research in which fetuses may be used as subjects of research funded by the federal government. "Additional Protections Pertaining to Research Development and Related Activities Involving Fetuses, Pregnant Women, and Human In Vitro Fertilization," 45 C.F.R. §46.201–211. Many states also prohibit nontherapeutic and some therapeutic research with fetuses. In December 1988, the Fetal Tissue Transplantation Research Panel recommended removing the ban on federal funding of research using fetal tissue for transplantation. See J. A. Robertson, "Rights, Symbolism, and Public Policy in Fetal Tissue Transplants," *Hastings Center Report* 18 (1988): 5–12; J. O. Mason, "Should the Fetal Research Ban be Lifted?," *Journal of NIH Research* 2 (1990): 17–18.

44. C. Levine, "Women and HIV/AIDS Research: The Barriers to Equity," *Evaluation Review* 14 (1990): 447–463.

CONCLUSION

17

Where Do We Go from Here?

GEORGE J. ANNAS
MICHAEL A. GRODIN

The contributors to this book, writing from a variety of professional and historical perspectives, have individually added a great deal to our understanding of the Nuremberg Code and its place in modern medical research. When we began this project, we assumed it would demonstrate the centrality of the Nuremberg Code in all ethical discussions involving human experimentation. The contributors seem to agree with this overall assessment. Nonetheless, although most discussions begin with Nuremberg, almost none end there, and there has been a consistent and insistent movement away from the directness of the Code toward more flexible forms of judging the conduct of human experimentation.

THE NATURE OF HUMAN EXPERIMENTATION

The modern movement away from the Nuremberg Code probably has to do with the nature of human experimentation itself. As Hans Jonas has noted, experimentation in the physical sciences involves small-scale models, such as balls rolling down inclined planes and atoms in supercolliders, in which the experimenter "extrapolates from these models and simulated conditions to nature at large."[1] In the physical sciences there is a substitute for the "real thing"; reality is extrapolated from a model that is itself the object of the experiment. In the medical arena, some modeling can be done by using animals for experiments. However, once the leap is made to human experimentation, subject and object merge. It is this merger of the subject and object of human experimentation that makes it problematic; the researcher uses the human "object" as her model for nature. Nonetheless the human subject retains humanity, and the experimenter is also obligated to respect the rights and welfare of this subject-object.

The Nazi concentration camp experiments demonstrate that once the subject is converted into a pure object, anything is possible, including experimentation without limitation. The Nuremberg Code's response is to prohibit the objectification of the subject by requiring the subject's voluntary, competent, informed, and understanding consent. The post-Nuremberg challenge has been to realize and protect the individual humanity of the human subject of medical research while permitting medical experimentation and, thus, progress.

Although there are many types of human experimentation, including psychological, educational, and motivational, by far the most pervasive and risky form is medical experimentation. Thus it is perfectly appropriate both to call the trial of Nazi experimenters the "Doctors' Trial" (even though 3 nonphysicians were among the 23 defendants). It was also perfectly appropriate for physicians, in the form of the World Medical Association, to try to codify the Nuremberg Code's principles in a way that applied to, and only to, medical experiments. While the division of experimentation into medical and nonmedical forms is reasonable, the further subdivision into therapy (treatment) and experimentation (research) is much more problematic.

Human experimentation can be functionally defined as the deviation from standard or accepted medical practice for the purpose of testing a hypothesis or obtaining new knowledge. Although this definition is generally accepted, attempts to avoid the regulations designed to protect research subjects have been made by arguing either (1) that the intervention is not a novel one or (2) that the *intent* of the researcher is not to gain new knowledge but rather to treat a patient. In this discussion, the line between experimentation and treatment, as illustrated in Chapter 16, has become almost hopelessly blurred in clinical medicine. The Nuremberg Code deals most directly with nontherapeutic experimentation, although its consent provisions apply to all competent subjects of experiments. Nonetheless, it does not deal with therapeutic experiments on subjects such as children and the mentally ill, who cannot consent themselves. This omission has led to the Code's marginalization in modern medicine.

The problem is that when the research subject can be considered a patient, and the researcher can be seen as the patient's physician, virtually all research can be transformed into treatment. Since the rules for informed consent are much more lax for treatment than for experimentation, much less attention is paid to consent than the Nuremberg Code demands.[2] On the other hand, physicians also engage in randomized clinical trials and other activities that even they would acknowledge constitute research. In the medical setting, consent has been supplemented (or replaced entirely) by prior ethical review by peers, usually in committees.

It is probably fair to say that modern physicians believe that *anything* they do to one of their patients is, by definition, treatment. This, of course, is consistent with the Hippocratic ethic of acting only for the benefit of one's patient. On the other hand, it makes the regulation of human research seem bureaucratic and unnecessary, since no physician would ever willfully harm her patient. In this regard, phase I cancer drug research, the world's first organ transplants, and the world's first temporary and permanent artificial hearts have all been described by the physicians involved as therapy.[3]

Currently, the most controversial and potentially far-reaching work in human experimentation is in the areas of genetics and genetic engineering. French Anderson, one of the leaders in the field, has argued that even the initial genetic experiments on humans should really be regarded as therapy:

> There exists a fundamental difference between the responses of clinicians and basic scientists to the question: Are we ready to carry out a human gene therapy clinical protocol? . . . The basic scientist objectively analyzes the preclinical data and finds it wanting. . . . Clinicians look at the situation from a different perspective. Every day they are expected to provide their patients with the *best treatments for disease*. When they deal with incurable diseases, they must watch their patients die. . . . The urge to do something, anything, if it might help is very strong. . . . A clinician's reaction to a new therapy protocol tends to be: If it is relatively safe, and it might work better, then let's try it. Historically, much of medical innovation has resulted from trial and error experimentation. . . . What's the rush? The rush is the daily necessity to help sick people. Their (our) illnesses will not wait for a more convenient time. We need help *when* we are sick.[4]

Anderson concludes his argument as follows: "It will take many years of clinical studies before gene therapy can be a widely used treatment procedure. The sooner we begin, the sooner patients will be helped." The distinction between experimentation and treatment is lost in this discussion, with the ethics of the doctor–patient treatment model dominating the scientist-subject model. Likewise, the use of a baboon heart in the Baby Fae transplant was considered lifesaving therapy by the surgeon, even though it was the first operation of its kind in the world. It should be obvious that the fact that the patient is dying does not transform experimental interventions into standard treatment modalities and does not eliminate the necessity for informed consent. It is the nature of the intervention and the data that support its use, not the medical status of the patient or the intent of the physician–researcher, that determine the nature of the intervention. This, of course, is clearest in the area of drugs and devices that are regulated in the United States by the Food and Drug Administration. Since there is no comparable regulation for medical or surgical procedures, the distinction is often operationally irrelevant to clinicians.

THE NUREMBERG CODE IN MODERN MEDICAL RESEARCH (THE U.S. PERSPECTIVE)

Does this mean that the Nuremberg Code has become irrelevant to modern medical research and thus has only historical significance? We think not. We believe the efforts to marginalize the Code rest primarily on a failure of physicians to take informed consent seriously and on a belief, perhaps a societal one, that when it is impossible or difficult to obtain consent, ways to get around this requirement should be found if the research is potentially important to society. This utilitarian view was in evidence, of course, in World War II Germany, but the Allies shared it as well. The U.S. government has always been deeply ambivalent about whether to consider experimentation without consent a crime, and thus to condemn it and its perpetrators publicly (as we did at Nuremberg), or to consider that human experimentation is necessary for our national welfare, and thus to excuse even criminal activity in this area if the national welfare can thereby be furthered.

This unfortunate ambivalence can be seen in two ironies of history. On August 8, 1945, the day the United States entered into the London Agreement with Russia, England, and France that established an International Military Tribunal for the trial of war criminals, the United States also dropped the second atomic bomb on Japan at Nagasaki. The use of nuclear weapons is now considered a major war crime by most countries.

This book recounts the Doctors' Trial at Nuremberg and records the eloquence of General Telford Taylor in proclaiming the significance of the trial for international justice. At the International War Crimes Trial in Tokyo, however, a far different scenario was played out. The United States had evidence that Japanese physicians had engaged in extensive lethal human experimentation on American prisoners of war in China at Unit 731. These experiments involved freezing, plague, gas gangrene, and other experiments of biological warfare not distinguishable in kind from those performed on concentration camp prisoners by the Nazi doctors. Nonetheless, the United States informed the Japanese physicians of Unit 731 that they would not be prosecuted if they agreed to turn over their records and findings to the United States.[5] At least part of the explanation for this decision seems to be that the United States did not want to reveal the results of the Japanese biological warfare studies to the Russians.[6]

Nor, as described in Chapter 11, are these examples of historical interest only. At the same time the U.S. government was talking about having a Nuremberg Trial for Saddam Hussein for war crimes, it was promulgating regulations that permitted the U.S. Defense Department to use experimental drugs and vaccines on U.S. military personnel involved in Operation Desert Shield (later Desert Storm) without their consent, informed or otherwise.[7] This direct violation of the Nuremberg Code was justified on the basis of military expediency. The irony of both endorsing and ignoring the Nuremberg War Crimes Trials was lost on both our government officials and the American public.[8]

On a more positive side, there have been recent moves in Congress to try to return at least some level of autonomy to U.S. military personnel regarding their medical treatment, and World War II experiments conducted by the U.S. military on its own troops continue to be exposed and compensation suggested. For example, in mid-1991 the Dept. of Veterans Affairs finally approved disability benefits for World War II veterans who, without their knowledge or consent, had been placed in a chamber at the Naval Research Laboratory in 1943 (prior to Nuremberg) where they thought they were engaged in the routine testing of protective clothing, but were actually exposed to mustard gas and poisonous arsenic gas. The subjects were not only severely injured, they were told that if they ever talked about the experiments they would be charged with espionage and imprisoned.[9]

THE NUREMBERG CODE IN MODERN MEDICAL RESEARCH (THE INTERNATIONAL PERSPECTIVE)

The manner in which the United States has dealt with the Nuremberg Code is important and instructive, but insofar as the Code was meant as a statement of international law, the manner in which it has been used by the international community is even more important. In this regard, the WHO writers of Chapter 8 have provided great insight. As they note, although the Nuremberg Code has not been adopted as a whole in the form of any United Nations document, its consent principle did become an important part of the United Nations International Covenant on Civil and Political Rights, which was promulgated in 1966 and adopted by the United Nations General Assembly in 1974. Article 7 of this covenant states:

> No one shall be subjected to torture or to cruel, inhuman or degrading treatment or punishment. In particular, no one shall be subjected without his free consent to medical or scientific experimentation.

Most physicians would, of course, be shocked at having anything they do to patients be considered "torture or cruel, inhuman or degrading treatment." They would thus view the Covenant's provisions much the same way they view the Nuremberg Code: as a criminal law document not applicable to anything done in the doctor–patient relationship. It should be noted, however, that in Nazi Germany no such distinction was possible, and even in the United Nations Convention Against Torture (1984) the definition of torture is broad enough to include medical experimentation done without consent:

> For the purpose of this Convention, the term "torture" means any act by which severe pain or suffering, whether physical or mental, is intentionally inflicted on a person for such purposes as obtaining from him or a third person information. . . .

However, because none of the existing conventions of the United Nations deal in a detailed manner with informed consent and the other conditions necessary for ethical and lawful human experimentation, M. C. Bassiouni has proposed that the United Nations adopt a specific criminal Covenant on Human Experimentation.[10] His draft Code provides:

Section 1. Acts of Unlawful Medical Experimentation

1.0 The crime of unlawful medical experimentation consists of any physical and/ or psychological alterations by means of surgical operations or injections, ingestion or inhalation of substances inflicted by or at the instigation of a public official, or for which a public official is responsible and to which the person subject to such experiment does not grant consent as described in Section 2.

Section 2. Defense of Consent

2.1 For the purpose of this Article a person shall not be deemed to have consented to medical experimentation unless he or she has the capacity to consent and does so freely after being fully informed of the nature of the experiment and its possible consequences.

2.2 A person may withdraw his or her consent at any time and shall be deemed to have done so if he or she is not kept fully informed within a reasonable time of the progress of the experiment and any development concerning its possible consequences.

In view of the increasingly international character of human experimentation, the dubious standing of the World Medical Association (since its failure to take a stance against apartheid in South Africa, it now has fewer than half the world's countries as members), and the movement of the Council of International Organizations of Medical Sciences (CIOMS) toward making broad exceptions for individual informed consent, we think that the United Nations is the only credible international body capable of articulating an international code of conduct for human experimentation. We accordingly endorse the proposal for an international Covenant on Human Experimentation based on the Nuremberg Code to cover all nontherapeutic research and all research, therapeutic or nontherapeutic, on competent individuals.

The last 45 years have taught us, however, that although a code is necessary, it is insufficient to safeguard human rights in human experimentation. In Chapter 9 Robert Drinan eloquently argues, in the context of war crimes, that we need an international tribunal to judge and punish those accused of such crimes. We believe the same arguments are applicable to human experimentation. The courts of individual countries, including the United States, have consistently proven incapable of either punishing those engaged in unlawful and unethical experimentation or compensating the victims of such experimentation.

Since criminal laws are almost exclusively state laws in the United States, a reasonable approach for the United States would be the adoption of a uniform state law that prohibited experimentation on competent adults without consent and provided for criminal and civil penalties for violation of the law. As Leonard Glantz notes in Chapter 10, it is striking that almost all of the criminal law that currently exists on human experimentation at the state level involves experimentation with fetuses. Although it is appropriate to have laws regulating experimentation on those vulnerable populations who are incapable of giving consent (fetuses, children, the mentally impaired, etc.), it is at least equally important to prohibit experimentation on competent adults, whether patients or not, without their informed, voluntary, competent, and understanding consent. We accordingly believe that a uniform state criminal law of human experimentation should be adopted. This would provide forums for remedies in the United States but would not, of course, meet the need for an international tribunal.

An international tribunal should be established and should have criminal as well as civil powers. As a beginning, and as an initial step in development, such a tribunal could be limited to civil sanctions, could be set up to enforce a United Nations-adopted Code, and could be financed with a small percentage of the human research budget of member states. This would go a long way toward making human rights in human experimentation a reality instead of a mere slogan.

The tribunal would also be responsible for developing an international common law on human experimentation and applying it to both therapeutic and nontherapeutic experimentation. The line between these types of experiments would be defined by the tribunal rather than by physicians, although physician groups can and should propose standards by which to judge therapeutic experiments. In this regard, the tribunal may find current documents, such as the Helsinki Declaration, the CIOMS proposal, and the U.S. federal regulations persuasive but would not be bound by them. This "internationalizing" of human experimentation may strike some as overly formalistic, but as Ruth Macklin notes in Chapter 13, there has been some movement toward the recognition of universal ethical principles, and enshrining these in law will help given them meaning and make the promise of the Nuremberg Code—the protection of individual dignity and autonomy in research through informed consent—a reality. And as Jay Katz correctly argues in Chapter 12, without the informed consent of the competent subject, there really is no defensible justification for using human beings as research subjects.

Another irony is noted by Leonard Glantz. In the United States, the practice of medicine is governed exclusively by state law, whereas human experimentation is regulated primarily by federal law. This same strange bifurcation exists on the international level: The practice of medicine is governed by the laws of individual countries, whereas codes for the conduct of human experimentation are mostly international. Nonetheless, as in the United States, so it is in the world community: There is virtually no enforcement of research rules, and therefore no penalties for those who violate them and no compensation for their victims. In Chapter 15 Marcia Angell rightly proposes that medical journals reject research that does not conform to international norms, but this does nothing to compensate its victims. Each nation can and should adopt criminal and civil laws to protect research subjects, but few have done so.

We need an international tribunal with authority to judge and punish violators of international norms of human experimentation. Without such a tribunal, we are left where we began: International norms of human experimentation are relegated to the domain of ethics. This is because without the possibility of judgment and punishment, there is no international law worthy of the name, only international ethics. We understand our proposal to be somewhat idealistic; but if the physicians and lawyers of the world unite to work for justice for the victims of unlawful experimentation, and work to prevent their future exploitation, we do not see it as unrealistic. The Nuremberg Code has already led to the virtual elimination of human experimentation on prisoners throughout the world. Is it too much to hope that it can guide us in eliminating all unconsented to research on competent persons throughout the world as well?

Elie Weisel has reminded us in his preface that we must never forget, for memory is part of our humanity. In Chapter 4, Holocaust survivor Eva Kor remembers: "The scientists of the world must remember that the research is being done for the sake of mankind and not for the sake of science; scientists must never detach themselves from the humans they serve. I hope with all my heart that our sad stories will in some special way impel the international community to devise laws and rules to govern human experimentation." We share her hope.

N O T E S

1. Hans Jonas, "Philosophical Reflections on Experimenting with Human Subjects," *Daedalus: Ethical Aspects of Experimentation with Human Subjects* 98 (Spring, 1969): 219.

2. See, e.g., George J. Annas, Leonard H. Glantz, and Barbara Katz, *Informed Consent to Human Experimentation: The Subject's Dilemma* (Cambridge, Mass.: Ballinger, 1977).

3. Ibid.; see also G. J. Annas, "Death and the Magic Machine: Informed Consent to the Artificial Heart," *Western New England Law Review* 9 (1987): 89–112.

4. French Anderson, "What's the Rush?," *Human Gene Therapy* 1 (1990): 109–110.

5. See, generally, Arnold C. Brackman, *The Other Nuremberg: The Untold Story of the Tokyo War Crimes Trials* (London: Collins, 1989), pp. 211–217.

6. Peter Williams and David Wallace, *Unit 731: The Japanese Army's Secret of Secrets* (London: Hodder & Stoughton, 1989).

7. See our Op/Ed piece, "Our Guinea Pigs in the Gulf," *New York Times* (January 8, 1991), p. A21, and the paper's response, "The Ethics of Troop Vaccination," *New York Times* (January 16, 1991), p. A22.

8. For a more detailed discussion of this regulation, reprinted in Appendix 5, *see* "Symposium on Treating the Troops," *Hastings Center Report*, March–April, 1991, pp. 21–29.

9. D. Moss, "Veterans get benefits for '43 gas tests," *USA Today*, June 13, 1991, p. 2A.

10. M. C. Bassiouni, Thomas G. Baffes, and John T. Evrard, "An Appraisal of Human Experimentation in International Law and Practice: The Need for International Regulation of Human Experimentation," *Journal of Criminal Law and Criminology* 72 (1981): 1597–1666.

APPENDIXES

1

Control Council Law No. 10
Punishment of Persons Guilty of War Crimes, Crimes Against Peace and Against Humanity

In order to give effect to the terms of the Moscow Declaration of 30 October 1943 and the London Agreement of 8 August 1945, and the Charter issued pursuant thereto and in order to establish a uniform legal basis in Germany for the prosecution of war criminals and other similar offenders, other than those dealt with by the International Military Tribunal, the Control Council enacts as follows:

Article I

The Moscow Declaration of 30 October 1943 "Concerning Responsibility of Hitlerites for Committed Atrocities" and the London Agreement of 8 August 1945 "Concerning Prosecution and Punishment of Major War Criminals of the European Axis" are made integral parts of this Law. Adherence to the provisions of the London Agreement by any of the United Nations, as provided for in Article V of that Agrement, shall not entitle such Nation to participate or interfere in the operation of this Law within the Control Council area of authority in Germany.

Article II

1. Each of following acts is recognized as a crime:
    a. *Crimes against Peace*. Initiation of invasions of other countries and wars of aggression in violation of international laws and treaties, including but not limited to planning, preparation, initiation or waging a war of aggression, or a war of violation of international treaties, agreements or assurances, or participation in a common plan or conspiracy for the accomplishment of any of the foregoing.

b. *War Crimes.* Atrocities or offences against persons or property constituting violations of the laws or customs of war, including but not limited to, murder, ill treatment or deportation to slave labour or for any other purpose, of civilian population from occupied territory, murder or ill treatment of prisoners of war or persons on the seas, killing of hostages, plunder of public or private property, wanton destruction of cities, towns or villages, or devastation not justified by military necessity.

c. *Crimes against Humanity.* Atrocities and offences, including but not limited to murder, extermination, enslavement, deportation, imprisonment, torture, rape, or other inhumane acts committed against any civilian population, or persecutions on political, racial or religious grounds whether or not in violation of the domestic laws of the country where perpetrated.

d. Membership in categories of a criminal group or organization declared criminal by the International Military Tribunal.

2. Any person without regard to nationality or the capacity in which he acted, is deemed to have committed a crime as defined in paragraph 1 of this Article, if he was (*a*) a principal or (*b*) was an accessory to the commission of any such crime or ordered or abetted the same or (*c*) took a consenting part therein or (*d*) was connected with plans or enterprises involving its commission or (*e*) was a member of any organization or group connected with the commission of any such crime or (*f*) with reference to paragraph 1 (*a*), if he held a high political, civil or military (including General Staff) position in Germany or in one of its Allies, co-belligerents or satellites or held high position in the financial, industrial or economic life of any such country.

3. Any person found guilty of any of the Crimes above mentioned may upon conviction be punished as shall be determined by the tribunal to be just. Such punishment may consist of one or more of the following:

   a. Death.

   b. Imprisonment for life or a term of years, with or without hard labour.

   c. Fine, and imprisonment with or without hard labour, in lieu thereof.

   d. Forfeiture of property.

   e. Restitution of property wrongfully acquired.

   f. Deprivation of some or all civil rights.

   Any property declared to be forfeited or the restitution of which is ordered by the Tribunal shall be delivered to the Control Council for Germany, which shall decide on its disposal.

4. a. The official position of any person, whether as Head of State or as a responsible official in a Government Department, does not free him from responsibility for a crime or entitle him to mitigation of punishment.

   b. The fact that any person acted pursuant to the order of his Government or of a superior does not free him from responsibility for a crime, but may be considered in mitigation.

5. In any trial or prosecution for a crime herein referred to, the accused shall not be entitled to the benefits of any statute of limitation in respect of the period from 30 January 1933 to 1 July 1945, nor shall any immunity, pardon or amnesty granted under the Nazi regime be admitted as a bar to trial or punishment.

Article III

1. Each occupying authority, within its Zone of occupation,
   a. shall have the right to cause persons within such Zone suspected of having committed a crime, including those charged with crime by one of the United Nations, to be arrested and shall take under control the property, real and personal, owned or controlled by the said persons, pending decisions as to its eventual disposition.
   b. shall report to the Legal Directorate the names of all suspected criminals, the reasons for and the places of their detention, if they are detained, and the names and location of witnesses.
   c. shall take appropriate measures to see that witnesses and evidence will be available when required.
   d. shall have the right to cause all persons so arrested and charged, and not delivered to another authority as herein provided, or released, to be brought to trial before an appropriate tribunal. Such tribunal may, in the case of crimes committed by persons of German citizenship or nationality against other persons of German citizenship or nationality, or stateless persons, be a German Court, if authorized by the occupying authorities.
2. The tribunal by which persons charged with offenses hereunder shall be tried and the rules and procedure thereof shall be determined or designated by each Zone Commander for his respective Zone. Nothing herein is intended to, or shall impair or limit the jurisdiction or power of any court or tribunal now or hereafter established in any Zone by the Commander thereof, or of the International Military Tribunal established by the London Agreement of 8 August 1945.
3. Persons wanted for trial by an International Military Tribunal will not be tried without the consent of the Committee of Chief Prosecutors. Each Zone Commander will deliver such persons who are within his Zone to that committee upon request and will make witnesses and evidence available to it.
4. Persons known to be wanted for trial in another Zone or outside Germany will not be tried prior to decision under Article IV unless the fact of their apprehension has been reported in accordance with Section 1 (*b*) of this Article, three months have elapsed thereafter, and no request for delivery of the type contemplated by Article IV has been received by the Zone Commander concerned.

5. The execution of death sentences may be deferred by not to exceed one month after the sentence has become final when the Zone Commander concerned has reason to believe that the testimony of those under sentence would be of value in the investigation and trial of crimes within or without his Zone.

6. Each Zone Commander will cause such effect to be given to the judgments of courts of competent jurisdiction, with respect to the property taken under his control pursuant hereto, as he may deem proper in the interest of justice.

Article IV

1. When any person in a Zone in Germany is alleged to have committed a crime, as defined in Article II, in a country other than Germany or in another Zone, the government of that nation or the Commander of the latter Zone, as the case may be, may request the Commander of the Zone in which the person is located for his arrest and delivery for trial to the country or Zone in which the crime was committed. Such request for delivery shall be granted by the Commander receiving it unless he believes such person is wanted for trial or as a witness by an International Military Tribunal, or in Germany, or in a nation other than the one making the request, or the Commander is not satisfied that delivery should be made, in any of which cases he shall have the right to forward the said request to the Legal Directorate of the Allied Control Authority. A similar procedure shall apply to witnesses, material exhibits and other forms of evidence.

2. The Legal Directorate shall consider all requests referred to it, and shall determine the same in accordance with the following principles, its determination to be communicated to the Zone Commander.

   a. A person wanted for trial or as a witness by an International Military Tribunal shall not be delivered for trial or required to give evidence outside Germany, as the case may be, except upon approval of the Committee of Chief Prosecutors acting under the London Agreement of 8 August 1945.

   b. A person wanted for trial by several authorities (other than an International Military Tribunal) shall be disposed of in accordance with the following priorities:

      (1) If wanted for trial in the Zone in which he is, he should not be delivered unless arrangements are made for his return after trial elsewhere;

      (2) If wanted for trial in a Zone other than that in which he is, he should be delivered to that Zone in preference to delivery outside Germany unless arrangements are made for his return to that Zone after trial elsewhere;

      (3) If wanted for trial outside Germany by two or more of the

United Nations, of one of which he is a citizen, that one should have priority;

(4) If wanted for trial outside Germany by several countries, not all of which are United Nations, United Nations should have priority;

(5) If wanted for trial outside Germany by two or more of the United Nations, then, subject to Article IV 2 (*b*) (3) above, that which has the most serious charges against him, which are moreover supported by evidence, should have priority.

Article V

The delivery, under Article IV of this Law, of persons for trial shall be made on demands of the Governments or Zone Commanders in such a manner that the delivery of criminals to one jurisdiction will not become the means of defeating or unnecessarily delaying the carrying out of justice in another place. If within six months the delivered person has not been convicted by the Court of the zone or country to which he has been delivered, then such person shall be returned upon demand of the Commander of the Zone where the person was located prior to delivery.

Done at Berlin, 20 December 1945.

JOSEPH T. McNARNEY
General
B. L. MONTGOMERY
Field Marshal
L. KOELTZ
General de Corps d'Armée
for P. KOENIG
General d'Armée
G. ZHUKOV
Marshal of the Soviet Union

2A

Military Government—Germany United States Zone Ordinance No. 7 *Organization and Powers of Certain Military Tribunals*

Article I

The purpose of this Ordinance is to provide for the establishment of military tribunals which shall have power to try and punish persons charged with offenses recognized as crimes in Article II of Control Council Law No. 10, including conspiracies to commit any such crimes. Nothing herein shall prejudice the jurisdiction or the powers of other courts established or which may be established for the trial of any such offenses.

Article II

a. Pursuant to the powers of the Military Governor for the United States Zone of Occupation within Germany and further pursuant to the powers conferred upon the Zone Commander by Control Council Law No. 10 and Articles 10 and 11 of the Charter of the International Military Tribunal annexed to the London Agreement of 8 August 1945 certain tribunals to be known as "Military Tribunals" shall be established hereunder.

b. Each such tribunal shall consist of three or more members to be designated by the Military Governor. One alternate member may be designated to any tribunal if deemed advisable by the Military Governor. Except as provided in subsection (*c*) of this Article, all members and alternates shall be lawyers who have been admitted to practice, for at least five years, in the highest courts of one of the United States or its territories or of the District of Columbia, or who have been admitted to practice in the United States Supreme Court.

c. The Military Governor may in his discretion enter into an agreement with one or more other zone commanders of the member nations of the Allied Control Authority providing for the joint trial of any case or cases. In such cases the tribunals shall consist of three or more members as may be provided in the agreement. In such cases the tribunals may include properly qualified lawyers designated by the other member nations.

d. The Military Governor shall designate one of the members of the tribunal to serve as the presiding judge.

e. Neither the tribunals nor the members of the tribunals or the alternates may be challenged by the prosecution or by the defendants or their counsel.

f. In case of illness of any member of a tribunal or his incapacity for some other reason, the alternate, if one has been designated, shall take his place as a member in the pending trial. Members may be replaced for reasons of health or for other good reasons, except that no replacement of a member may take place, during a trial, other than by the alternate. If no alternate has been designated, the trial shall be continued to conclusion by the remaining members.

g. The presence of three members of the tribunal or of two members when authorized pursuant to subsection (*f*) *supra* shall be necessary to constitute a quorum. In the case of tribunals designated under (*c*) above the agreement shall determine the requirements for a quorum.

h. Decisions and judgments, including convictions and sentences, shall be by majority vote of the members. If the votes of the members are equally divided, the presiding member shall declare a mistrial.

Article III

a. Charges against persons to be tried in the tribunals established hereunder shall originate in the Office of the Chief of Counsel for War Crimes, appointed by the Military Governor pursuant to paragraph 3 of the Executive Order Numbered 9679 of the President of the United States dated 16 January 1946. The Chief of Counsel for War Crimes shall determine the persons to be tried by the tribunals and he or his designated representative shall file the indictments with the Secretary General of the tribunals (see Article XIV, *infra*) and shall conduct the prosecution.

b. The Chief of Counsel for War Crimes, when in his judgment it is advisable, may invite one or more United Nations to designate representatives to participate in the prosecution of any case.

Article IV

In order to ensure fair trial for the defendants, the following procedure shall be followed:

a. A defendant shall be furnished, at a reasonable time before his trial, a copy of the indictment and of all documents lodged with the indictment, translated into a language which he understands. The indictment shall state the charges plainly, concisely and with sufficient particulars to inform defendant of the offenses charged.

b. The trial shall be conducted in, or translated into, a language which the defendant understands.

c. A defendant shall have the right to be represented by counsel of his own selection, provided such counsel shall be a person qualified under existing regulations to conduct cases before the courts of defendant's country, or any other person who may be specially authorized by the tribunal. The tribunal shall appoint qualified counsel to represent a defendant who is not represented by counsel of his own selection.

d. Every defendant shall be entitled to be present at his trial except that a defendant may be proceeded against during temporary absences if in the opinion of the tribunal defendant's interests will not thereby be impaired, and except further as provided in Article VI (c). The tribunal may also proceed in the absence of any defendant who has applied for and has been granted permission to be absent.

e. A defendant shall have the right through his counsel to present evidence at the trial in support of his defense, and to crossexamine any witness called by the prosecution.

f. A defendant may apply in writing to the tribunal for the production of witnesses or of documents. The application shall state where the witness or document is thought to be located and shall also state the facts to be proved by the witness or the document and the relevancy of such facts to the defense. If the tribunal grants the application, the defendant shall be given such aid in obtaining production of evidence as the tribunal may order.

Article V

The tribunals shall have the power

a. to summon witnesses to the trial, to require their attendance and testimony and to put questions to them;

b. to interrogate any defendant who takes the stand to testify in his own behalf, or who is called to testify regarding another defendant;

c. to require the production of documents and other evidentiary material;

d. to administer oaths;

e. to appoint officers for the carrying out of any task designated by the tribunals including the taking of evidence on commission;

f. to adopt rules of procedure not inconsistent with this Ordinance. Such rules shall be adopted, and from time to time as necessary, revised by the members of the tribunal or by the committee of presiding judges as provided in Article XIII.

Article VI

The tribunals shall
a. confine the trial strictly to an expeditious hearing of the issues raised by the charges;
b. take strict measures to prevent any action which will cause unreasonable delay, and rule out irrelevant issues and statements of any kind whatsoever;
c. deal summarily with any contumacy, imposing appropriate punishment, including the exclusion of any defendant or his counsel from some or all further proceedings, but without prejudice to the determination of the charges.

Article VII

The tribunal shall not be bound by technical rules of evidence. They shall adopt and apply to the greatest possible extent expeditious and nontechnical procedure, and shall admit any evidence which they deem to have probative value. Without limiting the foregoing general rules, the following shall be deemed admissible if they appear to the tribunal to contain information of probative value relating to the charges: affidavits, depositions, interrogations, and other statements, diaries, letters, the records, findings, statements and judgments of the military tribunals and the reviewing and confirming authorities of any of the United Nations, and copies of any document or other secondary evidence of the contents of any document, if the original is not readily available or cannot be produced without delay. The tribunal shall afford the opposing party such opportunity to question the authenticity or probative value of such evidence as in the opinion of the tribunal the ends of justice require.

Article VIII

The tribunals may require that they be informed of the nature of any evidence before it is offered so that they may rule upon the relevance thereof.

Article IX

The tribunals shall not require proof of facts of common knowledge but shall take judicial notice thereof. They shall also take judicial notice of official governmental documents and reports of any of the United Nations, including the acts and documents of the committees set up in the various Allied countries for the investigation of war crimes, and the records and findings of military or other tribunals of any of the United Nations.

Article X

The determinations of the International Military Tribunal in the judgments in Case No. 1 that invasions, aggressive acts, aggressive wars, crimes, atrocities or inhumane acts were planned or occurred, shall be binding on the tribunals established hereunder and shall not be questioned except insofar as the participation therein or knowledge thereof by any particular person may be concerned. Statements of the International Military Tribunal in the judgment of Case No. 1 constitute proof of the facts stated, in the absence of substantial new evidence to the contrary.

Article XI

The proceedings at the trial shall take the following course:
   a. The tribunal shall inquire of each defendant whether he has received and had an opportunity to read the indictment against him and whether he pleads "guilty" or "not guilty."
   b. The prosecution may make an opening statement.
   c. The prosecution shall produce its evidence subject to the cross examination of its witnesses.
   d. The defense may make an opening statement.
   e. The defense shall produce its evidence subject to the cross examination of its witnesses.
   f. Such rebutting evidence as may be held by the tribunal to be material may be produced by either the prosecution or the defense.
   g. The defense shall address the court.
   h. The prosecution shall address the court.
   i. Each defendant may make a statement to the tribunal.
   j. The tribunal shall deliver judgment and pronounce sentence.

Article XII

A Central Secretariat to assist the tribunals to be appointed hereunder shall be established as soon as practicable. The main office of the Secretariat shall be located in Nurnberg. The Secretariat shall consist of a Secretary General and such assistant secretaries, military officers, clerks, interpreters and other personnel as may be necessary.

Article XIII

The Secretary General shall be appointed by the Military Governor and shall organize and direct the work of the Secretariat. He shall be subject to the supervision of the members of the tribunals, except that when at least three tribunals shall be functioning, the presiding judges of the several tribunals may form the supervisory committee.

Article XIV

The Secretariat shall:
   a. Be responsible for the administrative and supply needs of the Secretariat and of the several tribunals.

b. Receive all documents addressed to tribunals.

c. Prepare and recommend uniform rules of procedure, not inconsistent with the provisions of this Ordinance.

d. Secure such information for the tribunals as may be needed for the approval or appointment of defense counsel.

e. Serve as liaison between the prosecution and defense counsel.

f. Arrange for aid to be given defendants and the prosecution in obtaining production of witnesses or evidence as authorized by the tribunals.

g. Be responsible for the preparation of the records of the proceedings before the tribunals.

h. Provide the necessary clerical, reporting and interpretative services to the tribunals and its members, and perform such other duties as may be required for the efficient conduct of the proceedings before the tribunals, or as may be requested by any of the tribunals.

Article XV

The judgments of the tribunals as to the guilt or the innocence of any defendant shall give the reasons on which they are based and shall be final and not subject to review. The sentences imposed may be subject to review as provided in Article XVII, *infra*.

Article XVI

The tribunal shall have the right to impose upon the defendant, upon conviction, such punishment as shall be determined by the tribunal to be just, which may consist of one or more of the penalties provided in Article II, Section 3 of Control Council Law No. 10.

Article XVII

a. Except as provided in (*b*) *infra*, the record of each case shall be forwarded to the Military Governor who shall have the power to mitigate, reduce or otherwise alter the sentence imposed by the tribunal, but may not increase the severity thereof.

b. In cases tried before tribunals authorized by Article II (*c*), the sentence shall be reviewed jointly by the zone commanders of the nations involved, who mitigate, reduce or otherwise alter the sentence by majority vote, but may not increase the severity thereof. If only two nations are represented, the sentence may be altered only by the consent of both zone commanders.

Article XVIII

No sentence of death shall be carried into execution unless and until confirmed in writing by the Military Governor. In accordance with Article III, Section 5 of Law No. 10, execution of the death sentence may be deferred by not to exceed one month after such confirmation if there is reason to believe that the testimony of the convicted person may be of value in the investigation and trial of other crimes.

Article XIX

Upon the pronouncement of a death sentence by a tribunal established thereunder and pending confirmation thereof, the condemned will be remanded to the prison or place where he was confined and there be segregated from the other inmates, or be transferred to a more appropriate place of confinement.

Article XX

Upon the confirmation of sentence of a death the Military Governor will issue the necessary orders for carrying out the execution.

Article XXI

Where sentence of confinement for a term of years has been imposed the condemned shall be confined in the manner directed by the tribunal imposing sentence. The place of confinement may be changed from time to time by the Military Governor.

Article XXII

Any property declared to be forfeited or the restitution of which is ordered by a tribunal shall be delivered to the Military Governor, for disposal in accordance with Control Council Law No. 10, Article II (3).

Article XXIII

Any of the duties and functions of the Military Governor provided for herein may be delegated to the Deputy Military Governor. Any of the duties and functions of the Zone Commander provided for herein may be exercised by and in the name of the Military Governor and may be delegated to the Deputy Military Governor.

This Ordinance become effective 18 October 1946.

BY ORDER OF MILITARY GOVERNMENT.

2B

Military Government—Germany
Ordinance No. 11
Amending Military Government Ordinance No. 7 of 18 October 1946, Entitled "Organization and Powers of Certain Military Tribunals"

Article I

Article V of Ordinance No. 7 is amended by adding thereto a new subdivision to be designated "(g)", reading as follows:

"(g) The presiding judges, and, when established, the supervisory committee of presiding judges provided in Article XIII shall assign the cases brought by the Chief of Counsel for War Crimes to the various Military Tribunals for trial."

Article II

Ordinance No. 7 is amended by adding thereto a new article following Article V to be designated Article V-B, reading as follows:

"a. A joint session of the Military Tribunals may be called by any of the presiding judges thereof or upon motion, addressed to each of the Tribunals, of the Chief of Counsel for War Crimes or of counsel for any defendant whose interests are affected, to hear argument upon and to review any interlocutory ruling by any of the Military Tribunals on a fundamental or important legal question either substantive or procedural, which ruling is in conflict with or is inconsistent with a prior ruling of another of the Military Tribunals.

"b. A joint session of the Military Tribunals may be called in the same manner as provided in subsection (*a*) of this Article to hear argument upon and to review conflicting or inconsistent final rulings contained in the decisions or judgments of any of the Military Tribunals on a fundamental or important legal question, either substantive or procedural. Any motion with respect to such final ruling shall be filed within ten (10) days following the issuance of decision or judgment.

"c. Decisions by joint sessions of the Military Tribunals, unless thereafter altered in another joint session, shall be binding upon all the Military Tribunals. In the case of the review of final rulings by joint sessions, the judgments reviewed may be confirmed or remanded for action consistent with the joint decision.

"d. The presence of a majority of the members of each Military Tribunal then constituted is required to constitute a quorum.

"e. The members of the Military Tribunals shall, before any joint session begins, agree among themselves upon the selection from their number of a member to preside over the joint session.

"f. Decisions shall be by majority vote of the members. If the votes of the members are equally divided, the vote of the member presiding over the session shall be decisive."

Article III

Subdivisions (*g*) and (*h*) of Article XI of Ordinance No. 7 are deleted; subdivision (*i*) is relettered "(*h*)"; subdivision (*j*) is relettered "(*i*)"; and a new subdivision, to be designated "(*g*)" is added, reading as follows:

"g. The prosecution and defense shall address the court in such order as the Tribunal may determine."

This Ordinance becomes effective 17 February 1947.

3

Declaration of Helsinki Recommendations Guiding Doctors in Clinical Research

Declaration I, 18th World Medical Assembly, Helsinki, June 1964
Declaration II, 29th World Medical Assembly, Tokyo, October 1975
Declaration III, 35th World Medical Assembly, Venice, October 1983
Declaration IV, 41st World Medical Assembly, Hong Kong, September 1989

WORLD MEDICAL ASSOCIATION

DECLARATION OF HELSINKI I
18TH WORLD MEDICAL ASSEMBLY
HELSINKI, FINLAND, JUNE 1964

It is the mission of the doctor to safeguard the health of the people. His knowledge and conscience are dedicated to the fulfillment of this mission.

The Declaration of Geneva of the World Medical Association binds the doctor with the words, "The health of my patient will be my first consideration"; and the International Code of Medical Ethics which declares that "Any act or advice which could weaken physical or mental resistance of a human being may be used only in his interest."

Because it is essential that the results of laboratory experiments be applied to human beings to further scientific knowledge and to help suffering humanity, the World Medical Association has prepared the following recommendations as a guide to each doctor in clinical research. It must be stressed that the standards as drafted are only a guide to physicians all over the world. Doctors are not relieved from criminal, civil, and ethical responsibilities under the laws of their own countries.

In the field of clinical research a fundamental distinction must be recognized between clinical research in which the aim is essentially therapeutic for a patient, and clinical research the essential object of which is purely scientific and without therapeutic value to the person subjected to the research.

I. BASIC PRINCIPLES

1. Clinical research must conform to the moral and scientific principles that justify medical research, and should be based on laboratory and animal experiments or other scientifically established facts.
2. Clinical research should be conducted only by scientifically qualified persons and under the supervision of a qualified medical man.
3. Clinical research cannot legitimately be carried out unless the importance of the objective is in proportion to the inherent risk to the subject.
4. Every clinical research project should be preceded by careful assessment of inherent risks in comparison to foreseeable benefits to the subject or to others.
5. Special caution should be exercised by the doctor in performing clinical research in which the personality of the subject is liable to be altered by drugs or experimental procedure.

II. CLINICAL RESEARCH COMBINED WITH PROFESSIONAL CARE

1. In the treatment of the sick person the doctor must be free to use a new therapeutic measure if in his judgment it offers hope of saving life, re-establishing health, or alleviating suffering.

   If at all possible, consistent with patient psychology, the doctor should obtain the patient's freely given consent after the patient has been given a full explanation. In case of legal incapacity consent should also be procured from the legal guardian; in case of physical incapacity the permission of the legal guardian replaces that of the patient.
2. The doctor can combine clinical research with professional care, the objective being the acquisition of new medical knowledge, only to the extent that clinical research is justified by its therapeutic value for the patient.

III. NON-THERAPEUTIC CLINICAL RESEARCH

1. In the purely scientific application of clinical research carried out on a human being it is the duty of the doctor to remain the protector of the life and health of that person on whom clinical research is being carried out.

2. The nature, the purpose, and the risk of clinical research must be explained to the subject by the doctor.

3a. Clinical research on a human being cannot be undertaken without his free consent, after he has been fully informed; if he is legally incompetent the consent of the legal guardian should be procured.

3b. The subject of clinical research should be in such a mental, physical, and legal state as to be able to exercise fully his power of choice.

3c. Consent should as a rule be obtained in writing. However, the responsibility for clinical research always remains with the research worker; it never falls on the subject, even after consent is obtained.

4a. The investigator must respect the right of each individual to safeguard his personal integrity, especially if the subject is in a dependent relationship to the investigator.

4b. At any time during the course of clinical research the subject or his guardian should be free to withdraw permission for research to be continued. The investigator or the investigating team should discontinue the research if in his or their judgment it may, if continued, be harmful to the individual.

WORLD MEDICAL ASSOCIATION

DECLARATION OF HELSINKI II
29TH WORLD MEDICAL ASSEMBLY
TOKYO, JAPAN, OCTOBER 1975

INTRODUCTION

It is the mission of the medical doctor to safeguard the health of the people. His or her knowledge and conscience are dedicated to the fulfillment of this mission.

The Declaration of Geneva of the World Medical Association binds the doctor with the words, "The health of my patient will be my first consideration", and the International Code of Medical Ethics declares that, "Any act or advice which could weaken physical or mental resistance of a human being may be used only in his interest".

The purpose of biomedical research involving human subjects must be to improve diagnostic, therapeutic and prophylactic procedures and the understanding of the aetiology and pathogenesis of disease.

In current medical practice most diagnostic, therapeutic or prophylactic procedures involve hazards. This applies *a fortiori* to biomedical research.

Medical progress is based on research which ultimately must rest in part on experimentation involving human subjects.

In the field of biomedical research a fundamental distinction must be recognized between medical research in which the aim is essentially diagnostic or therapeutic for a patient, and medical research, the essential object of which is purely scientific and without direct diagnostic or therapeutic value to the person subjected to the research.

Special caution must be exercised in the conduct of research which may affect the environment, and the welfare of animals used for research must be respected.

Because it is essential that the results of laboratory experiments be applied to human beings to further scientific knowledge and to help suffering humanity, the World Medical Association has prepared the following recommendations as a guide to every doctor in biomedical research involving human subjects. They should be kept under review in the future. It must be stressed that the standards as drafted are only a guide to physicians all over the world. Doctors are not relieved from criminal, civil and ethical responsibilities under the laws of their own countries.

I. BASIC PRINCIPLES

1. Biomedical research involving human subjects must conform to generally accepted scientific principles and should be based on adequately performed laboratory and animal experimentation and on a thorough knowledge of the scientific literature.

2. The design and performance of each experimental procedure involving human subjects should be clearly formulated in an experimental protocol which should be transmitted to a specially appointed independent committee for consideration, comment and guidance.

3. Biomedical research involving human subjects should be conducted only by scientifically qualified persons and under the supervision of a clinically competent medical person. The responsibility for the human subject must always rest with a medically qualified person and never rest on the subject of the research, even though the subject has given his or her consent.

4. Biomedical research involving human subjects cannot legitimately be carried out unless the importance of the objective is in proportion to the inherent risk to the subject.

5. Every biomedical research project involving human subjects should be preceded by careful assessment of predictable risks in comparison with foreseeable benefits to the subject or to others. Concern for the interests of the subject must always prevail over the interest of science and society.

6. The right of the research subject to safeguard his or her integrity must always be respected. Every precaution should be taken to respect the privacy of the subject and to minimize the impact of the study on the subject's physical and mental integrity and on the personality of the subject.

7. Doctors should abstain from engaging in research projects involving human subjects unless they are satisfied that the hazards involved are

believed to be predictable. Doctors should cease any investigation if the hazards are found to outweigh the potential benefits.

8. In publication of the results of his or her research, the doctor is obliged to preserve the accuracy of the results. Reports of experimentation not in accordance with the principles laid down in this Declaration should not be accepted for publication.

9. In any research on human beings, each potential subject must be adequately informed of the aims, methods, anticipated benefits and potential hazards of the study and the discomfort it may entail. He or she should be informed that he or she is at liberty to abstain from participation in the study and that he or she is free to withdraw his or her consent to participation at any time. The doctor should then obtain the subject's freely-given informed consent, preferably in writing.

10. When obtaining informed consent for the research project the doctor should be particularly cautious if the subject is in a dependent relationship to him or her or may consent under duress. In that case the informed consent should be obtained by a doctor who is not engaged in the investigation and who is completely independent of this official relationship.

11. In case of legal incompetence, informed consent should be obtained from the legal guardian in accordance with national legislation. Where physical or mental incapacity makes it impossible to obtain informed consent, or when the subject is a minor, permission from the responsible relative replaces that of the subject in accordance with national legislation.

12. The research protocol should always contain a statement of the ethical considerations involved and should indicate that the principles enunciated in the present Declaration are complied with.

II. MEDICAL RESEARCH COMBINED WITH PROFESSIONAL CARE (Clinical Research)

1. In the treatment of the sick person, the doctor must be free to use a new diagnostic and therapeutic measure, if in his or her judgment it offers hope of saving life, reestablishing health or alleviating suffering.

2. The potential benefits, hazards and discomfort of a new method should be weighed against the advantages of the best current diagnostic and therapeutic methods.

3. In any medical study, every patient — including those of a control group, if any — should be assured of the best proven diagnostic and therapeutic method.

4. The refusal of the patient to participate in a study must never interfere with the doctor-patient relationship.

5. If the doctor considers it essential not to obtain informed consent, the specific reasons for this proposal should be stated in the experimental protocol for transmission to the independent committee (I, 2).

6. The doctor can combine medical research with professional care, the objective being the acquisition of new medical knowledge, only to the extent that medical research is justified by its potential diagnostic or therapeutic value for the patient.

III. NON-THERAPEUTIC BIOMEDICAL RESEARCH INVOLVING HUMAN SUBJECTS (Non-clinical biomedical research)

1. In the purely scientific application of medical research carried out on a human being, it is the duty of the doctor to remain the protector of the life and health of that person on whom biomedical research is being carried out.

2. The subjects should be volunteers — either healthy persons or patients for whom the experimental design is not related to the patient's illness.

3. The investigator or the investigating team should discontinue the research if in his/her or their judgment it may, if continued, be harmful to the individual.

4. In research on man, the interest of science and society should never take precedence over considerations related to the wellbeing of the subject.

WORLD MEDICAL ASSOCIATION

DECLARATION OF HELSINKI III
35TH WORLD MEDICAL ASSEMBLY
VENICE, ITALY, OCTOBER 1983

INTRODUCTION

It is the mission of the physician to safeguard the health of the people. His or her knowledge and conscience are dedicated to the fulfillment of this mission.

The Declaration of Geneva of the World Medical Association binds the physician with the words, "The health of my patient will be my first consideration," and the International Code of Medical Ethics which declares that, "A physician shall act only in the patient's interest when providing medical care which might have the effect of weakening the physical and mental condition of the patient."

The purpose of biomedical research involving human subjects must be to improve diagnostic, therapeutic and prophylactic procedures and the understanding of the aetiology and pathogenesis of disease.

In current medical practice most diagnostic, therapeutic or prophylactic procedures involve hazards. This applies especially to biomedical research.

Medical progress is based on research which ultimately must rest in part on experimentation involving human subjects.

In the field of biomedical research a fundamental distinction must be recognized between medical research in which the aim is essentially diagnostic or therapeutic for a patient, and medical research, the essential object of which is purely scientific and without implying direct diagnostic or therapeutic value to the person subjected to the research.

Special caution must be exercised in the conduct of research which may affect the environment, and the welfare of animals used for research must be respected.

Because it is essential that the results of laboratory experiments be applied to human beings to further scientific knowledge and to help suffering humanity, the World Medical Association has prepared the following recommendations as a guide to every physician in biomedical research involving human subjects. They should be kept under review in the future. It must be stressed that the standards as drafted are only a guide to physicians all over the world. Physicians are not relieved from criminal, civil and ethical responsibilities under the laws of their own countries.

I. BASIC PRINCIPLES

1. Biomedical research involving human subjects must conform to generally accepted scientific principles and should be based on adequately performed laboratory and animal experimentation and on a thorough knowledge of the scientific literature.
2. The design and performance of each experimental procedure involving human subjects should be clearly formulated in an experimental protocol which should be transmitted to a specially appointed independent committee for consideration, comment and guidance.
3. Biomedical research involving human subjects should be conducted only by scientifically qualified persons and under the supervision of a clinically competent medical person. The responsibility for the human subject must always rest with a medically qualified person and never rest on the subject of the research, even though the subject has given his or her consent.
4. Biomedical research involving human subjects cannot legitimately be carried out unless the importance of the objective is in proportion to the inherent risk to the subject.
5. Every biomedical research project involving human subjects should be preceded by careful assessment of predictable risks in comparison with foreseeable benefits to the subject or to others. Concern for the interests of the subject must always prevail over the interests of science and society.
6. The right of the research subject to safeguard his or her integrity

must always be respected. Every precaution should be taken to respect the privacy of the subject and to minimize the impact of the study on the subject's physical and mental integrity and on the personality of the subject.

7. Physicians should abstain from engaging in research projects involving human subjects unless they are satisfied that the hazards involved are believed to be predictable. Physicians should cease any investigation if the hazards are found to outweigh benefits.

8. In publication of the results of his or her research, the physician is obliged to preserve the accuracy of the results. Reports of experimentation not in accordance with the principles laid down in this Declaration should not be accepted for publication.

9. In any research on human beings, each potential subject must be adequately informed of the aims, methods, anticipated benefits and potential hazards of the study and the discomfort it may entail. He or she should be informed that he or she is at liberty to abstain from participation in the study and that he or she is free to withdraw his or her consent to participation at any time. The physician should then obtain the subject's freely given informed consent, preferably in writing.

10. When obtaining informed consent for the research project the physician should be particularly cautious if the subject is in a dependent relationship to him or her or may consent under duress. In that case the informed consent should be obtained by a physician who is not engaged in the investigation and who is completely independent of this official relationship.

11. In case of legal incompetence, informed consent should be obtained from the legal guardian in accordance with national legislation. Where physical or mental incapacity makes it impossible to obtain informed consent, or when the subject is a minor, permission from the responsible relative replaces that of the subject in accordance with national legislation. Whenever the minor child is in fact able to give a consent, the minor's consent must be obtained in addition to the consent of the minor's legal guardian.

12. The research protocol should always contain a statement of the ethical considerations involved and should indicate that the principles enunciated in the present declaration are complied with.

II. MEDICAL RESEARCH COMBINED WITH PROFESSIONAL CARE (Clinical research)

1. In the treatment of the sick person, the physician must be free to use a new diagnostic and therapeutic measure, if in his or her judgement it offers hope of saving life, reestablishing health or alleviating suffering.

2. The potential benefits, hazards and discomfort of a new method should be weighed against the advantages of the best current diagnostic and therapeutic methods.
3. In any medical study, every patient — including those of a control group, if any — should be assured of the best proven diagnostic and therapeutic method.
4. The refusal of the patient to participate in a study must never interfere with the physician-patient relationship.
5. If the physician considers it essential not to obtain informed consent, the specific reasons for this proposal should be stated in the experimental protocol for transmission to the independent committee (I, 2).
6. The physician can combine medical research with professional care, the objective being the acquisition of new medical knowledge, only to the extent that medical research is justified by its potential diagnostic or therapeutic value for the patient.

III. NON-THERAPEUTIC BIOMEDICAL RESEARCH INVOLVING HUMAN SUBJECTS (Non-clinical biomedical research)

1. In the purely scientific application of medical research carried out on a human being, it is the duty of the physician to remain the protector of the life and health of that person on whom biomedical research is being carried out.
2. The subjects should be volunteers — either healthy persons or patients for whom the experimental design is not related to the patient's illness.
3. The investigator or the investigating team should discontinue the research if in his/her or their judgment it may, if continued, be harmful to the individual.
4. In research on man, the interest of science and society should never take precedence over considerations related to the wellbeing of the subject.

WORLD MEDICAL ASSOCIATION

DECLARATION OF HELSINKI IV
41ST WORLD MEDICAL ASSEMBLY
HONG KONG, SEPTEMBER 1989

INTRODUCTION

It is the mission of the physician to safeguard the health of the people. His or her knowledge and conscience are dedicated to the fulfillment of this mission.

The Declaration of Geneva of the World Medical Association binds the physician with the words, 'The health of my patient will be my first consideration,' and the International Code of Medical Ethics declares that, 'A physician shall act only in the patient's interest when providing medical care which might have the effect of weakening the physical and mental condition of the patient.'

The purpose of biomedical research involving human subjects must be to improve diagnostic, therapeutic and prophylactic procedures and the understanding of the aetiology and pathogenesis of disease.

In current medical practice most diagnostic, therapeutic or prophylactic procedures involve hazards. This applies especially to biomedical research.

Medical progress is based on research which ultimately must rest in part on experimentation involving human subjects.

In the field of biomedical research a fundamental distinction must be recognized between medical research in which the aim is essentially diagnostic or therapeutic for a patient, and medical research, the essential object of which is purely scientific and without implying direct diagnostic or therapeutic value to the person subjected to the research.

Special caution must be exercised in the conduct of research which may affect the environment, and the welfare of animals used for research must be respected.

Because it is essential that the results of laboratory experiments be applied to human beings to further scientific knowledge and to help suffering humanity, the World Medical Association has prepared the following recommendations as a guide to every physician in biomedical research involving human subjects. They should be kept under review in the future. It must be stressed that the standards as drafted are only a guide to physicians all over the world. Physicians are not relieved from criminal, civil and ethical responsibilities under the laws of their own countries.

I. BASIC PRINCIPLES

1. Biomedical research involving human subjects must conform to generally accepted scientific principles and should be based on adequately performed laboratory and animal experimentation and on a thorough knowledge of the scientific literature.
2. The design and performance of each experimental procedure involving human subjects should be clearly formulated in an experimental protocol which should be transmitted for consideration, comment and guidance to a specially appointed committee independent of the investigator and the sponsor provided that this independent committee is in conformity with the laws and regulations of the country in which the research experiment is performed.
3. Biomedical research involving human subjects should be conducted only by scientifically qualified persons and under the supervision of

a clinically competent medical person. The responsibility for the human subject must always rest with a medically qualified person and never rest on the subject of the research, even though the subject has given his or her consent.

4. Biomedical research involving human subjects cannot legitimately be carried out unless the importance of the objective is in proportion to the inherent risk to the subject.

5. Every biomedical research project involving human subjects should be preceded by careful assessment of predictable risks in comparison with foreseeable benefits to the subject or to others. Concern for the interests of the subject must always prevail over the interests of science and society.

6. The right of the research subject to safeguard his or her integrity must always be respected. Every precaution should be taken to respect the privacy of the subject and to minimize the impact of the study on the subject's physical and mental integrity and on the personality of the subject.

7. Physicians should abstain from engaging in research projects involving human subjects unless they are satisfied that the hazards involved are believed to be predictable. Physicians should cease any investigation if the hazards are found to outweigh the potential benefits.

8. In publication of the results of his or her research, the physician is obliged to preserve the accuracy of the results. Reports of experimentation not in accordance with the principles laid down in this Declaration should not be accepted for publication.

9. In any research on human beings, each potential subject must be adequately informed of the aims, methods, anticipated benefits and potential hazards of the study and the discomfort it may entail. He or she should be informed that he or she is at liberty to abstain from participation in the study and that he or she is free to withdraw his or her consent to participation at any time. The physician should then obtain the subject's freely-given informed consent, preferably in writing.

10. When obtaining informed consent for the research project the physician should be particularly cautious if the subject is in a dependent relationship to him or her or may consent under duress. In that case the informed consent should be obtained by a physician who is not engaged in the investigation and who is completely independent of this official relationship.

11. In case of legal incompetence, informed consent should be obtained from the legal guardian in accordance with national legislation. Where physical or mental incapacity makes it impossible to obtain informed consent, or when the subject is a minor, permission from the responsible relative replaces that of the subject in accordance with national legislation.

Whenever the minor child is in fact able to give a consent, the minor's consent must be obtained in addition to the consent of the minor's legal guardian.

12. The research protocol should always contain a statement of the ethical considerations involved and should indicate that the principles enunciated in the present Declaration are complied with.

II. MEDICAL RESEARCH COMBINED WITH PROFESSIONAL CARE (Clinical research)

1. In the treatment of the sick person, the physician must be free to use a new diagnostic and therapeutic measure, if in his or her judgment it offers hope of saving life, reestablishing health or alleviating suffering.

2. The potential benefits, hazards and discomfort of a new method should be weighed against the advantages of the best current diagnostic and therapeutic methods.

3. In any medical study, every patient — including those of a control group, if any — should be assured of the best proven diagnostic and therapeutic method.

4. The refusal of the patient to participate in a study must never interfere with the physician-patient relationship.

5. If the physician considers it essential not to obtain informed consent, the specific reasons for this proposal should be stated in the experimental protocol for transmission to the independent committee (I, 2).

6. The physician can combine medical research with professional care, the objective being the acquisition of new medical knowledge, only to the extent that medical research is justified by its potential diagnostic or therapeutic value for the patient.

III. NON-THERAPEUTIC BIOMEDICAL RESEARCH INVOLVING HUMAN SUBJECTS (Non-clinical biomedical research)

1. In the purely scientific application of medical research carried out on a human being, it is the duty of the physician to remain the protector of the life and health of that person on whom biomedical research is being carried out.

2. The subjects should be volunteers — either healthy persons or patients for whom the experimental design is not related to the patient's illness.

3. The investigator or the investigating team should discontinue the research if in his/her or their judgment it may, if continued, be harmful to the individual.

4. In research on man, the interest of science and society should never take precedence over considerations related to the wellbeing of the subject.

4

Memorandum for the
Secretary of the Army
Secretary of the Navy
Secretary of the Air Force

TOP SECRET

26 Feb. 1953

SUBJECT: Use of Human Volunteers in Experimental Research

1. Based upon a recommendation of the Armed Forces Medical Policy Council, that human subjects be employed, under recognized safeguards, as the only feasible means for realistic evaluation and/or development of effective preventive measures of defense against atomic, biological or chemical agents, the policy set forth below will govern the use of human volunteers by the Department of Defense in experimental research in the fields of atomic, biological and/or chemical warfare.

2. By reason of the basic medical responsibility in connection with the development of defense of all types against atomic, biological and/or chemical warfare agents, Armed Services personnel and/or civilians on duty at installations engaged in such research shall be permitted to actively participate in all phases of the program, such participation shall be subject to the following conditions:

  a. The voluntary consent of the human subject is absolutely essential.

    (1) This means that the person involved should have legal capacity to give consent; should be so situated as to be able to exercise free power of choice, without the intervention of any element of force, fraud, deceit, duress, over-reaching, or other ulterior

form of constraint or coercion; and should have sufficient knowledge and comprehension of the elements of the subject matter involved as to enable him to make an understanding and enlightened decision. This latter element requires that before the acceptance of an affirmative decision by the experimental subject there should be made known to him the nature, duration, and purpose of the experiment; the method and means by which it is to be conducted; all inconveniences and hazards reasonably to be expected; and the effects upon his health or person which may possibly come from his participation in the experiment.

(2) The consent of the human subject shall be in writing, his signature shall be affixed to a written instrument setting forth substantially the aforementioned requirements and shall be signed in the presence of at least one witness who shall attest to such signature in writing.

    (a) In experiments where personnel from more than one Service are involved the Secretary of the Service which is exercising primary responsibility for conducting the experiment is designated to prepare such an instrument and coordinate it for use by all the Services having human volunteers involved in the experiment.

(3) The duty and responsibility for ascertaining the quality of the consent rests upon each individual who initiates, directs or engages in the experiment. It is a personal duty and responsibility which may not be delegated to another with impunity.

b. The experiment should be such as to yield fruitful results for the good of society, unprocurable by other methods or means of study, and not random and unnecessary in nature.

c. The number of volunteers used shall be kept at a minimum consistent with item b., above.

d. The experiment should be so designed and based on the results of animal experimentation and a knowledge of the natural history of the disease or other problem under study that the anticipated results will justify the performance of the experiment.

e. The experiment should be so conducted as to avoid all unnecessary physical and mental suffering and injury.

f. No experiment should be conducted where there is an a priori reason to believe that death or disabling injury will occur.

g. The degree of risk to be taken should never exceed that determined by the humanitarian importance of the problem to be solved by the experiment.

h. Proper preparation should be made and adequate facilities provided to protect the experimental subject against even remote possibilities of injury, disability, or death.

i. The experiment should be conducted only by scientifically qualified persons. The highest degree of skill and care should be required through all stages of the experiment of those who conduct or engage in the experiment.

j. During the course of the experiment the human subject should be at liberty to bring the experiment to an end if he has reached the physical or mental state where continuation of the experiment seems to him to be impossible.

k. During the course of the experiment the scientist in charge must be prepared to terminate the experiment at any stage, if he has probable cause to believe, in the exercise of the good faith, superior skill and careful judgment required of him that a continuation of the experiment is likely to result in injury, disability, or death to the experimental subject.

l. The established policy, which prohibits the use of prisoners of war in human experimentation, is continued and they will not be used under any circumstances.

3. The Secretaries of the Army, Navy and Air Force are authorized to conduct experiments in connection with the development of defenses of all types against atomic, biological and/or chemical warfare agents involving the use of human subjects within the limits prescribed above.

4. In each instance in which an experiment is proposed pursuant to this memorandum, the nature and purpose of the proposed experiment and the name of the person who will be in charge of such experiment shall be submitted for approval to the Secretary of the military department in which the proposed experiment is to be conducted. No such experiment shall be undertaken until such Secretary has approved in writing the experiment proposed, the person who will be in charge of conducting it, as well as informing the Secretary of Defense.

5. The addresses will be responsible for insuring compliance with the provisions of this memorandum within their respective Services.

/signed/
C. E. WILSON

Copies furnished:
Joint Chiefs of Staff
Research and Development Board

TOP SECRET   Downgraded to UNCLASSIFIED
22 Aug 75
per S. Clements
DDR&E OSD (PA)

5

Department of Defense
Request for Exemption from
Informed Consent Requirements for
Operation Desert Shield and
Food and Drug Administration Response

· · ·

The Assistant Secretary of Defense (Health Affairs) set forth DoD's request in his October 30, 1990 letter to the Assistant Secretary for Health of the Department of Health and Human Services as follows:

> This is to follow up on discussions of DoD and HHS personnel over the past weeks. As you know, the memorandum of understanding between DoD and the Food and Drug Administration recognizes "special DoD requirements to meet national defense considerations." Operation Desert Shield presents such special DoD requirements.
>
> Our contingency planning in Desert Shield has had to take into account endemic diseases in the area and the well-publicized capabilities of the Iraqi military with respect to chemical and biological weapons. For some of these risks, we have determined that the best preventive or therapeutic treatment calls for the use of products now under "investigational new drug" (IND) protocols of the FDA.
>
> These are not exotic new drugs; these drugs have well-established uses (although in contexts somewhat different from our requirements) and are believed by medical personnel in both DoD and FDA to be safe. For example, one product consists of a very commonly used drug packaged in a special intramuscular injector to make it readily useable by soldiers on the battlefield. Another example involves a vaccine long recognized by the Centers for Disease Control as the

From 55 *Federal Register* 52813-17, Dec. 21, 1990

primary preventive treatment available for a particular disease, but the relative infrequency of its use has slowed the accumulation of sufficient immunogenicity data to yet support full licensing of the product. Still another example involves a drug in common use at a particular dosage level, but to preserve alertness of the soldiers, we prefer a lower-dosage table, which is not an FDA approved product. FDA personnel have been extremely cooperative and supportive in reviewing our proposed protocols for these products, quickly providing favorable responses to all of our submissions to date.

FDA assistance is also needed on the issue of informed consent. Under the Federal Food, Drug and Cosmetic Act, the general rule is that, regardless of the character of the medical evidence, any use of an IND, whether primarily for investigational purposes or primarily for treatment purposes, must be preceded by obtaining informed consent from the patient. The statue authorizes exceptions, however, when the medical professionals administering the product "deem it not feasible" to obtain informed consent.

Our planning for Desert Shield contingencies has convinced us that another circumstance should be recognized in the FDA regulation in which it would be consistent with the statute and ethically appropriate for medical professionals to "deem it not feasible" to obtain informed consent of the patient – that circumstance being the existence of military combat exigencies, coupled with a determination that the use of the product is in the best interest of the individual. By the term "military combat exigencies", we mean military combat (actual or threatened) circumstances in which the health of the individual, the safety of other personnel and the accomplishment of the military mission require that a particular treatment be provided to a specified group of military personnel, without regard to what might be any individual's personal preference for no treatment or for some alternative treatment.

In all peacetime applications, we believe strongly in informed consent and its ethical foundations. In peacetime applications, we readily agree to tell military personnel, as provided in FDA's regulations, that research is involved, that there may be risks or discomforts, that participation is voluntary and that refusal to participate will involve no penalty. But military combat is different. If a soldier's life will be endangered by nerve gas, for example, it is not acceptable from a military standpoint to defer to whatever might be the soldier's personal preference concerning a preventative or therapeutic treatment that might save his life, avoid endangerment of the other personnel in his unit and accomplish the combat mission. Based on unalterable requirements of the military field commander, it is not an option to excuse a non-consenting soldier from the military mission, nor would it be defensible militarily – or ethically – to send the soldier unprotected into danger.

To those familiar with military command requirements, this is, of course, elementary. It is also very solidly established in law through a number of Supreme Court cases establishing that special military exigencies sometimes must supersede normal rights and procedures that apply in the civilian community. Consistent with this, long-standing military regulations state that military members may be required to submit to medical care determined necessary to preserve life, alleviate suffering or protect the health of others.

Such special military authority carries with it special responsibility for the well-being of the military personnel involved. Thus, we propose specific procedural limitations on the "not feasible" waiver of informed consent based on military combat exigencies. We propose that decisions on waiving informed consent be made on a case-by-case basis by the Commissioner, assuring an objective review outside of military channels of all pertinent information and an independent validation of the special circumstances presented. Further, we propose the following specific limitations: (1) That drug-by-drug requests for waiver be accompanied by written justification based on the intended uses and the military circumstances involved; (2) that no satisfactory alternative treatment is available; (3) that available safety and efficacy data support the proposed use of the drug or biologic product; (4) that each such request be approved by the applicable DoD Institutional Review Board; and (5) that the waivers be time-limited.

To recap, we have nothing exotic in the works. We are methodically planning for a range of medical treatment contingencies in Operation Desert Shield corresponding to the predictable medical problems that might arise. Some of these contingencies require the availability of products now under IND protocols. For products that will be in the best interests of the patients, military combat exigencies may justify deeming it not feasible to obtain informed consent. FDA's regulation should provide the mechanism, subject to appropriate limitations, for DoD to request on a drug-by-drug basis, and the Commissioner to decide, that a waiver be granted in cases in which it is established that military combat exigencies make that necessary.

Your cooperation and assistance in this regard is appreciated.

III. PROVISIONS OF THIS REGULATION

FDA continues to recognize its responsibility in protecting the human subjects exposed to investigational drugs and the central role that informed consent plays in ensuring that protection. Because of the paramount importance of informed consent, only the narrowest exceptions to this requirement are consistent with FDA's responsibilities and consistent with the best interests of human subjects. Nevertheless, FDA has determined that, in the special circumstances that may be created by the use of troops in combat and consistent with its obligations under sections 505(i) and 507(d), FDA may narrowly expand the circumstances in which the Commissioner may determine that obtaining informed consent is not feasible. FDA agrees with DOD's judgment that, in certain combat-related situations, it may be appropriate to conclude that obtaining informed consent from military personnel for the use of investigational drugs is not feasible and withholding treatment would be contrary to the best interests of military personnel involved. DOD has the right and responsibility to make command decisions that expose troops to the possibility of combat and has the concomitant responsibility to protect the welfare of these troops both individually and as a group. DOD has stated that traditional informed consent, based on the right of the individual to choose his or her own treatment, may not be appropriate under the circumstances of specific combat-related conditions. FDA respects DOD's obligation and commitment to do everything possible to protect military personnel who may be exposed to potentially hazardous conditions.

FDA further appreciates that this protection may include medical treatment or prevention with an investigational drug considered necessary to protect not only the health of individual soldiers but to ensure the welfare of the remaining forces. FDA will consider investigational products proposed for military use on a case-by-case basis, and the agency is prepared to waive the requirement of informed consent where it can be documented that use of these agents in combat-related situations serves the best interests of individual soldiers and the military combat units in which they serve. Since these individual soldiers may be required to be exposed to combat, permitting them to choose whether to receive an investigational product that is the only available satisfactory protection against life-threatening conditions, is contrary to their individual best interests and to the welfare of the other soldiers involved. FDA therefore believes that such an exercise of the Commissioner's discretion is ethically justified. Moreover, all the products at issue would be reviewed by FDA for safety and expanded availability, and their use would be monitored by DOD and reported to and reviewed by FDA. DOD and FDA do not expect that all combat-related situations will create a situation of the kind that would obviate obtaining informed consent. DOD and FDA must determine that there is justification for a waiver of informed consent for a particular drug, following the approval of the use and the waiver by a duly constituted IRB, and a conclusion that the circumstances surrounding the anticipated distribution and use of the drug meet the limited circumstances recognized in the regulations. DOD and FDA also emphasize that accepted ethical principles permit waiver of informed consent only where the preventive or treatment is in the best interests of the individuals involved. Therefore, it is not sufficient as an ethical matter to waive informed consent in the military context where obtaining informed consent is "not feasible," unless it is also the case that withholding the treatment would be contrary to the best interests of the individuals involved. FDA is therefore amending 21 CFR 50.23 to add limited conditions under which the Commissioner may find that it is not feasible to obtain informed consent in the proposed use of an investigational drug. Under the amended regulation, the Commissioner will make any such determination on a product-by-product basis. In determining whether obtaining informed consent is not feasible and withholding treatment would be contrary to the best interests of the military personnel, the Commissioner must find that there is no available satisfactory alternative therapy for the intended diagnosis, prevention, or treatment of the disease or condition. The Commissioner will also consider other factors, including the extent and strength of the evidence of the safety and effectiveness of the investigational drug for the intended use. Other factors that the Commissioner will consider include the nature of the information provided to the recipients of the investigational drug concerning the potential risks and benefits of the drug, known adverse effects of the drug, and risks of not taking such a product in combat-related situations, whether the disease or condition to be treated is life-threatening or highly contagious and debilitating, and the setting in which the drug is to be administered. For example, it may be more feasible to obtain informed consent in a hospital than on the battlefield or when it is administered by a health professional rather than self-administered. FDA recognizes, however, that there may be combat-related circumstances in which obtaining informed consent is not feasible and withholding treatment would be contrary to the best interests of military personnel even outside battlefield conditions.

When DOD seeks a determination by FDA that obtaining informed consent would not be feasible in the proposed use of a specific investigational drug and withholding treatment would be contrary to the best interest of the military personnel, DOD must submit a written request. The request must be for use of a specific investigational drug in a specific protocol under an IND sponsored by DOD, in a specific combat-related setting. The request will also include a written justification supporting the conclusions of the physician(s) responsible for the medical care of the military personnel involved and the investigator(s) identified in the IND that a military combat exigency exists because of special military combat (actual or threatened) circumstances in which, in order to facilitate the accomplishment of the military mission, preservation of the health of the individual and the safety of other personnel require that a particular treatment be provided to a specified group of military personnel, without regard to what may be any individual's personal preference for no treatment or for some alternative treatment.

The request must further contain a statement that the duly constituted IRB has reviewed and approved the proposed use of the investigational drug and concluded that it may be administered without obtaining informed consent under the criteria set forth in this document. The request must be submitted with the original IND submission or as an amendment to the IND.

The Commissioner may consult with appropriate experts, including those responsible for the protection of human subjects, before reaching a determination on a DOD request under this regulation.

To ensure that the period in which informed consent is not obtained does not exceed that necessary to deal with the actuality or threat of combat, the Commissioner's determination regarding informed consent will automatically expire at the end of 1 year or when DOD informs FDA that the specific military operation creating the need for the investigational drug has ended, whichever is earlier. If, at the end of 1 year, United States military forces are still engaged in the military operation, DOD may seek to renew the determination. This provision does not preclude the Commissioner from revoking or otherwise modifying the determination at any time based upon changed circumstances. In particular, consistent with DOD's responsibilities under the IND's under which these products will be administered, DOD will collect data on any use of these products without informed consent. FDA will review these data and will revoke or modify the determination if the review indicates that the determination is no longer appropriate.

This amendment applies only to the use of investigational drugs. It does not apply to other clinical investigations to which 21 CFR part 50 applies.

. . .

2. Section 50.23 is amended by adding new paragraph (d) to read as follows:

§ 50.23 Exception from General Requirements

. . . . .

(d)(1) The Commissioner may also determine that obtaining informed consent is not feasible when the Assistant Secretary of Defense (Health Affairs) requests such a determination in connection with the use of an investigational drug (including an antibiotic or biological product) in a specific protocol under an investigational new drug application (IND) sponsored by the Department of Defense (DOD). DOD's request for a determination that obtaining informed consent from military personnel is not feasible must be limited to a specific military operation involving combat or the immediate threat of combat. The request must also include a written justification supporting the conclusions of the physician(s) responsible for the medical care of the military personnel involved and the investigator(s) identified in the IND that a military combat exigency exists because of special military combat (actual or threatened) circumstances in which, in order to facilitate the accomplishment of the military mission, preservation of the health of the individual and the safety of other personnel require that a particular treatment be provided to a specified group of military personnel, without regard to what might be any individual's personal preference for no treatment or for some alternative treatment. The written request must also include a statement that a duly constituted institutional review board has reviewed and approved the use of the investigational drug without informed consent. The Commissioner may find that informed consent is not feasible only when withholding treatment would be contrary to the best interests of military personnel and there is no available satisfactory alternative therapy.

(2) In reaching a determination under paragraph (d)(1) of this section that obtaining informed consent is not feasible and withholding treatment would be contrary to the best interests of military personnel, the Commissioner will review the request submitted under paragraph (d)(1) of this section and take into account all pertinent factors, including, but not limited to:

(i) The extent and strength of the evidence of the safety and effectiveness of the investigational drug for the intended use;

(ii) The context in which the drug will be administered, e.g., whether it is intended for use in a battlefield or hospital setting or whether it will be self-administered or will be administered by a health professional;

(iii) The nature of the disease or condition for which the preventive or therapeutic treatment is intended; and

(iv) The nature of the information to be provided to the recipients of the drug concerning the potential benefits and risks of taking or not taking the drug.

(3) The Commissioner may request a recommendation from appropriate experts before reaching a determination on a request submitted under paragraph (d)(1) of this section.

(4) A determination by the Commissioner that obtaining informed consent is not feasible and withholding treatment would be contrary to the best interests of military personnel will expire at the end of 1 year, unless renewed at DOD's request, or when DOD informs the Commissioner that the specific military operation creating the need for the use of the investigational drug has ended, whichever is earlier. The Commissioner may also revoke this determination based on changed circumstances.

James S. Benson,
Deputy Commissioner of Food and Drugs.

Louis W. Sullivan,
Secretary of Health and Human Services.

Dated: December 18, 1990.

Index